UNDERSTANDING CANCER

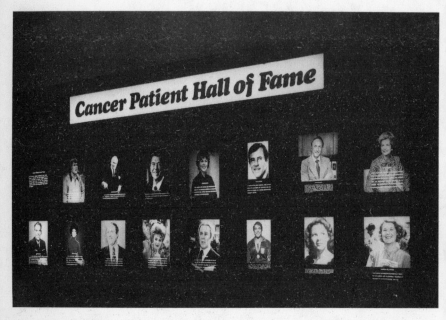

The famous people pictured in this exhibit at Roswell Park Memorial Institute in Buffalo, New York, were all treated for cancer and continued to lead active lives. They are heroes of the struggle against cancer and living proof that it can be beaten. (Photo kindly provided by Mr. Dante Terrana and Dr. E. Mirand)

UNDERSTANDING CANCER

John Laszlo, M.D.

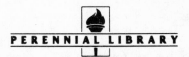

PERENNIAL LIBRARY

HARPER & ROW, PUBLISHERS, New York
Cambridge, Philadelphia, San Francisco, Washington
London, Mexico City, São Paulo, Singapore, Sydney

Grateful acknowledgment is made for permission to reprint:

Table on page 159 from "Insights on How to Quit Smoking: A Survey of Patients with Lung Cancer" by Nancy Knudsen, et al. Reprinted from *Cancer Nursing* 8:3 (1985):145–50 by permission of Raven Press, Publishers.

Figures and tables on pages 58, 140, 141, and 163 from *Cancer Research* 45 (1985): front cover; 44 (1984):5940; and 37 (1977):4608. Reprinted by permission of *Cancer Research.*

Table on page 214. Reprinted courtesy of Alice B. Nily of Nily Realty Inc., Easton, MD.

Photograph on page 253, © 1983 Marilynne Herbert. Reproduced by permission of Victor Herbert, M.D.

Frontispiece and photograph on pages 160–61. Reproduced by permission of Dr. Edwin A. Mirand.

Figure on page 256 from article by Dr. C. G. Moertel, *New England Journal of Medicine* 312 (1985):137. Reprinted by permission of the *New England Journal of Medicine.*

Figure on page 88 by Dr. Edwin Cox and table 2 on pages 110–11 by Dr. Joseph Fraumeni from Cecil's *Textbook of Medicine,* 17th ed. (Philadelphia: W. B. Saunders, 1985). Reprinted by permission of the publisher.

Figure on page 199 from "The Epidemiology of AIDS: Current Status and Future Prospects" by J. Curran, et al., from *Science* 229, no. 4720, pp. 1352–(7), September 27, 1985. Copyright 1985 by the AAAS. Reprinted by permission of AAAS and the author.

Figure and tables on pages 99, 100, 101, 175, and 178–79 from the American Cancer Society. Reprinted by permission of American Cancer Society.

Excerpt on pages 270–71 from *The Road Back to Health: Coping with the Emotional Side of Cancer* by Neil A. Fiore, Ph.D. Copyright © 1984 by Neil A. Fiore, Ph.D. Reprinted by permission of Bantam Books Inc. All rights reserved.

First PERENNIAL LIBRARY edition published 1988

Designed by Gayle Jaeger

Library of Congress Cataloging-in-Publication Data

Laszlo, John, 1931–
    Understanding cancer.

    "Perennial Library."
    Bibliography: p.
    Includes index.
    1. Cancer—Popular works.   I. Title.
RC263.L356   1988   616.99'4   86-46079
ISBN 0-06-091491-2 (pbk.)

88 89 90 91 92 FG 10 9 8 7 6 5 4 3 2 1

Dedicated to our children

Rebecca, Jennifer and Daniel Walter

CONTENTS

PREFACE xiii

1
THE STARTING POINT 1

2
LEARNING ABOUT CANCER 6
What Brings the Patient to the Doctor? 7   Diagnostic
Procedures 9   The Second Opinion (and How to Get It) 14
Where Are the Best Places to Get Care? 20

3
COMMUNICATION IS THE SECRET OF SUCCESS 22
Setting Up Goals 23   "My Doctor Won't Tell Me Anything"
26   "You Can Tell Me, but Don't Tell . . ." 31   "What Are
My Chances, Doctor?" 34

4
CANCER TREATMENT 35

Treatment with Curative Intent 35 Surgery 40 Radiation Therapy 46 Chemotherapy 51 Interferon and Other Types of Immunotherapy 71 Nutrition 73 Attitude and Imagery 77

5
WHAT IS CANCER AND HOW DOES IT KILL? 80

Definitions and Biology of Cancer 81 How Does Cancer Kill? 89 Pain 90 Nutrition 92 Infection 94

6
CANCER STATISTICS: THE BIG PICTURE 95

Lung Cancer 102 Breast Cancer 102 Cancer of the Uterus 103 Cancer of the Colon and Rectum 104 Skin Cancer 104 Oral Cancer 105 Leukemia 105 Childhood Cancer 105 If We Could Cure Cancer and Heart Disease, Then Would We Live Forever? 106

7
THE CAUSES AND PREVENTION OF CANCER 108

Studies of Causation—Epidemiology 108 Hazards of Lifestyle—Diet, Obesity, Alcohol, Radiation 113 Sexual Lifestyle 122 Occupational and Environmental Hazards—Asbestos, Vinyl Chloride, Air and Water 123 Drugs That May Cause Cancer 126 Viruses, Cancer and Onco-genes 128 Excerpt from *Nutrition and Cancer: Cause and Prevention* 132

8
TOBACCO AND CANCER: THE BLIGHT AMONG US 137

Relationship to Smoking 137 Is There Any Relationship Between the Amount a Person Smokes and the Risk of

Developing Lung Cancer? 139 Are There Really
Cancer-causing Chemicals in Cigarette Smoke, or Are the
Relationships Described Above Merely Coincidental? 142 Are
There Any Beneficial Effects of Smoking As Far As Cancer Is
Concerned? 144 What Is the Role of Nicotine? 145 What
about Filter Cigarettes? Are They Safe? 145 Warning
Labels—Everyone's Friend 147 Advertising and Social
Concerns 148 Quit-Smoking Programs—The How To's 153
Passive Smoking—A New Public Controversy 164
Recommendations for Public Policy 165 Smokeless Tobacco
166 Economics of Smoking and Lung Cancer 168

9
CANCER SCREENING AND DETECTION: HOW USEFUL ARE PERIODIC EXAMINATIONS? 172

Principles of Screening for Cancer 173 Pap Test 174 Breast
Cancer Screening 176 Testicular Cancer 181 Lung and
Bowel Cancer—The "Tough" Problems 181 Mouth and
Skin—The "Easy" Problems 185 Cancer Detection 186
Summary 189

10
MARIJUANA AND THC: FROM POT TO PRESCRIPTION 191

11
CANCER AND AIDS: A DOUBLE WHAMMY 198

The Clinical Syndrome and Its Causes 198 Treatment 203
Immunity and Cancer 204 Serendipity—Preparing for Luck
205

12
ON REDUCING THE ENORMOUS ECONOMIC BURDEN OF CANCER: PERSONAL AND NATIONAL 207

Overview 207 What Can We Do to Help Reduce Costs? 208
THE BILL 213 What the Doctor Can Do to Reduce Costs

216 Hospice and Home Care—When? 223 Societal Issues
225 What Cost Cure? 228 Paying for Research on Yourself
229 Lessons 231 Is There a Better Way? 234

13
EXPERIMENTAL THERAPY OR QUACKERY: WHAT'S THE DIFFERENCE? 239

Testing of New Drugs in Humans 239 Testing of Compound
"X"—The Story of Krebiozen 246 Other Miracle
Drugs—Litmus Tests for Intelligent Consumers 251 Laetrile,
Serum Therapy, Vitamin C 252

14
ATTITUDE: THE ISSUE OF MIND-BODY UNITY 257

15
CANCER RESEARCH: THE CUTTING EDGE 274

Understanding How Cancer and Normal Cells Differ 275
New Technologies and New Insights 277 Monoclonal
Antibodies for Diagnosis and Treatment 280 Killing by
Lymphocytes—The Interleukin-2 Story 283 Turning Cancer
Cells Back Toward Normal 285 Experimental Chemotherapy
287

16
HOPE FOR TOMORROW 293

Summary of Year 2000 (and Some 1990) Objectives from NCI
298

EPILOGUE: VIEW FROM THE OTHER SIDE—A PERSONAL EXPERIENCE 306

APPENDIX 1: HELP IS FOR THE ASKING 313

American Cancer Society 313 National Cancer Institute 318
Candlelighters 320 National Hospice Organization 321

Contents

Leukemia Society of America, Inc. 322   Reach to Recovery
323   Comprehensive Cancer Centers 324   Other Cancer
Centers 326   Canadian Cancer Society 328   European Groups
329   Cancer Programs Approved by the American College of
Surgeons 329   Additional Sources of Information 330

APPENDIX 2: LEGAL ASPECTS (MONEY, WILLS, ESTATES,
          ORGAN DONATION, FUNERALS) 331
Where to Get Legal Services 332   What Are Your Social
Security Benefits? 333   Managing the Affairs of Someone Else
335   Wills 337   Living Wills 340   Planning for Family
Security 342   Anatomical Gifts 343   Planning a Funeral 344
When Death Occurs 346   Settling an Estate 349

GLOSSARY 353

BIBLIOGRAPHY 367

INDEX 373

PREFACE

Cancer kills some 483,000 Americans annually, and it is now impossible to live in this society and not have a family member or friend afflicted by cancer. Yet there is much that we are not doing at present but that we *can* do to protect ourselves from getting it, to find it early and to cope with its manifestations if it does strike. This book discusses the overall problem from the viewpoint of a cancer specialist (oncologist), and tries to see the particular anxieties, fears and difficulties through the eyes of the patient.

This is my first book for a lay audience in a career of practicing medicine, doing research and writing articles and books for scientists. This book was not planned; it virtually erupted while I was away from my work and contemplating volcanos during a lecture tour in Hawaii. Having just finished a book for physicians about the care of patients with cancer, it occurred to me that it is far more difficult for people who are not health professionals to get the information they might need on this broad subject "cancer"—such as how to evaluate the latest treatment "breakthrough" (what an awful term!) or the latest food that is implicated in the causation or prevention of cancer, and how to separate fact from fancy about new treatments.

I owe my initial interest in helping patients with cancer to my father, Daniel Laszlo, M.D., who started the first separate department of oncology in a general hospital at Montefiore Hospital in The Bronx, New York, in the 1940s. (An oncologist is a doctor who is specially trained first in a major field such as Medicine, Surgery, Pediatrics, Gynecology or Radiology and then becomes further specialized in caring for patients with cancer. As a medical oncologist I combine the tools of medical care of adults with knowledge about the special problems of patients with cancer, such as the use of chemical treatment or chemotherapy.) I spent many weekends accompanying my father on house calls to walkup apartments to see poor patients who had been discharged from the hospital because they preferred to be cared for and to die at home. He and his dedicated medical colleagues and bright administrators started the home care program in New York as an outgrowth of this experience. (Sadly, both he and my mother died of cancer.)

My later medical training exposed me to many excellent scientists and students at Harvard Medical School, then to the excitement of working at a young National Cancer Institute and, for over twenty-six years, teaching and researching at Duke Medical Center and its Comprehensive Cancer Center. I have just started a "second career" as a senior leader at the American Cancer Society, a position that permits me to reflect on the totality of issues related to cancer. However, the views expressed are my own, and in some controversial areas there is no "right" or "wrong" way. For simplicity I use the masculine pronoun in most contexts where "he or she" would be more accurate but cumbersome.

My gratitude goes to many friends and colleagues who have taught me, argued with me and collaborated with me over the years, and to the patients whom we were privileged to treat. I would especially like to acknowledge my gratitude for her generous assistance in the preparation of this manuscript to Connie Fennema, and to the American Cancer Society and numerous authors and publishers for permitting the use of authoritative illustrative material in this book. I appreciate helpful suggestions for various chapters from Drs. Charles Moertel, James Holland, C.Y. Tso, Pat Cotanch, Gustavo Montana, Andrew Huang, Edwin A. Mirand, Saul B. Gusberg and Victor Herbert, and from Mr. Edwin Silverberg and Mr. Ralph Hawkins. Judith Weber, Elizabeth Tornquist and Carol Cohen provided constructive editorial advice. My heartfelt thanks go to Ian and Betty Ballantine, who believed in the importance of this book and helped in many ways to make it a reality.

THE STARTING POINT

Cancer the Crab lies so still that you might think he was asleep if you did not see the ceaseless play and winnowing motion of the feathery branches round his mouth. That movement never ceases. It is like the eating of a smothering fire into rotten timber in that it is noiseless and without haste.
—RUDYARD KIPLING, "The Children of the Zodiac"

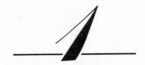

This book is neither a doomsday message nor a fairy tale—it does not promise what cannot be delivered. It is about real problems, people, progress and opportunity. Its message is simply that we can and must arm and defend ourselves against this great scourge of mankind, which has killed more Americans than all wars, which often causes pauperization and degradation in its victims and which strikes terror by mere mention of its name. And there is much that we can do to help ourselves, for in this case to have knowledge is to have power. Indeed, I believe that an informed patient is the doctor's best friend and strongest partner in the battle to win the war against cancer.

Much of the material contained here was inspired by questions that patients and their families have asked me during my thirty-year career as a cancer researcher and physician. While many of the topics covered are unique to cancer, many apply equally to other serious diseases: how to choose a doctor, how to get a second opinion without offending the doctor, how to get information from the doctor, whom to tell what about the illness, how to minimize the costs of medical care, how to assess your nutritional needs, how to understand immune deficiency conditions such as AIDS, and what is the nature (and attraction) of quackery—to mention but a handful. There is a tremendous amount of information in this book, and some opinions about highly controversial issues—not all of the latter will prove to be correct, of course. There is more information in the book than is needed for practical usage, some of which, interesting and instructive though it may be, readers may want to skip temporarily to get at the "meat," or what most immediately concerns them. Obviously there is also less than we all need to know about some key areas of prevention and treatment. However, this book is overall a current and probably fair representation of the state of professional knowledge, its power and its limitations. In addition, readers will find some radical suggestions on how to help both themselves and society to cope with the loss of control, dehumanization and despair that often accompany a major illness such as cancer, and on how to build a better system of "caring." It is in this area that each and every one can play a very significant part once the subject matter is understood—it is my job to present the information and at least some choices.

The past three decades have brought tremendous technological changes into our daily lives—but too often there has not been an adequate counterbalance at the human level. Indeed, the technology itself tends to dehumanize—witness the profound effect of television on the fabric of the American family. Medicine, with its intensive-care units, test-tube babies, organ transplantation and advanced life-support systems, has not always kept an equal balance in nurturing the afflicted person and family. In his very clear exposition of the concept of "high tech/high touch," John Naisbitt *(Megatrends)* proposes that whenever new technology is introduced into society there must be a counterbalancing human response, called high touch, or the technology will be rejected. Medical educators, hospital administrators and particularly the popular press have not understood this clearly. On the contrary, they have stood on the sidelines and been amazed at the extraordinary public interest in family practitioners, home deliveries of babies and hospice programs. These public interests are predictable responses to the gaps and voids in medical care that are created by fallout from the technological explosion. A prominent medical center recently tried to close its Community Medicine program only to be forced to reverse the decision because of the great public outcry! I cannot imagine even a whimper of protest from the public had the decision been to close the Department of Biochemistry or Physiology. The message is clear—the medical community must keep human values right up there with technological achievements or we cannot effect the full potential of our own expertise.

A subject as broad as cancer can be examined on at least three distinct levels. First, there is a rich and rapidly expanding scientific body of knowledge dealing with many aspects of this disease, and this can profitably be studied for its pure intellectual and biological interest. There is even a certain beauty to scientific discovery, regardless of the subject matter. Second, cancer is one of the world's major killers, at least in those areas of the world where people are likely to live long enough to enter the high-risk group. Certainly it is a major killer in the industrialized nations of the world and wherever public health measures and economic conditions have eliminated major parasitic infections and starvation. Concerned people in these countries want information about the disease and its causes in order to minimize the risk of developing cancer for themselves and for their family. They are also interested in learning how to detect cancer early enough that it can be cured by simple surgical removal.

Finally, those who have, or suspect that they have, cancer obviously have a special interest: they want to know how they can get the best information and medical care available. There are many fears and misconceptions about cancer, and the patient often does not know where to turn to ask about second opinions, or how to find a caring and knowledgeable specialist or generalist or what the different kinds of treatment entail—their advantages, disadvantages and particularly their potential side effects. Finding the best path through the health-care maze in our country is difficult at best and almost impossible under conditions of fear and stress. There are dangerous extremes to be avoided, such as the overuse of technology on the one hand and too much pessimism as to what can be accomplished by modern medicine on the other.

We must admit that there are serious impediments to learning about cancer. First and foremost, the information base is vast and rapidly evolving. At the same time, many key questions are still unanswerable. Indeed, the lack of complete information can erode interest and motivation to learn more about the subject—the temptation is to avoid the issue entirely and say, "I'll be back when you find the cure." Also, while the subject of cancer may be viewed from a detached perspective, often it hits close to home on some very sensitive issues that are easier to deny than to resolve. That is part of the reality to be faced. How much do we want to be reminded of possible disaster to our health; will it worry us more than it will help? And there is the cynical view—which I have heard expressed at cocktail parties but never at the hospital— that doctors cannot be bothered to explain what they do (why else would they write so illegibly), nor will they expose their ignorance on *any* subject. And to be honest, I have met such doctors and medical students. Although it is not a prevailing or new viewpoint, there exists an element of mistrust toward doctors (epitomized in the extreme by George Bernard Shaw's play *The Doctor's Dilemma*), and often this mistrust stands in the way of learning and of effective action. Finally, even some cancer experts are extremely competent only in a small area of the problem and are not sufficiently knowledgeable about or comfortable in providing a broad overview of various treatment options.

In this book I hope to provide the reader with one "expert" distillation of the many aspects of cancer as it affects us or may affect us, our family and friends in the future. It will be addressed to you, the reader, as though you were a person sitting in my office having just learned that you may have cancer, or as though you were the loved one sitting next to this patient. We will speak about other diagnostic tests, discuss the treatments that lie ahead and then talk more generally about cancer as a disease and about the relevant questions that you, as a patient or interested party, may want to ask me. We will delineate the limits of present knowledge and candidly and critically review common practices, dogmas and myths. There are a distressing number of pseudoscientific books that offer magical solutions to currently unsolvable problems. I offer no quick-fix of a diet, immune stimulation or mind-body cure of advanced cancer; the only magic is knowledge and truth. The public wants and demands no less of its scientists. (And in taking a stand on many controversial issues, I will undoubtedly express some opinions that will prove to be incorrect as further information becomes available.) This book contains practical information about health and doctor-patient relationships, cancer's economic impact, the psychosocial issues and the importance of attitude in chronic illnesses, the need for a humane approach and the nature of basic and clinical research—which, it is to be hoped, will not only change practices in the field of cancer but will also be applicable to many other areas of medicine.

LEARNING ABOUT CANCER

For a start, let us take a couple of typical patients with cancer, and follow them as closely as possible, step by step.

You are a woman in your late fifties, and you have gone to see your doctor for a routine annual physical. You have no history of cancer in the family, your checkups have been good, but this time your doctor finds a small lump in your right breast and recommends a mammogram. The mammogram tells the doctor enough to decide that he definitely wants to perform further tests, such as a biopsy and some x-rays. This could involve a hospital visit, even minor surgery. Or the visit might be more protracted and more serious, depending on the size of the lump, the findings of the biopsy and/or other factors. The test cannot be done until next week.

Right away, your mind races full of frightening complications and uncertainties. And you haven't even gotten to a diagnosis yet. So much to do at home and at work—this is not a good time for this to happen.

But what you *have* done is to encounter the nature of cancer: *it* is individual and complex and impersonal; *you,* however, as a creature of emotions, are now in a state of acute anxiety. You wonder how you should act, how other women you know would handle this problem. And meanwhile, your doctor has gone to full alert.

Now let's suppose you are a male in your late fifties. You are having trouble urinating; it's hard to start, the flow is slow, and you have to go frequently—particularly at night. What you are having is what is known vaguely and somewhat shamefacedly as "prostate trouble." It is an extremely common affliction, but without tests your doctor cannot tell you whether your particular trouble is minor and benign or cancerous, or whether it might require surgery now or at some time in the future and what such surgery will mean to your bodily functions, including your ability to have sex. Indeed, nothing will become clear unless and until your doctor measures, tests, gets results and evaluates. You too are now in a state of extreme anxiety, close to panic. The tests must be taken. The wait for the verdict is going to seem very long.

Once again (and always), diagnosis becomes the first important step in your cancer experience. It is worth examining the process of diagnosis in greater detail so that you will know what is happening to you.

WHAT BRINGS THE PATIENT TO THE DOCTOR? You, as the patient (or as loving friend or relative), are almost certainly concerned about only one form of cancer. But for me it is necessary to cover as many forms as possible and indicate how doctors at present detect their presence. You may, if you wish, skip those that don't immediately concern you. But I recommend nevertheless that you read all the way through this chapter and all the subsequent chapters in logical order, because the better understanding you have of the overall picture, the better able you will be to cope with your particular problem.

We want to detect cancer when it is still at an early stage and before it has produced any symptoms, because clearly it is far more treatable at that point. The screening programs designed for detection purposes are described in Chapter 9. Unfortunately, the usual story is that cancer is first detected only after the patient comes to the doctor with a specific complaint, which then leads to the diagnosis. There are so many different ways of discovering cancer that it is impossible to describe them all here; briefly (and arbitrarily), however, there are three major methods that lead to the diagnosis. In the first, a patient comes to the doctor complaining of some symptom such as a lump or a nonhealing sore, a changing mole, persistent cough or coughing up of blood or bleeding in the stools or urine which, while possibly due to other causes, may lead the physician quickly to diagnose cancer.

In the second type of situation you go in for an unrelated medical problem, or one that seems unrelated, and in the course of the examination the doctor finds a suspicious lesion—such as a mass in the rectum or vagina, enlarged lymph glands, an enlarged liver, et cetera. Sometimes the clue comes from the history obtained from the patient, which reveals some important symptoms such as excessive weight loss, lack of energy, difficulty swallowing, frequent infections, change in bowel habits, nonhealing sores in the mouth or a variety of other symptoms that physicians are trained to inquire about. A laboratory test may reveal the problem, as with an elderly man who came to the hospital for cataract surgery, had a routine preoperative blood test and was found to have leukemia. From the doctor's point of view, it happens sometimes that a patient comes in for an unrelated or trivial complaint and while in the office casually mentions the problem that really concerns her, such as a question of a mass in the breast. Cancer is held in such dread that a patient may not be psychologically able to make an appointment specifically to check this serious concern. For the doctor, too, cancer and its detection are emotionally complex matters.

Finally, there is the patient who comes in for a routine checkup without any symptoms whatever; the doctor finds no suspicious abnormality from the history or physical examination, but the laboratory tests or x-ray may show abnormalities that lead to a diagnosis of malignancy. For example, a patient who has no cough, chest pain, sputum production or other symptoms of lung cancer may be found by a routine chest x-ray to have a mass in the lung. Or the patient who has no constipation or abdominal pain and has not seen any blood in the stools still tests positive for blood in the stools, and this leads, on further study, to a diagnosis of colon cancer. This is the type of situation that often leads to an early diagnosis and good possibility of cure.

DIAGNOSTIC PROCEDURES

Biopsies All right. It has been established that suspicious circumstances exist. What next? Whatever the presenting circumstances—and as you see, they vary tremendously—certain steps will be taken to find out whether the suspicious abnormality has cancer cells in it and, if it does, to define its size and the extent to which the cancer has spread. The most important part of the process is to establish whether the cells are cancerous by doing a biopsy and sending it to the pathology laboratory for analysis. This involves taking out a piece of tissue, either by a small surgical procedure or by using a thin, hollow biopsy needle to cut and remove a small core of tissue; either of these procedures can be done very simply and painlessly under local anesthesia. Sometimes the tumor is not very accessible and the biopsy has to be performed through a flexible tube called an endoscope. Such instruments can be passed up into the colon through the rectum or down into the esophagus or stomach through the mouth; similarly, they can be used to look into the bronchial passages through the main windpipe (trachea) or into the bladder through the urinary passage (urethra). These procedures are somewhat uncomfortable, as I can attest from personal experience, yet they can be performed without much difficulty when the patient is adequately prepared and sedated or lightly anesthetized.

With these techniques the physician actually looks at the suspicious lesion and then is able to take a piece of it and make slides, which are stained and analyzed by a pathologist who is trained to recognize abnormal cells such as cancer, or other types of diseases that may be located in those areas. Depending on the type of tissue, some of it may also have to be sent off to other laboratories that will analyze it for specific findings, such as for the presence of female hormone (estrogen) receptors that may be present on the surface of breast cancer cells. This analysis can give critical information for predicting the results of treatment (see Chapter 4).

Often the entire tumor mass may be removed for purposes of diagnosis. For example, a suspicious mass in the breast or an enlarged lymph gland will be removed in its entirety and sent for examination. Sometimes cancer is found first in the lymph glands, since that is a favored site for spread. Then the physician has to go back to try to find the place of origin. For example, one might first find in the lymph glands a cancer that has spread there from the lung, thyroid or bowel. Occasionally the original tumor is so small that it can never be found. However, once the diagnosis is clear, it is important to determine the extent to which the disease has spread (metastasized), both in the area in which it originated (assuming that it is known) and in more distant tissues. The reason that so many studies (x-rays, scans, blood tests) are often used to establish the extent of disease involvement is that *planning of treatment* depends upon those findings. A cancer that is truly localized in one area may be removable in its entirety by surgery, particularly if it is small and does not involve vital tissues; but if the cancer is found to have spread to distant tissues, then surgery alone will not cure the patient. If the tumor is located in a place where to remove it surgically would cause irreparable damage, say to the brain or heart, then even a localized tumor may be treated without surgery, often by radiation therapy (see Chapter 4).

If the process of diagnosis seems to you like initial bad news followed by an escalating series of worse shocks, remember that the doctor, of necessity, is learning as the results come through, at least as much as the patient. There is nothing he would rather do than give you good news, and he would be both inhuman and a fool to give you firm bad news based on uncertainties. The doctor really *is* on your side. There are times in the treatment of cancer when this is very hard to believe. You may become angry with the doctor at times, and I hope you will have enough trust to tell him so, and to talk about how you really feel. If the doctor is good, he will hang in there with you, understand and respect your feelings and be really supportive.

Blood Tests *A great many types of blood tests can be useful in diagnosing cancer, but there is no single test that detects all types of early cancers—it would be a great boon if there were.* A few tests are very sensitive for certain types of cancer because they involve measuring potent biological substances that are produced by those cancer cells. For example, the hormone called "human chorionic gonadotropin" (HCG) is produced by cells that originate from the placenta, and high levels of HCG can indicate a rapidly growing cancer of young women called choriocarcinoma; fortunately this is now curable in about 95 percent of cases.

High levels of other hormones such as steroids, insulin or thyrocalcitonin help indicate endocrine (glandular) tumors of adrenals, pancreas or thyroid; other substances will signal certain rare tumors if we are smart enough to think of the possibility and order the right test.

The presence in the blood of a cell wall substance that is an antigen derived from the bowel (chorioembryonic antigen [CEA]) was once thought to detect colon cancer at an early stage, but it is not very specific in that it can be present in other conditions as well. Nonetheless, when it is elevated, a CEA level is useful for following the progress of a colon cancer or to see if cancer has recurred after surgical removal, because a rising CEA level will indicate recurrent or advancing disease. In other words, a high blood CEA level can be due to cancer or to some other conditions, but when due to cancer it is helpful to see whether it goes higher or lower after treatment since the change in level usually corresponds with whether the tumor is shrinking or growing.

Prostate cancer cells often produce a unique enzyme (acid phosphatase), and when levels of this are elevated, it is usually a signal that a cancer of the prostate has spread outside the prostate gland into distant tissues. There are other enzymes that are characteristically increased in liver cancer or other cancers, and these have to be considered by the physician in ordering diagnostic blood tests. Such tests can be very useful, but we are aware that they are not always accurate, as will be discussed in the chapter on cancer screening.

Blood counts and bone marrow examination can also be extremely helpful in evaluating a patient with cancer. Anemia is common in many forms of cancer, but also in numbers of benign conditions such as iron deficiency caused by bleeding hemorrhoids or excessive menstrual or other blood loss. However, the appearance of certain types of abnormal red blood cells and white blood cells can typically suggest that there is cancer involving the bone marrow—a condition physicians call myelophthisic anemia. When such cells appear on a blood slide, it is important to follow that lead with a bone marrow test to find the cancer cells. For example, I have had many patients with prostate or breast cancer who have immature and abnormal red and white blood cells in their blood; this makes it quite certain that their cancer has spread to the bone marrow—an important factor that can readily be documented by further examination.

Leukemia is of course a special case because it is a malignancy that involves the blood-forming organs and is easily detected by direct examination of these materials.

Radiological Imaging Various types of x-rays are extremely important in determining the areas of cancer spread; different types of structures are separated by their varying density (fat, air spaces, bone) and thus show up differently upon exposure to x-rays. Certain areas can also be highlighted by changing their density with dyes or contrast material such as barium.

There was a time not so long ago when exploratory surgery was almost always required to examine the abdominal contents, but now this can usually be accomplished by means of special computerized axial tomograph (CT or CAT) scans without discomfort to the patient and without the need for an operation: this type of surgery is now restricted to defining the extent of disease and taking a tissue sample (biopsy). This remarkable technology also separates images on the basis of density, but it provides far greater clarity than conventional x-rays. Magnetic resonance imaging (MRI) is the latest computer-enhanced way of visualizing tumors within the body, for example within the brain. MRI uses a combination of radio waves and a strong magnetic field to penetrate the body; it does not use x-rays. In addition, radioisotope scanning techniques permit detection of lesions in liver, bone and brain that will not show up on standard x-rays. In this case, when a radioactive substance is injected into the blood, it becomes concentrated in or around the cancer and provides energy from that location, which is detected by radioisotope counters; these are then converted into visual images or pictures.

Another special radiologic procedure is called angiography. In this procedure a radiopaque (dense) liquid substance is injected into the artery that supplies blood to the part of the body that one wishes to study. This method is particularly useful for large and deep-seated cancers such as those of the kidney or liver. These and various other techniques represent a very great medical advance, although the technology is very costly. Sometimes CAT scans, ultrasound tests, or angiograms locate suspicious masses deep within the abdomen or chest; in the past those masses surely would have called for major surgery, but now a needle biopsy can be directed to the precise area of abnormality, the tissue can be sampled without surgery, and a definitive diagnosis can be reached. It is certainly much easier on the patient and also less costly than having surgery.

It will be evident even from this brief summary that considerable expertise is required to make the diagnosis and determine the extent of disease in order to plan treatment. In the depth of anxieties that these tests mean for you, bear in mind that *knowledge* is their special contribution, and knowing, having hard information, is far better than not knowing. It is also true that some patients don't want to know. But you are not numbered among them or you would not be reading this book.

The tests serve a vital function for the doctor—and for you. Unfortunately, many of the tests are quite expensive, but they can often be done on an outpatient basis, thereby eliminating expensive hospital costs. Indeed, the new reimbursement regulations for Medicare-eligible patients virtually require that these tests be done on an outpatient basis, although this is not always in the best interest of the patient. Exceptions do arise where it is better to have the test in the hospital. I'm thinking of frail and elderly patients who need to have laxatives and enemas and then bowel x-rays and other tests that are quite exhausting. For financial reasons these now need to be done on an outpatient basis, and that is certainly not ideal.

Sometimes a great deal of testing is required, sometimes very little. You should be aware that unnecessary tests not only lead to unnecessary costs, they also lead to confusion and generate still further costs as the confusion is sorted out. So it is important for *you* to know what the tests are about and why they are being done. This is where your oncologist (cancer specialist) is of immense help. Planning an efficient yet appropriate evaluation is what oncologists do regularly; with appropriate consultation, these matters can also be dealt with by other physicians who do not specialize in cancer. Certain types of problems clearly require specialists from the start, and a patient who has leukemia or a brain tumor, for instance, might just as well be sent to the proper specialist right away.

Whatever the particular outcome of the tests you have been undergoing, you now have a diagnosis. You have cancer. You might be in a state of shocked disbelief—you haven't really allowed yourself to think, "What if the tests are positive?"—or you may immediately despair, or become resigned or be mad as hell. Or you may have been able to put yourself on "hold": decide to wait, don't decide anything else, see what the next step must be. And that would probably be the second opinion.

THE SECOND OPINION (AND HOW TO GET IT) When a medical diagnosis is serious, and the suggested therapy hard to accept (e.g., need for surgery, intensive chemotherapy, etc.), it is almost always wise to seek a second opinion, not necessarily because one questions the diagnosis but because surgery and chemotherapy are very serious matters for you and your body and it is simply sensible to proceed with cautious speed. Often there is the question of whether one's own general doctor is the best person to give the care. He or she might very well prefer to get a second opinion also. In particular, if the primary physician is a surgeon or a general practitioner or an internist, one must ask whether this is the best-qualified person to weigh the worth of alternative treatments. The problem many patients face is how to get answers to those questions without offending the doctor, who probably seems competent, is eager to proceed and has confidence in his own judgment. To the uninvolved observer or helpful friend it may seem reasonable, indeed obvious, that before undergoing something as serious as radical surgery, all other options should be considered. But it is often very difficult for the patient to decide to seek other advice, often not knowing that it can be beneficial (even if it merely confirms the original suggestion), and to work out a plan to transfer summaries, x-rays and pathology slides to the consultant. Most of us have experience to show that it is particularly difficult to be efficient in following through with important details if one is ill, depressed or both.

Let us suggest some practical tips, all of which derive from three basic premises:

☐ No one is as concerned with your health as you are.

☐ Doctors are there to serve patients (and not the other way around).

☐ Getting a second opinion is not only legitimate but is often a relief and a tangible help to your doctor.

Reasons for Obtaining Second Opinions There is no set formula for what constitutes the need to obtain a second opinion. If you feel insecure or unsure about what you have been told and about accepting treatments that seem dangerous or radical, then you probably need a second opinion. If your doctor is not a specialist in oncology, a consultation by an oncologist (cancer specialist) would seem appropriate. If there is disagreement within your family whether the right course of action is being taken, getting a second opinion may relieve you of the stress of defending your doctor's suggestions. Family and friends, no matter how well-intentioned, can often bring unnecessary grief by trying to be helpful without understanding how your medical situation differs from that of a friend who was "cured" by a totally different type of treatment. If this is the reason for a consultation, then you will want that person(s) present during the discussion following your evaluation so that any questions can be answered by the specialist.

Arranging Your Priorities Try to itemize the questions that you want the consultant to answer. Are you questioning whether the tests that were done really add up to what you have been told, or whether there might be an error in the diagnosis? Do you want to avoid the surgery that may have been recommended if you can find another treatment that appears equally effective? Are you questioning whether less extensive surgery might be a good alternative—for example, a "lumpectomy" instead of modified radical mastectomy for breast cancer? Are you concerned about the type of chemotherapy being recommended and how to minimize side effects? Are you concerned about being sterile or sexually impotent after cancer treatment? Do you want to learn more about newer, experimental therapy? These are all reasonable questions to ask of a consultant, and you are more likely to get the answers if you can frame the questions in advance. Write down the questions, since it is easy to get nervous in these circumstances, and be sure to tell your doctor that you have some specific points that you want to cover before leaving the office.

Whom Would You Like to See? Depending on the circumstances (and your degree of medical sophistication), you may already have a good idea about whom you would like to see or where you want to be seen. If you have no idea, then it is safest to be seen by an oncologist at a major cancer center or university medical center if one is accessible to you. *Remember that the key is the individual expert who will work with you and not the reputation of the place or its size.* I have seen a few very poor doctors in highly respected centers and many outstanding ones in private practice. Thus, there is no single formula for finding the right person. Sometimes the experts with the "big names" are the best people to see if you can, but they may also be so busy that there will not be time to have all of your questions answered. If your questions are of a general nature, a medical oncologist is the person to see; if you have technical questions such as what is the right kind of surgery or radiation therapy, then see a specialist in those fields (surgical and radiation oncologist, respectively). By and large it is a good idea to start the consultations by seeing a medical oncologist for an adult or a pediatric oncologist for a child and let that person be the center of coordination if other consultants are needed, as they often are. Perhaps this is my bias, being a medical oncologist myself, but these are often the experts who deal most broadly with cancer problems and who will usually take the necessary time to explain the various procedures and options. If they won't take the time you had better find another doctor.

What Are the Most Important Qualities for Your Consultant to Have? Some very knowledgeable doctors (including oncologists) seem to be gruff or distant; they spend little time answering questions, leaving this to their junior colleagues or assistants. At the other end of the spectrum are oncologists who are great communicators but are not up to date on the latest treatments or are too conservative to mention them as options, even if they might appeal to the patient. Still others may want to treat all patients aggressively (that is, in the sense of using maximum treatment even if the individual circumstances make that a questionable decision). From my point of view, an aggressive form of treatment is most appropriate to recommend to a patient who knows that despite the risk, this offers the only chance of major benefit. Yet a treatment that is very toxic and not likely to cause a lasting benefit may be anathema to the individual who prefers a better quality of life. *The doctor has to be willing and able to explain the choices and let the patient decide.* Very often the patient passes the decision back to the doctor by saying, in effect, "You're the doctor and you know best," and that's all right, too! That is a positive decision on the part of the patient. I was shocked a few years ago when I was on a panel at a postgraduate seminar and a physician in the audience asked a noted breast cancer surgeon what he would do if a patient of his refused to have a conventional modified radical mastectomy and preferred a "lumpectomy"—the surgeon said he would tell her to find another doctor because he would not engage in malpractice! First, that is not malpractice, and second, the medical profession has an obligation to take patients' wishes seriously and to try to accommodate them if it is at all reasonable to do so. I told this particular doctor he would never have to worry about seeing any patients of mine: fortunately the breast cancer surgeons at our institution were not so rigid in their approach. In my view, malpractice is not caring about what the patient wants, and so my recommendation was, and will always be, that the patient go to see another surgeon. In fact, on one or two occasions I have even supervised the giving of a quack remedy (krebiozen, laetrile) that a patient wanted, simply because the patients would then not drop out of sight of proper medical care. After they had their try and it failed, they were satisfied to take conventional treatment.

Oncologists who are highly specialized, particularly if they work in a large medical center, spend most of their time seeing only patients who have lymphoma or leukemia, urologic malignancy or some other particular type of cancer. Such doctors can be tremendously useful if the diagnosis has already been established and the question is what therapy to employ. For example, if a person has head and neck cancer, for which there are many treatment options, a specialized multidisciplinary clinic where all specialists are present at once is the ideal place to go. I wish all of our work were organized in this way, but it is difficult to get specialists who have different training to work together in a single clinic.

Other oncologists are more general in their orientation, and they can be very helpful if there are some diagnostic questions or some coexisting medical complications that might influence therapeutic decisions. Broad experience and wisdom are the qualities that serve best in this capacity—knowledge about the latest experience at some other institution is not as relevant as the capacity to sort out the medical issues and complications and to synthesize an individualized approach to management.

Where Do You Find This Consultant? By all odds this is the most difficult question to answer. One way to start is to ask your personal physician and perhaps another physician whom you may know to give you a list of their three top choices for oncologists whose expertise is in the area of your problem. Ask them to discuss with you the pros and cons of each, being sure to cover the points that are important to you, such as those discussed above. *In the course of discussing the pros and cons of several candidates you will become clearer in your own mind about what is most important to you.* Also, if your physician is a surgeon, you may want to have some medical as well as surgical oncologists recommended to you.

By *involving your personal doctor* in the process of choosing a consultant, rather than going it alone, without help, you automatically enlist your doctor's cooperation in sending summaries, slides and x-rays (without which the consultant usually cannot function), and you also set in motion the feedback of information and recommendations to your doctor, who can then take full advantage of the second opinion. Sometimes in a small community group practice your doctor will suggest his partner or close colleague because that is familiar and comfortable, and that is useful. My advice, however, would be to get other suggestions as well by going outside your local area for the consultant.

What Happens If the Opinions Differ Significantly? Sometimes the problem of differing opinions is more apparent than real. It usually disappears if the consultant and primary physician communicate with each other after talking with you. For example, if my second opinion differs from that of the referring physician, I am perfectly willing to call (if my patient so wishes) and discuss the key issues to see if we are working from different perceptions of the same data or if our database differs in some significant way. Sometimes I have found something that was missed in an earlier examination, and that may cause the referring physician to change his opinion, or vice versa. When differences of opinion do occur, it is always in the patient's best interest to get all of the concerned parties together if that is at all feasible, even if only by telephone hookup.

We must recognize that at times the patient is not satisfied by the second opinion or the opinions differ greatly, and then it may be necessary to get another opinion, preferably from a nationally recognized expert. While there is nothing minor about their cost, these consultations are not nearly as expensive as liver scans or other technical procedures, and they can be moneysaving by eliminating unnecessary further testing; at times they may also be lifesaving. *The most common benefit is to have the peace of mind of knowing that you have done what you could to inform yourself and that you are in the best of hands.*

How Do You Accept Advice? Sometimes the advice of the primary doctor and of the consultant will be the same, but still it is difficult to accept—in some instances you may even want a third opinion if you are confused. For example, a woman called me from another state to ask me to give her interferon for breast cancer. Now I obviously don't practice medicine over the telephone, but it turned out after my questioning her that she had localized breast cancer and both of her doctors had advised surgery. Since she had a high chance of cure from surgery, it would have been quite inappropriate to give her interferon, which had no chance to cure her, and I explained this to her. Her problem had to be faced at a different level, and we put her in touch with professionals who could help deal with those emotional issues.

WHERE ARE THE BEST PLACES TO GET CARE? This is another very difficult question to answer because it depends upon so many individual factors. Health care in this country is arranged around personal physicians, who have differing interests and training. A woman may consider her gynecologist-obstetrician to be her primary care physician, which places a somewhat unfamiliar responsibility on that physician to diagnose a brain tumor, for example. It would be advisable for everyone, all of us in fact, to have a very competent general physician (internist, general or family practitioner) who can coordinate any consultants or specialists as circumstances require and who has the resources to follow up on recommendations if long-term care is required. *Excellent care is provided by excellent people, and they can be found everywhere—in cancer institutes, in medical centers and in community hospitals.* Having been at a major cancer center throughout my career, I can see advantages of having a team of highly skilled specialists who are used to working together. There is a time to use such facilities, and there is a time to use the more convenient and economical facilities of the community hospital. Moreover, there is an ever-increasing reason to use home care, particularly in the terminal phase of an illness. The time for hospice care arises when the goals of treatment are to make life as comfortable as possible rather than to extend it by aggressive means when there is no expectation of improvement. Major medical centers are often not very good at recognizing when it is time to stop being so aggressive, although that generalization is subject to exceptions, to be sure. But that decision, if it should have to be made, is a "fur piece" down the road of treatment.

It may help you to know that each and every graduating doctor has taken the ancient Oath of Hippocrates. These words still do have meaning for us today.

THE OATH OF HIPPOCRATES

I do solemnly swear by whatever I hold most sacred, that I will be loyal to the profession of medicine and just and generous to its members.

That I will lead my life and practice my Art in uprightness and honor.

That into whatsoever home I shall enter it shall be for the good of the sick and the well to the utmost of my power and that I will hold myself aloof from wrong and from corruption and from the tempting of others to vice.

That I will exercise my Art, solely for the cure of my patients and the prevention of disease and will give no drugs and perform no operation for a criminal purpose and far less suggest such thing.

That whatsoever I shall see or hear of the lives of men which is not fitting to be spoken, I will keep inviolably secret.

These things I do promise and in proportion as I am faithful to this oath, may happiness and good repute be ever mine, the opposite if I shall be forsworn.

COMMUNICATION IS THE SECRET OF SUCCESS

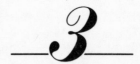

As we have seen, a great deal occurs before patient and doctor together decide what to do, even before the diagnosis has been made. A very great deal more must now take place in evolving treatment, and this immediately brings into focus a perennial two-way concern, that of communication. Communication is so vital to the course of good treatment that it deserves, at this point, a special chapter to itself. It may not even be too much to say that the effectiveness of everything that follows—that is to say, your mutual understanding with your doctor of the problem you are now fighting together—may depend on getting this one *right.*

Experience has taught me that whenever there is a problem with patients, families, staff and students, the overwhelming likelihood is that it can be solved by improving communication. It can be taken as a given that each party comes to a particular situation with a unique background and point of view, and with unique concerns—this literally can mean that everyone is right but the situation is not working well! Numerous books have been written from the perspective of patients who are coping with cancer, which serve to illustrate how their perceptions and needs may often not be seen or met by the medical staff. By contrast, little information is available about this from the medical perspective. Let us examine some common problems and see how the individual can best deal with the complexities that arise within the system (often referred to by health professionals as the nonsystem) of medical care.

SETTING UP GOALS When you go to see a doctor, you do so out of choice and with some specific objective in mind—whether it is to obtain reassurance from a regular checkup or to obtain care for a specific complaint or disease. Your doctor needs to know *your* wishes, although as your professional caregiver he may delve into many areas beyond those you think are relevant. The need to do so will usually be fully explained as you go along, since you are the one who must bear the inconvenience, discomfort (if any) and cost. Certain points that at first seem distant or even unrelated to the matter at hand may turn out to be important and even central to your care. At the end of the evaluation there should be a summing up in which the physician presents you with the findings and gives you a chance to ask questions and seek advice. If there are major new findings or decisions that need to be made, this is the time when a plan should be set up in a way that suits you—even if you find that your only option is to select the best from among a series of unattractive choices. This is the first really clear point for you to ask a host of questions. You need to make up the same *pattern* of questions that are outlined for hospital use later in this chapter. But now is the time, in the privacy and leisure of your own doctor's office, to *ask.* There may be questions you will find yourself asking again, later, of your oncologist, or an intern, a radiologist, a nurse—it doesn't matter: remember, you are learning, and what you are learning is literally far more important to you than to anybody else in the world. So questioning will never—and *should* never—stop.

Depending on the complexity of the problem, the process of setting out the goals and objectives may require more than one session. It may involve getting some more tests or a second opinion, time for private thought and reflection and discussion with family members. Remember, in the final analysis *the decision to be made is yours,* with the help and support of your physician. You need not be embarrassed to ask what may seem like "silly" questions if you do not understand something. You need not fear hurting the doctor's feelings by questioning his advice or reasoning; you should not even fear discharging (yes, I mean firing) your doctor if there seems to be a serious problem in working together. *For you the term "working together" must mean working for your best interests; for the doctor it must mean doing for you what he believes to be in your best interest—given all the known facts.* Most of the time this does not prove to be difficult, but since these two points of view are different, it is not surprising that occasionally problems do arise.

To illustrate these different perspectives, let us briefly examine the concerns that arise when a diagnosis of cancer is first made. The doctor wants to check over all the slides to make sure the diagnosis is certain, to obtain additional x-rays or scans to see whether the cancer has spread, to do other special blood tests that give some indication of how aggressive the disease is and then perhaps to bring in some consultants to help devise a treatment plan.

The patient, on the other hand, is hoping that the diagnosis is wrong or worrying about whether the disease will be painful, whether there is any possibility of a cure, how long he will live, whether some other hospital has a more advanced treatment and whether the treatments cause hair loss, nausea and vomiting or other side effects, as they did with an acquaintance who may have been unsuccessfully treated for cancer. Clearly, some of these concerns overlap with those of the physician, but others are unique to the patient; all of them are legitimate and must be satisfactorily explored. Let me emphasize here that there are a wide variety of cancers and an equally wide variety of possible treatments. Both areas will be covered later in this book. For now we are concerned with the *how* of conveying information.

If there is an aggressive course of treatment available that has a high chance of curing a patient, the patient needs to learn how often the treatment needs to be given and what its side effects are and possibly also to be given the statistics that show *why* it is so important to proceed with the treatment. If there is a good chance to achieve a cure but the patient chooses not to pursue the necessary treatment, then the doctor is in a most uncomfortable position, and under certain circumstances may recommend that the patient go where staff may cater to that particular point of view. For example, if someone with religious convictions against receiving a blood transfusion comes to me for help with a bleeding problem, and in my best judgment there is no substitute for using blood transfusion for lifesaving purposes, then I may choose not to become that person's doctor but will help the person find other care. Good medical care is hard enough to render without having your hands tied from the outset—which is not to say that I would refuse the patient if there was any possible alternative to transfusion. For example, many years ago I was treating leukemia in an elderly man whose religion forbade blood transfusions, and blood substitutes were not available. His leukemia was in remission and the man was quite well when he developed a hemolytic anemia in which his spleen was rapidly destroying his red blood cells. Unable to remove his spleen because of inability to give blood transfusions, we tried him on high doses of steroids as a last-ditch alternative treatment, and this stopped the breakdown of his blood cells. Later we were able to reduce the dosage of the drug to an acceptable maintenance level. We did not advise using steroids at first because he was already susceptible to infection and this made it more likely—but we got through it satisfactorily. He expected the Lord would provide for him and he was rewarded! (It may be blasphemous to say, but things usually do not work out that well!)

What we are recommending is a kind of unwritten contract—the technical term is "therapeutic alliance"—in which goals are acceptable and can be agreed upon by the patient and the doctor. If that kind of relationship can be established mutually from the outset, it will serve as a strong foundation or bond for all future dealings and be supportive even during times of extreme difficulty and stress. This is very important because *almost* any doctor-patient relationship can be acceptable as long as the patient is doing well—the hard part is to have a sustaining and trusting relationship if and when the going gets rough.

"MY DOCTOR WON'T TELL ME ANYTHING" "My doctor won't tell me anything" is a frequently heard complaint when people are struggling to cope with a serious problem such as cancer (or any other problem, for that matter). That statement may be an accurate answer to a question from a friend, or it may be a cry for help. It is important to try to understand the true nature of the problem because those words have many possible meanings and they may point to widely different needs and actions.

First let us consider the statement at face value and assume that our patient has indicated to the physician that he wants to be given all the pertinent information as soon as possible. There are physicians who find it hard to talk to patients about "bad news"—such as a new and serious diagnosis, a dire prognosis based on evidence of disease progression or the need for major surgery, whether it be life threatening or disfiguring (e.g., amputation). In a hospital situation the telltale signs about these doctors are often that they make rounds quickly (sometimes very early in the morning when the patient is sleeping or washing), exchange pleasantries and trivial information about sleep and food or ration out incomplete bits of information and disappear with their entourage before the patient has a chance to ask any sensitive questions. Such doctors often do not initiate discussion even when there is news, and if a question is not quickly forthcoming, they feel they have given the patient every opportunity to ask—they may even instruct their students or staff that it is not necessary to overwhelm patients with dreaded news, for when patients are ready they will ask. When I was a resident one of my senior attending physicians refused to awaken his private patients when he made ward rounds in the early morning; he told his students that "a sleeping patient is a happy patient." However, that was not what the patient would tell me later in the day! This doctor was a brilliant man who could have succeeded in many things, but he got into the wrong profession, or stayed at it too long.

In or out of a hospital such doctors make it extremely difficult to ask them questions, and when asked, their response often seems curt and insensitive. They may never have learned how to communicate with their patients; more often, they may simply find it personally painful since, believe it or not, they may identify you, the patient, with their spouse, sibling, parent or child for reasons obscure to everyone, particularly themselves. Manifestly, this is not your problem. Medical school admission committees do a very good job of screening applicants for intelligence, diligence and scientific aptitude—but unfortunately, the crucial question of whether the candidate has the potential to become a compassionate physician often cannot be answered on the basis of test scores, grades, a brief interview or enthusiastic letters of recommendation. Regardless of the reason (and we are not here to make excuses for doctors), the task of exchanging difficult and sometimes painful information in a clear and easily understandable manner is in many cases not carried out because the doctor does not provide a warm, open and supportive environment. In such a situation, seeking a second and third opinion is vital, and must be done promptly.

The words "my doctor won't tell me anything" can also have a very different meaning, requiring a very different response. The patient may be using denial as a coping strategy, meaning that he avoids asking questions when genuine opportunities exist. In fact, the patient may indicate a need *not* to be told ("I can take anything as long as it isn't cancer"). It is also possible that having been told, the patient doesn't "hear" or, more precisely, isn't properly able to process, store and recall the painful information that has been given. The spouse or another person who was in the room when the information was communicated may occasionally have comparable problems, illustrated by repeatedly asking whether the doctor is sure of the diagnosis and then, upon hearing that it is just barely a possibility that it is a benign lesion, recalling only that possibility, later to be "shocked" to learn the truth. More often than not, however, the other person understands the information even when the patient doesn't, and then that person has the difficult task of trying to explain to other family members, or to the patient, what actually was said if that differs from the patient's perceptions. If this task makes people sufficiently uncomfortable, they may choose to remain silent and thereby compound the confusion. There are many things that can go wrong with the complexity of conveying unwelcome, frightening information. The most common way to cope is to shut down, stop receiving input and become depressed.

How can these important communication problems be minimized? Although there is no single formula for all circumstances, the patient and family can improve the odds of a successful encounter by considering the following steps:

1   *Choose a doctor who is not only technically competent, but who is also recommended as warm, easy to talk to and compassionate.* This is not as simple as it sounds—it is a general problem in choosing physicians.

2   *Discuss with your spouse or other loved one what you expect to learn from the doctor, and do this before going to see the doctor the first time.* If you make it clear that you want full information and total honesty as soon as the information is available, and then ask the doctor if he will abide by that request, your wish will generally be respected. The more knowledge you have the better able you are to ask questions, and to follow up on developments. Don't expect absolutes. Very often, the best your doctor can give you is an educated guess. For your own peace of mind (and to give your body a better fighting chance), understand the differences when your doctor(s) is telling hard fact and when he is only guessing or speculating. This process is part of the larger process of developing a therapeutic alliance with the physician.

3   It is often helpful to have your spouse or significant other(s) in the room when major news is expected. This can be very important and comforting because it ensures that this person is given the news and has a chance to ask questions too, and it minimizes the need for time-consuming repetition. It does

place responsibility on you for making an appointment to have your "other" present—and sometimes these encounters are difficult to arrange or may even have to be canceled, especially in a hospital, because of the timing of ward rounds, the occurrence of unexpected emergencies and the like. It is often useful to have your nurse in the room during the conference in the hospital to clarify certain points after the doctor leaves—I find that very few patients avail themselves of this opportunity, and very few doctors think to ask the nurse to be present. If the nurse is not present, this opportunity for communication can be lost.

4   *Ask questions if you do not understand the information or the terminology. There is no reason to be intimidated because you do not comprehend technical terms.* By the same token, try to grasp the big picture and don't be afraid to ask the same question in several ways, either in this encounter or a subsequent one. You do not have a medical degree, so take your time; you may not think of all the questions on the first occasion. You may not realize that you didn't completely grasp your doctor's explanation until you try to explain it to someone else.

5   If you have specific questions or concerns and if intimidating encounters on hospital rounds or clinic visits cause you to forget to ask them, *make a list in advance, ask the questions and check off the list.* This may seem sophomoric or make you feel that the doctor finds you bothersome, but *do it anyway and get on with the job!*

6   Try not to play "games" with important medical information—whether you are the patient or the spouse. Honesty and open communication are important in primary relationships, never more so than when dealing with situations that may involve medical crises. This is discussed further below.

7   You should, however, understand that the physician often cannot stop rounds long enough to give long, detailed explanations on the spur of the moment. Other patients need to be seen, and other duties are tightly scheduled. Therefore, *it is preferable to indicate on rounds that you have questions, and request that time be specifically scheduled for you (and for all others whom you*

wish to have present). From personal experience I can tell you that it is very discouraging for a doctor to spend thirty to forty-five minutes explaining a problem and various options to the patient, repeat the process later with the spouse and then have a relative appear the next day to get "the full story" or even to get "just a minute of your time." Those "minutes" can be particularly long because this self-appointed spokesperson often has a particular point of view to express—such as, what about using megavitamins because they cured a friend who suffered from the "same problem." As a patient you may find yourself "assaulted" by well-meaning friends or relatives who really care about you and are having the very human reaction of wanting to help.

There are various ways to handle such suggestions; perhaps the most direct one is to say that your doctor is responsible for the medical aspects of your case and you would be glad if this friend wants to discuss his ideas with the physician and then you and your doctor will discuss it in turn. Explain that since no two people are alike, a treatment that may be appropriate for another patient may not be right for you and that you trust your doctor can listen to and evaluate any such suggestion. Then alert your doctor to expect a visit from your friend: you can assume that this may not be met by enthusiasm but it can certainly be accepted gracefully if adequate notice is given. From my own experience it is very rare for anything useful to come from such outside sources, but there is always a possibility that there might be something to look into further, and it does relieve *you* to know that the information has been properly evaluated and in turn your friend feels his responsibility to deliver the suggestion has been fulfilled. If a new idea emerges and you want it investigated further, ask your doctor to make the necessary calls, get the information and then discuss it with you. *That makes positive use of your doctor's ability to make contacts not open to you, to consider the new information in view of your particular medical circumstances and then act as your resource and advocate using all available means.* This is much more sensible than going around your doctor to do it all on your own. See if this point of view makes sense to you.

"YOU CAN TELL ME, BUT DON'T TELL . . ." One of the problems most frequently faced by patients and families, one that is almost guaranteed to cause consternation and anguish, is the question of who to tell what information. Physicians and nurses who have the information are often put into the uncomfortable position of being asked by their patients to restrict access to it in a manner that seems counterproductive to the very goals they are trying to achieve. Many times I have been asked by a patient to tell him everything, but not to tell his spouse if the news was bad because "she can't take it"; then that request has been followed by the same request from the spouse to tell her everything, but not him because "he is already so severely depressed." Or an entire family, particularly adult children and their spouses, have begged their doctor to withhold key medical information from an aged parent, even though that person was in full control of his faculties.

Perhaps there are no absolute truths—but honest, open and what we may call realistically optimistic communication makes it much easier to deal not only with the immediate situation, but also with the difficult events that will inevitably ensue during the course of active anticancer therapy or the course of incurable cancer. Patients usually know when there is something seriously wrong, and when the family or doctor tells them otherwise, this does not reassure and comfort them but, rather, it undermines trust and confidence in the very individuals who are most needed to provide emotional support, and possibly survival. And if a question is asked directly and the physician dances around the answer, then the patient surmises, usually correctly, that the news is bad. And that scenario can be repeated frequently if the disease progresses. This is tough on everyone!

Before we ask to protect our loved ones from bad news, we must first ask if we are really protecting ourselves, because it is hard for us to comfort them or find the right thing to say or do when the news is bad. It is my observation that the more severe the conflict that arises about sharing the information, the more impaired communications were likely to have been previously, even during times of good health. Our friend Uncle Louie, the long-lost relative who suddenly appears on the scene and who wants to direct the flow of information or offer dramatic advice about what to do next, is an especially destructive force with whom the rest of the family must contend at a time when they are already maximally strained and have depleted emotional reserves. (And don't be an "Uncle Louie" yourself if the situation is reversed—the temptation can be hard to resist.)

The best way to avoid these problems is to have the patient and significant other(s) (spouse, parent, child, friend) all be in the room with the physician at the same time, as discussed earlier. The patient or spouse can make particular concerns known to the doctor in advance so that some thinking can be done before confronting an emotionally charged situation with a divided family, or one that contains hostile members. And do not underestimate the possibility that flagrant hostility can exist in your family, as it can in the best of families! The group of conferees selected by the patient will then share the same information and there will be no need to have secrets from each other, nor will there be nearly as much chance for confusion (there is always some). They will also decide who, if anyone else, should be told the medical information.

Are there any good reasons to make exceptions to forthright discussions such as we have suggested? Yes, in some situations the most forthright approach may indeed be an inappropriate course of action. There are some patients whose mechanism of coping with a serious illness is to deny its seriousness—*they do not want to discuss it* and they make it clear to the doctor that they want to be treated in the best possible manner but not bothered with the details. It is wise for all concerned to respect this denial mechanism, and not assault the patient with information which he is not prepared to receive at that time. The physician should explain this to the spouse separately and then, in joint meetings with the patient and spouse, offer to answer any questions the patient may have—then or at any later time. We try to impress young doctors not to assault patients with news that they are not yet ready to hear—we can proceed more deliberately than that. We want to provide the patient with the opportunity to control the flow of information that must be processed. The person who needs to get the information slowly, or in small packages, is like the swimmer who prefers to enter a very cold lake inches at a time, while someone else strides in or dives in to "get it over with." There is also a middle ground of going slowly up to the point of decision and then getting it over with—there are an infinite number of individual variations.

Information may also be held back in the case of a young child, or a very aged person who may already have numerous other illnesses and whose mental capacities are impaired. With an elderly patient the physician may need to tread lightly in divulging the news if there is not a surviving spouse, no critical decisions to be made and the children feel strongly that their parent cannot handle the news. If, on the other hand, the aged patient is in command of his faculties and demands to be told, the physician needs to explain to the family that his primary obligation is to serve the patient, unless that person proves to be mentally incompetent.

In thinking about legitimate exceptions to what we believe is a wise policy of making information available as the patient is ready to receive it, we must recall that this type of approach is relatively new in American medicine, and even more so in Europe. Until recently, it was generally not the practice to tell the patient about the diagnosis of cancer. Why has there been such a drastic change in the approach? First, the days of the paternalistic relationship between doctor and patient are past; patients want more control over their destiny than they were previously afforded. Then, too, there are often far more therapeutic choices available than in the past, and patients have a legal right to participate fully in the decisions about them. Furthermore, from a purely practical point of view, it is virtually impossible to recommend complex and potentially uncomfortable treatment programs, in which the patients may have to have blood counts weekly and intravenous drugs every three weeks, without telling the patients more than that they have some minor illness. It is difficult (as well as illegal and unethical) to deceive an intelligent, mentally competent patient who wants to know, and it is crucial for patients' trust and mental well-being that they not be manipulated by well-meaning relatives or doctors!

"WHAT ARE MY CHANCES, DOCTOR?" This may be the most frequently asked question and the one that is most emotionally charged. If the answer is an unhappy one, it is often emotionally charged for the doctor as well (yes, we certainly do have feelings). Sometimes the question is technically easy to answer if the odds are extremely good or bad, but usually it is very difficult to predict what an individual patient will do, since no two people are the same or react in the same way to medication. Overall statistics, which are discussed later in this book, do not really apply to the individual—because each person is a "series of one" and whatever the outcome is, it will be 100 percent for that patient. So statistics can be useful only as generalized guidelines, never as absolute end results. True, we are increasingly using sophisticated computer-ized data systems to try to predict more precisely than we might do otherwise. Still, there are people alive today whose doctors gave them "six months to live" many years ago, and it is the doctor who has since died. Thus, there is a real difficulty in predicting outcome, and failure to get a clear answer to this question is *not necessarily an ominous sign.* In fact, it may be a sign of a cautious and wise doctor. So go for the facts, understand the overall picture, learn all about the particular problem you have to cope with and deal with it step by step as you go along.

CANCER TREATMENT

TREATMENT WITH CURATIVE INTENT There are three major forms of treatment for cancer: surgery, radiation therapy and chemotherapy, and they can be used singly, in sequence or in combination. There is also the newly emerging and exciting field of immunotherapy with drugs such as interferons, interleukins and monoclonal antibodies—though immunotherapy is not yet a well-established technique for treating most types of cancers. *Selecting the type of initial treatment is a matter of paramount importance because it is widely accepted that the best opportunity to cure a patient is the first opportunity,* and if a cure is not effected at that time, the disease will recur. Consultation is important because this is the point at which understanding the full range of alternatives is vital to the patient, and because this is the point at which the oncologist is probably most valuable. The best moment at which to attack a cancer is the time when a permanent cure is most likely to be successful. Once cancer recurs it is less likely to be curable, although further treatment may cause notable shrinkage of tumor and extension of life.

To delay getting on with potentially curative treatment may be to miss the "chance of a lifetime." Why is it that even highly educated people turn to quack remedies such as laetrile, krebiozen, megavitamins and serum therapy? Why do people turn to well-meaning but medically ignorant friends and relatives for medical information when they are in distress, and what has happened to their trust in doctors as guardians of health care? I suppose the answers are different for different people.

It may surprise you to learn that two people who have the same type of cancer may be treated very differently. Let me explain why this may have to occur for both patients to be treated properly. In addition to evaluating a suspicious lesion and determining whether it is cancer and, if so, the extent to which it has spread, the physician needs to look for other medical conditions that may have a bearing on the type of treatment that can best be used. For example, a patient who has cancer and severe lung disease or heart disease may be treated differently from one who does not. Thus, information about other medical conditions needs to be obtained as part of the initial planning of treatment because some types of treatment are not feasible for people who have impairment of certain organs.

A cancer that occurs in a localized area of the body is treated by surgical removal, provided that surgery can be done without causing irreparable harm to nearby normal vital structures such as brain, spinal cord or heart. At times a localized cancer can be treated equally well with radiation therapy, as in the case of cancer of the larynx, some cancers of the prostate and selected others. In some circumstances radiation therapy is preferable to surgery, for example, for Hodgkin's disease and other malignant lymphomas. If doctors fail to recognize the unique characteristics and opportunities of the initial situation, they may lose valuable time that can mean the difference between cure and no cure—the most vital distinction of all. *Although time is important, it is even more important not to rush in with a treatment program before thinking it through carefully,* and taking a week or so to develop the best initial approach can be time very well spent. Sometimes it is hard for the patient to wait that long before getting the breast lump removed, but from a medical standpoint a week is usually not a consequential delay. In acute leukemia, on the other hand, or some other type of cancer-related emergency, treatment may need to be started on the same day. You, as the patient in whom a particular cancer has been diagnosed, need to ask right away what the expected time sequences for your decisions might be.

The term "five-year cure" is used in describing the results of cancer treatment, although the word "cure" is difficult to define in an absolute sense. For example, a five-year-old child who is treated for acute leukemia may have a remission in the first three months and then either may relapse despite continuing treatment or not relapse for many years. We know that the likelihood of relapse is greatest in the first few years and that if relapse does not occur within five years, it is very unlikely it will ever occur. *Theoretically* one would have to wait the entire life of the individual before one could draw the conclusion that the patient had actually been cured—obviously it is impractical to wait for seventy years to make that judgment, and so we *operationally* decide that a child free of leukemia for five years is "cured." Or, for instance, a child who has cancer of the bone and is treated with a combination of surgery and chemotherapy will either relapse within one or two years following the initial treatment or is unlikely ever to relapse; thus at the end of five years we consider that individual to be cured. One major exception to this kind of definition of the term five-year cure is in the case of cancer of the breast, which has a peculiar natural history in that the chance of having a recurrence of disease never fully reaches a plateau and thus the cancer may recur at five, ten or even fifteen years, although a recurrence certainly becomes progressively less likely with the passage of time. In other types of cancer it is also possible, although unlikely, for disease to recur after five years.

There are other aspects of the use of the term "cure" that bear discussion for they explain, in part, why there are no legitimate instant "miracle" treatments. A new experimental treatment that is to be proven successful will first be curative for only a small group of patients at one hospital. These results need to be verified by larger studies conducted at several institutions, with sufficient numbers of patients treated so that statistically significant results can be achieved. Also, the patients obviously need to be followed for a long enough period to confirm the earlier results. These data are then reported to the community of scientists and physicians at large, and if a new drug is involved, the sponsoring pharmaceutical company will then apply to the government for licensing to market the product. Only physicians who are participating in a research study can prescribe an experimental drug before the granting of federal approval, which essentially permits packaging and marketing. (This can be a real bottleneck if there is a known effective drug that the Food and Drug Administration has not yet approved, as discussed in a later chapter.) Thereafter physicians are free to prescribe the medication; there is a variable period of time for this so-called technology transfer to take place, during which physicians learn about the new advance and how to use it for their own patients. (The period of time required to inform practicing oncologists about effective new treatments is much shorter than is generally perceived. There are now many well-informed oncologists who read journals and attend postgraduate meetings to learn about the latest advances. Basically, news travels fast!) Then a significant number of the nation's patients must be treated by the drug and followed for years in order for the mortality statistics to begin gradually to show a decline in deaths from that particular disease.

The entire process can take a decade or so (after the basic studies of the drugs are completed). Obviously, we must begin to think about the possibility of cure long before that period is over, if in fact we have a successful new treatment. A good example of this process is the curative combination chemotherapy for Hodgkin's disease, which was first reported in 1963; it was 1970 before the patients had been followed sufficiently long that the probable cure of Hodgkin's disease by chemotherapy could be announced. It was not until the mid-1970s that it became generally known that patients with widespread Hodgkin's disease could potentially be cured by chemotherapy, and only after that could one discern a significant drop in the mortality figures for Hodgkin's disease based on nationwide statistics. There are no shortcuts to good clinical research, as has been learned time and again from premature announcements of "pseudo-breakthroughs." Unfortunately, there are frustrating delays in the course of drug development.

The cure of cancer of the testis did not take as long to be reflected in the national statistics that marked the event with a rapid decline in deaths from that illness. Nonetheless, it is clear that we are always at least somewhat behind in recognizing successful treatment, and we cannot yet fully appreciate advances that have occurred from experimental treatments started during the past few years since too little time has passed to establish that the disease is not going to recur. We know that Hodgkin's disease is a type of malignant lymphoma that now is curable in a high percentage of patients. There is a large group of patients who have other types of lymphomas, some of which are curable with combination chemotherapy and some of which are not; the types of treatment that are used with patients who have these conditions depend upon the microscopic appearance plus certain other technical features of the disease. Diffuse histiocytic lymphoma is one variety of non-Hodgkin's lymphoma that used to kill patients within a few months, but now the cure rate for it is in the neighborhood of 50 percent. Burkitt's lymphoma is also potentially curable by chemotherapy; for the most part these and other malignant lymphomas are treated with combinations of active drugs. For those forms of lymphoma that have not been found to be curable by currently available drug programs, better drug or immunologic treatments are sorely needed.

One point to remember is that successful treatment of cancer, unlike that of many other chronic illnesses, often restores patients to a state of health where they can resume a normal lifestyle and occupation. Indeed, I have rarely met healthy people who can achieve the degree of happiness that is experienced by a patient with cancer who has been successfully treated. Recently I have been impressed that even elderly patients who are treated with interferon for their hairy cell leukemia will improve dramatically in a few weeks to months, and they manage to achieve a state of well-being that they had not known for years. Those naysayers who argue against vigorous treatment of elderly people need to see this remarkable example! Unfortunately, patients with chronic kidney disease who are on dialysis programs or those who have chronic heart failure are rarely able to achieve this degree of rehabilitation. Nevertheless, one very important social side effect of cure is to convince employers that people who have been cured of cancer are employable: in fact, such people are generally so thrilled to be alive that their work record is at least as good as that of people who have not had to face such devastating illness. The right to be employed is a matter of no small importance to the ever-growing ranks of cured patients who wish to resume their place in society but who may suffer job discrimination.

SURGERY Surgery is, of course, the oldest form of treatment for cancer—it can be traced back to antiquity. *Planning the strategy for the operation is at least as important as its technical aspects;* in some situations large portions of organs can be removed without damage to the patient, while in others surgery can be detrimental to the patient's long-term interests. Knowing how much to do and the circumstances under which to do it requires considerable expertise in surgical oncology. In some instances these decisions are of life-threatening importance; in others the questions are of vital psychological importance—for example, the question of whether to amputate or do a limited resection of a leg in a young patient with bone cancer, or how much surgery (mastectomy or lumpectomy) to do in a patient with a breast tumor or how much surgery to do in a patient with a cancer involving the jaw. The consequences of those decisions are enormous, for the surgery often necessitates subsequent rehabilitative services, for both physical and emotional disability.

For some tumors, the less surgery the better; this is particularly true when surgery is required to make a diagnosis but not for treatment. Hodgkin's disease is an example of that principle. The wise surgeon knows the limitation of his tools; at the other extreme, the unwise surgeon may perform heroic surgery to attempt to remove a cancer that is clearly incurable and thereby needlessly add to the patient's disability and reduce the quality of remaining life. This can often be avoided by getting a second opinion, and it is worth avoiding unnecessary surgery. But if there is any doubt about a particular situation, I think the decision should go in the direction of the more aggressive treatment in order to give the patient the best possible chance for improved survival or cure.

Some of the current controversies about surgical treatments have to do with just how much surgery should be done. There is no argument about surgery that is done to establish the diagnosis by biopsy procedure, or to remove a localized primary tumor and effect a cure. And there are at least two other circumstances in which surgery may be a useful treatment for a patient with cancer. Surgeons may remove a large primary tumor, say in the kidney, and even a single metastasis (a cancer that has "traveled") in a distant area, for reasons of "debulking" the patient. The large primary tumor is removed not only to reduce the threat of this tumor to surrounding areas, but also, and even more important, to increase the effectiveness of chemotherapy to the metastases. It is a curious phenomenon in using chemotherapy that the drugs will kill only a certain fraction of the cancer cells and that fraction is constant, regardless of how many cells there are to begin with. Thus, if there is a large tumor, weighing say a pound or there-abouts, there are literally billions of cancer cells that need to be killed, and even drugs that kill 99.99 percent of the tumor cells can still leave millions of cells in the primary tumor. If that tumor is surgically removed first, then the chemotherapy will sometimes be able to reduce the small metastases so much that the immune system of the body may be able to eradicate the remaining cancer cells.

Under the right circumstances the combined use of surgery and chemotherapy will not only effect a higher cure rate, but also can reduce the amount of surgery that is required. There are two really striking examples of this. The first is the addition of chemotherapy to surgery for cancer of the bone (osteosarcoma), a cancer predominantly affecting young people. Not only does this greatly improve the chances of cure, which in itself is gratifying, but investigators at several major cancer centers have also found that they could decrease the amount of surgery that had to be performed to the point that, with the addition of chemotherapy, they can actually save the limb! So a patient who in the past would have had to have an entire leg or arm amputated may now have the tumor in the bone removed and perhaps receive a bone graft and use chemotherapy after or before and after surgery. Thus, the patient not only lives but also retains a functional limb—the *ultimate* goal of treatment. The multidisciplinary teams of surgical, medical and pediatric oncologists who have worked in this area of cancer research deserve a great deal of credit for their attention to the quality, as well as to the quantity, of life of their patients. Hippocrates, who admonished young physicians to *above all do no harm,* would have been very proud!

A second example is in the use of chemotherapy following surgery for breast cancer in patients who have cancer not only in the breast, but also in the lymph glands underneath the arm (axillary nodes). The likelihood of recurrence depends upon the location and number of lymph glands that are involved with the cancer, and the best time to minimize the chances for recurrence are right after surgery. In this case chemotherapy is used as an adjunct to surgery. A number of programs of chemotherapy have been tried, many of them variations on the theme of the so-called Cooper regimen, which uses combinations of three to five chemotherapeutic drugs given at monthly intervals for six to twelve months. Also, a collaborative series of studies by surgical oncologists led by Dr. Bernard Fisher of Pittsburgh have used chemotherapy with a single drug called melphalan (Alkeran). It has been well demonstrated that women who are so treated have a lesser likelihood of developing recurrent disease and a greater interval before recurrence if it does occur. This is a very important finding, which is particularly true for premenopausal women.

Chemotherapy appears to be far less effective in postmenopausal women with breast cancer, and there has been a great deal of speculation as to why there is such a difference. To explore the reasons for this, a team of investigators from Milan, led by Dr. Giovanni Bonadonna, compared the treatment that was actually given to postmenopausal women with that of premenopausal women who were supposed to be treated in an identical manner. It turned out that the former were far less likely than the latter to receive the full course of treatment, presumably because of their age. As you might expect, doctors tended to treat older patients less aggressively than younger patients (this is not the first time this phenomenon has been observed in medicine, as we noted earlier). Furthermore, Bonadonna's group found that the older patients who completed the prescribed course of treatment did as well as the younger women who completed the course of treatment; thus, failure to treat aggressively might well be the explanation for the poorer results in older patients. In any event, the use of chemotherapy after surgery for patients who have small areas of remaining disease, or in whom disease is likely to recur, is being tried in a variety of other types of cancers, although mostly with far less success than with the examples mentioned. In particular, adjuvant (a helper, a substance added to assist or heighten effectiveness) chemotherapy has not been very useful for patients with cancers of the bowel or lung, at least not in the studies reported to date. That does not mean that it is inappropriate for an individual patient, since, as we will see in Chapter 6, the application of statistics derived from research studies to the care of the individual can be quite misleading at times. That is another reason why it is useful to get treatment advice from an expert who has read, thought about and really understood the available information.

The question of how much surgery should be done is a very difficult one, and the problem is perhaps best illustrated by the case of breast cancer. Traditional teaching about cancer surgery is to remove as wide a margin of normal tissue as possible around the cancer to minimize the risk of leaving tumor cells behind; and thus for many years radical surgery has been emphasized for breast cancer, as well as for colon cancer, lung cancer, pancreatic cancer et cetera. While that point of view may seem logical, the number of studies that bear out the usefulness of radical surgery is really limited. Specifically, mastectomy (removal of the breast with preservation of some underlying chest muscles) has been called into question in recent studies by the National Surgical Adjuvant

Breast Program (NSABP) in which a large group of surgeons, again headed by Dr. Bernard Fisher, compared local removal of the tumor and conservation of the breast with more conventional modified radical mastectomy. In both operations the lymph glands under the arm are removed to see if they are involved with tumor. Although some pioneering cancer surgeons had earlier thought that more limited surgery is as effective as more aggressive methods, and additionally creates a far more acceptable cosmetic effect, properly randomized controlled studies are only now being completed by the NSABP. Thus, contrary to the belief of many noted cancer surgeons, the "lumpectomy" or "tylectomy," as it is medically called, is now being shown to give therapeutic results comparable to modified radical mastectomy.

Furthermore, Dr. Fisher argues that instead of having two surgical procedures performed under anesthesia if the biopsy is positive (one biopsy and one mastectomy), the patient need have only a single surgical procedure. If prior to surgery the indications are strong that the lump in the breast will be malignant, then the patient is informed that the surgeon will not only remove the local tumor but will also make a separate incision and remove the lymph glands under the arm to test them for the presence of tumor. In recent years it has been the practice to do a biopsy first and, if cancer is diagnosed, to discuss the options with the patient before doing a second and larger cancer operation. This procedure was followed because the majority of women operated on for lumps in the breast turn out not to have cancer. Thus, it seemed far less traumatic to approach the patient with the idea of removing the lump and examining it and then making a decision about the need for further surgery than to propose a possible mastectomy without discussing it in detail. Controversy will undoubtedly continue to exist in this area, but at least it is useful to know that there are alternatives that take into consideration the psychological needs of the woman, including the alternative of breast reconstructive surgery following a mastectomy, if that is deemed necessary, or the possible use of radiation treatment as an alternative to surgery.

I believe that patients who are suspected to have breast cancer who wish to have a second opinion should obtain that opinion before *any* operation is performed; they should not wait until an initial biopsy has been done and they have been told it is cancer. (That would not necessarily be true for other types of biopsies.) After surgery it is very difficult for the second physician to make an intelligent assessment because the breast tissue is substantially distorted in the acute postoperative phase. As we have just learned, the latest data seem to argue in favor of having a lumpectomy if it is technically feasible (it is not always feasible). If the surgeon is unwilling to do that procedure under any circumstances, then perhaps the patient should request a second opinion before anything is done (see Chapter 2). Sometimes a modified radical mastectomy to remove the entire breast and lymph glands under the arm is the operation of choice, as with Nancy Reagan, and sometimes radiation is added. (It was most encouraging to hear Dr. Fisher, when he received an award recently from the American Cancer Society, predict that it may not be very long before breast cancer surgery becomes replaced by less drastic procedures. Clearly we are not at that point yet, but the day is coming.)

There are all kinds of nuances to surgery for cancer of the breast, and my personal feeling is that a general surgeon who was trained twenty-five years ago and who has not kept up with recent advances in the management of patients with breast cancer should not assume sole responsibility (without consultation) for the care of these patients. It is too important to do all the right things, including preparing the tumor immediately after removal, not only for pathologic study but also for analysis of hormone receptors. The presence or absence of tumor receptors for female hormones (estrogen and progesterone) makes a great deal of difference in how the disease is dealt with if it recurs, since the presence of receptors on these cancer cells gives the patient a 55 percent or better chance that the cancer will respond to hormone treatment alone, whereas the lack of these receptors drops the likelihood of response to this treatment to about 5 percent. Proper preparation of the tissue sample and proper analysis of the tissue are essential to obtaining this very important information, as most surgeons are aware. In the case of women who have lumps in the breast, the primary physician who raises the possibility of cancer may be an obstetrical-gynecological surgeon and that person may operate on women with lumps in the breast no more than once or twice a year. Although this is a judgment call, I am not sure that this is optimal from the standpoint of the patient, and my patients will be referred to surgeons who are making such decisions and doing such operations frequently.

In patients who cannot be cured by removal of their cancer, surgery may also be useful for *palliation,* a term used to describe the relief of symptoms or complications due to the tumor mass. For example, a patient with cancer may be getting along relatively well, but one of the lesions is pressing on the spinal cord causing weakness with loss of motor function in the legs. If the tumor is not removed surgically or shrunk promptly with radiation, the patient is destined to be permanently paralyzed—this is truly an emergency. Removal of the tumor from a critical area can restore the patient to the previous health status even though there is the continuing presence of tumor in less sensitive areas. Sometimes when surgeons remove tumor masses that are obstructing organs such as the bowel or bile ducts, the mere removal of those tumors can give the patient immense relief and provide for additional good quality of life.

There are many things that can happen to patients who have cancer, and it is very important to consider each new problem on its own merits and not assume it is due to cancer. It is a tragedy to lose a patient to appendicitis or to a ruptured gall bladder when these problems are curable if only they are thought about and treated as though they occurred in a patient who did not have a history of cancer.

RADIATION THERAPY Another form of localized treatment of cancer is radiation therapy, which kills tumor cells by damaging vital molecules such as the DNA and proteins. Different types of cancer vary in their sensitivity to radiation; some are exquisitely sensitive and others are relatively resistant, requiring exceedingly high doses to eradicate them. Since cancer cells exist around and among normal cells it is impossible to isolate them totally and give radiation treatments without injuring some normal cells. Sometimes this has no harmful consequences, but it can be dangerous when high doses of radiation are required to treat tumors involving or near to vital organs. For example, radiation therapy to a lung cancer may cause extensive inflammation followed by scarring of nearby normal lung, thus damaging normal lung function even if the tumor is completely eradicated. Naturally, the larger the dose of radiation or the larger the volume treated, the more danger there is of side effects.

Depending upon the site treated, large doses of radiation can cause nausea and vomiting, loss of appetite and reduction in bone marrow function. (Some of these same problems exist with chemotherapy as will be described below.) Paradoxically, radiation can destroy a radiosensitive tumor very rapidly and efficiently, and when the tumor is involving an organ such as the stomach or the intestine, a perforation may occur. Should this perforation happen, peritonitis would develop and this constitutes an emergency requiring surgery for removal of that portion of the bowel or closure of the perforation.

Radiation therapy is used in some instances to cure patients as an alternative to surgery. By way of illustration, a patient with cancer of the vocal cords (larynx) can undergo a partial or total laryngectomy (removal of a portion or the entire larynx, the "voice box") or can be treated with radiation therapy. Following total laryngectomy a patient requires some type of artificial device to speak or has to develop the so-called esophageal speech, whereas with radiation therapy the vocal cords are spared and the person retains the ability for relatively normal speech. Partial laryngectomy does affect speech to a greater or lesser degree, depending upon the extent and nature of the procedure. Since the cure rate for appropriately selected patients who have this form of cancer is extremely high with both forms of treatment, radiation is a very good treatment option and it is generally preferred. It must be emphasized, however, that treating with radiation is not merely a matter of pointing a radiation beam at a tumor mass and turning on the machine. This form of treatment is far more complex than that. Furthermore, the patient has no way of knowing how accurately and appropriately the treatment is being administered. It takes exquisite care to calculate the treatment dose, to set up the appropriate field or fields of treatment to deliver the desired dose to a tumor, particularly tumors lying deep in the body, and to minimize the exposure of adjacent normal tissues.

Sometimes the best way of giving radiation is to insert hollow needles or devices containing radioactive sources in tissue or cavities containing the tumor. These sources are left in place for a specific period of time to deliver a certain amount of radiation to the tumor in close proximity to the device. This technique of placing radioactive sources in the tissues or cavities is called brachytherapy and is particularly suited for the treatment of patients with cancer of the cervix. Modeling of the treatment fields so that the best possible approach is used for a specific patient requires a great deal of expertise in physics and dosimetry, adequate personnel support and the availability of costly equipment. Once again, when one is trying for a cure, the initial course of treatment is the most important because once the tumor recurs it is usually no longer curable, although there are certainly exceptions to this rule.

Radiation therapy may be used in conjunction with surgery or chemotherapy. For example, surgical removal of a cancer in the head and neck region may result in removal of the vast majority of the tumor but there may remain areas of microscopic disease. If not treated successfully, these areas will be an Achilles heel and eventually grow and cause recurrence of the tumor. The approach of using radiation therapy directed specifically at the area or areas of remaining tumor is a very effective one and combines the beneficial effects of radiation with those of surgery and can enhance the chance for cure. Radiation therapy is also often used after limited breast cancer surgery to reduce the likelihood of local recurrence.

Radiation therapy can be combined with chemotherapy in many different ways, such as in the growing field of bone marrow transplantation. This aggressive therapy is aimed at killing large numbers of cancer cells that are resistant to standard doses of chemotherapy. Unfortunately in the process such combined therapy also wipes out the normal bone marrow cells and requires a transplant of normal bone marrow from a compatible donor such as an identical twin or a matched sibling. If the cancer has not invaded the bone marrow, then the patient's own marrow can be removed, stored under special frozen conditions and given back *after* the chemotherapy is completed. One of the remarkable properties of bone marrow cells is that they can be infused intravenously and, like migratory birds, they will find their home in the marrow cavity. To cure patients with certain forms of leukemia it may be necessary to kill all of the bone marrow cells (we cannot separate the normal cells from the leukemic ones), and this can be achieved by combining massive doses of chemotherapy with total body radiation. The bone marrow transplant is therefore necessary to restore the patient's ability to form normal blood cells, which are essential for survival. This is still not a common practice, but it is a case in which radiation therapy is used on the total body instead of being targeted at specific tumor masses.

A common use of radiation therapy is for palliation of symptoms like those of women with breast cancer who may have tumor metastasis involving several bones. When a bone is weakened to the point that it may fracture spontaneously or with minor stress, this is called a *pathological fracture.* Sometimes the areas of bone metastases are very painful even before they fracture. Radiation therapy can destroy the tumor cells in that region and thus alleviate the pain and help to stabilize the bone. Multiple bone lesions, however, are generally not treated with radiation therapy because so much normal bone marrow would have to be radiated that the patients could experience more complications than benefits from this treatment. Another common example of palliation is the use of radiation to shrink a tumor involving a vital organ such as the brain, spinal cord or lung. Tumors in the lung may obstruct the great blood vessels to the heart; however, in a very high percentage of cases the obstruction of the blood vessels can be reversed with radiation therapy.

Radiation therapy is painless, of course, and it is similar in that respect to having a diagnostic x-ray taken. Once the initial treatment planning has been done, the course of x-ray therapy can be started. Treatments are usually given on a daily basis, five days per week, and they last only a few minutes every day. The entire course of therapy can last from a few days to several weeks depending upon the area treated and the goal of the therapy. Palliative courses of treatment, in general, are given over shorter periods of time than curative courses, which generally require much higher doses. There is no need for the patient to remain in the hospital during this time, and most radiation treatments are given on an outpatient basis provided that there are no complications or other problems that require hospitalization. The usual schedule of five treatments per week with a rest usually on the weekends evolved as a convenience to the health care team and sometimes to the patients as well. However, it has been found that this schedule allows the patients to recover, partially, from the side effects of radiation during the two days of rest and that if the treatment were to be given continuously, seven days per week, the treatment would have to be shortened or the daily dose reduced. Currently there is a great deal of investigation of the importance of different treatment schedules, particularly using more than one treatment per day.

Radiation therapy is an expensive form of treatment because it involves a highly skilled team and extremely expensive facilities. Some types of lesions are relatively simple to treat but others require a great deal of expertise and resources in order to achieve the maximum possible benefit. For some tumors there is a difference of opinion on whether the patient may be best treated with surgical removal of the tumor or by radiation. For example, as mentioned earlier, some surgeons would argue that surgical removal of a tumor in the vocal cords is still preferable to radiation therapy because it might give a slightly higher cure rate. As a general rule, when more than one treatment option is available doctors are more comfortable in recommending treatments they give or are familiar with. But clearly this is an instance where the patient's *preference* for quality of life should be of major concern. This is not unique to oncology, of course.

An example of an area of significant controversy regarding

whether radiation therapy is as effective as surgery is the treatment of prostate cancer. Urologic surgeons are convinced that surgery gives a higher cure rate for localized prostate cancer than does radiation, while radiation therapists cite studies that indicate that the cure rates are entirely comparable. The arguments favoring surgery are that not only is the cancer removed once and for all along with the gland itself, but also that there is the opportunity to examine the adjacent lymph glands, which can be used as an indicator of what will happen or what to do next. Surgical exploration of the lymph glands can also lead to the detection of tumors outside of the prostate gland area that cannot be removed but, if appropriately identified, can be treated with postoperative radiation therapy. One disadvantage of surgery is that prostatic cancer usually occurs in elderly men who generally have a high surgical risk even with modern anesthesia. Furthermore, the incidence of sexual impotence following prostatectomy is very great; fortunately new surgical techniques will be better in this regard. The importance of this used to be overlooked. Impotence was once considered (by the medical profession) to be a small price to pay for a potentially life-saving procedure, but we have increasingly come to appreciate the emotional impact of impotence even in older age groups. A patient who has been sexually active prior to radical prostatectomy and wishes to maintain potency after surgery has to have a penile prosthesis. Although radiation therapy for prostatic cancer can also lead to impotence, the likelihood of this happening is somewhere around 30 to 50 percent. It should be noted that radiation therapy can cause, in a small percentage of patients, damage to nearby normal tissues like the bladder and the rectum. Therefore, both of these forms of therapy are not without potential side effects that are unwanted, unpleasant and sometimes dangerous.

CHEMOTHERAPY Chemotherapy is the most rapidly developing field of cancer treatment. Recalling the biblical admonition to turn swords into plowshares, chemotherapy began with the discovery that some drugs (so-called alkylating or "mustard" agents) that were being studied by the Army for use in germ warfare in World

War II caused destruction of lymph glands (nodes) in animals. Some bright pharmacologists asked themselves whether that effect could be exploited specifically for treatment of tumors such as malignant lymphomas that originated in lymph glands; happily, this turned out to be the case! At about the same time the antimetabolites were developed—chemicals that are designed by chemists to mimic closely vital building blocks of normal body metabolism, but that have significant differences such as that once they are incorporated into a rapidly growing tissue, a tumor, for example, they destroy it. Thus, in taking up a critical amount of this type of drug, a cell essentially commits suicide!

Many different types of chemicals have been synthesized or found in nature and studied for their anticancer effects, and literally tens of thousands of compounds have been evaluated against tumors in mice and rats. Some of the ideas and syntheses have been brilliantly conceived by chemists to interfere with certain essential processes of the cell. Naturally, it is not possible to test more than a tiny fraction of promising drugs in patients, so a great deal of thought and animal experimentation must precede this step. *We would not be curing any children or adults with chemotherapy were it not for research on animals,* as current supporters of the antivivisectionist groups need to know. The other research methods (tissue culture, computer modeling, etc.) urged by these groups are simply not adequate alternatives to animal research that is carefully conducted under humane conditions.

The first cure of a cancer that had metastasized (spread) widely was achieved in the late 1950s at the National Cancer Institute (NCI), when young women with a highly malignant form of cancer called choriocarcinoma were found to be curable with the use of one of the first antimetabolites, methotrexate. I trained at the NCI during that time and was privileged to be exposed to Drs. Roy Hertz and M. C. Li, who pioneered in this treatment, and imagine my excitement at curing the first patient with choriocarcinoma at Duke, shortly after joining the staff in 1960. A young black woman with two children who worked as a maid to support her family was admitted to our hospital because she was coughing up blood. Her chest x-ray showed widespread tumor masses in the lung (Figure 1), and the pelvic examination revealed a large tumor mass in the uterus. When the mass was removed it established a diagnosis of choriocarcinoma and we began giving her methotrexate, a drug that is still in use today. Without this treatment her life expectancy was only a matter of weeks. Happily, her tumors literally disappeared from her lungs and elsewhere in a matter of weeks. I have followed her progress over the last twenty-six years (and presented her to many groups of medical students). Deciding to further her education, she later became a nurse and still practices; her nursing sometimes brings her into contact with other young women who suffer from this same formerly rapidly fatal cancer, which now is curable in well over 90 percent of cases. In the old days I often thought that one needs some spectacular successes like that to get through the rough times of working in this field!

Childhood acute leukemia, Hodgkin's disease, certain forms of malignant lymphoma and various other types of malignancies in children have also been found to be curable in the majority of cases. The major advances in chemotherapy have come from the discovery of active compounds, and from the skillful design of dose schedules and combinations of different drugs designed to maximize the killing of tumor cells and minimize toxicity to normal cells.

Medical oncologists are primarily the people who use cancer chemotherapy, but depending on the complexity of the problem, chemotherapy may also be used by other physicians. For example, when chemotherapy is used as an "adjuvant" to follow up after breast cancer surgery in otherwise healthy women, the chemotherapeutic program is sufficiently standard so that internists and/ or other medically and surgically trained physicians are perfectly capable of administering this type of therapy.

Chemotherapy disseminates cancer-killing chemicals throughout the body in order to kill tumor cells wherever they may be, whether in sizable lumps or in tiny nests of cells that may be visible only by the use of the microscope. There is no doubt that the smaller the amount of tumor present, the better the outcome of treatment is likely to be; but there is tremendous variability in

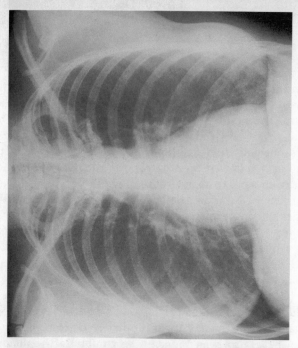

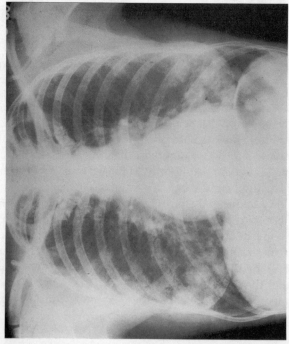

the sensitivity of different kinds of cancer to the effects of chemotherapy. For example, testicular cancer and choriocarcinoma are highly sensitive to chemotherapy, whereas cancers that originate in the pancreas or bowel or brain are notoriously insensitive to the effects of our current drugs. Between these extremes are quite a number of cancers that vary in their responsiveness; sometimes excellent responses can be achieved, but in other cases no beneficial effect occurs. However, before we can decide that chemotherapy does not have a beneficial role in the management of a patient with a particular type of cancer, it is necessary to "push" the dose to the maximum tolerated level, because some cancers may be insensitive to low doses of chemotherapy but respond very dramatically if the dose of those very same chemicals is doubled. One has to be willing to try the treatment, at least for two or three courses, to see if it is working. If it is, then the benefit can be tremendous—if not, then another decision needs to be made, depending on what other options are available.

The problem is that when we push onward to the maximum tolerated dose, there are generally side effects that are uncomfortable for the patient, and some that may be very dangerous as well. That is because chemotherapeutic drugs, regardless of how they are given (by mouth or by injection), circulate throughout the entire body, and obviously, normal cells are exposed to the potentially harmful effects of chemotherapy. Rapidly growing normal cells such as bone marrow and intestinal lining cells are especially vulnerable to being destroyed by chemotherapeutic agents, but these usually recover within weeks. In the meantime the treatments can temporarily make you feel bad, raise your chances of becoming infected, cause hair loss, nausea and vomiting, sores in the mouth, diarrhea, injuries to organs (liver, lungs, kidney, etc.). The dilemma then is that the only way to be sure of not having complications is not to take any treatment. However, we are learn-

Figure 1 Chest x-ray showing tumor masses in the lung. In November 1960 (left) the chest x-ray showed many white nodules of cancer in the lungs (between the ribs). In October 1962 (right) these had all disappeared and the chest x-ray was normal, and it remained normal thereafter.

ing a great deal about how to anticipate and minimize these complications of cancer chemotherapy—the techniques are rapidly improving. Often we can take measures that will keep these problems to a minimum—and we are steadily getter better at doing that, and at individualizing the treatment for any given circumstances. There are now many former patients who are leading normal lives who are glad that they opted for treatment, regardless of how vigorous it may have been over the short haul. Wouldn't it be nice if we could tell in advance if a drug is likely to work? There are some new laboratory techniques that may be helpful at least in predicting whether a drug has the potential to kill that particular kind of cancer, and they may become very useful in the future—the techniques remain experimental for now.

Cure of Childhood Leukemia It is instructive to examine the types of discoveries and other advances that are necessary to make progress in the treatment of a particular kind of cancer and the need to construct a series of building blocks that solve particular parts of the problem before final solutions can be reached. The best-studied form of cancer has been acute lymphocytic leukemia of children, and what has been learned in this disease has often been of practical importance in studies of other types of malignancy. In fact, that experience was so important that Dr. Joseph Burchenal of Memorial Sloan-Kettering, one of the pioneers in treatment of leukemia, called childhood leukemia the "stalking horse" for cancer chemotherapy. The first chemotherapy that proved useful in treating acute leukemia employed antimetabolites of folic acid; these are fraudulent building blocks that closely resemble this normal factor needed for growth and development. That chemotherapy was introduced in 1947 by Dr. Sidney Farber and colleagues in Boston, and its use led to brief remissions in some children. During these remissions the leukemic cells disappeared from the blood and the leukemic child was restored to normal health until the disease recurred. Additional chemotherapeutic drugs that have proven to be important in the management of this disease include steroid hormones, developed in 1951; 6-mercaptopurine, another antimetabolite, developed in 1953; two different drugs, vincristine and cyclophosphamide, in 1961; and since that time several other agents, named asparaginase, anthra-cycline drugs and cytosine arabinoside, all of which have anti-leukemic effects.

Quantitative research methods for comparing different drug treatments were introduced at the National Cancer Institute in the mid-1950s under the leadership of Dr. C. Gordon Zubrod, and included standard scientific techniques of developing a hypothe-sis, selecting suitable patients, developing specific treatment strategies, developing criteria for measuring a favorable response, randomly assigning treatments to patients and controlling the quality of data collection, with major biostatistical consultation for analysis of data. These quantitative techniques really did not exist within any of the medical disciplines before that time, with the possible exception of the drug development program to com-bat malaria during World War II, and the lessons learned have been invaluable not only in oncology but also in the development of any new treatment. (In friendly debates, I sometimes find that the cardiologists believe that they invented quantitative clinical trials, which is about as accurate as Russian claims to invention of the telephone!)

One of the most important early discoveries with leukemia was that the use of chemotherapy could result in complete remissions, as we have said, and that the length of these remissions was directly correlated with the length of survival. *This meant that extend-ing survival while the patient was sick was not a question of prolonging the period of illness but of restoring a period of wellness—adding life to years rather than just years to life.* That knowledge led to greater emphasis upon achieving more frequent and lengthier complete remissions, since that was the most powerful determinant of life span, and gradu-ally the complete remission rate improved from the neighborhood of 5 to 10 percent for single chemotherapy agents to 20 to 30 percent with combinations of the early agents, and on up to 80 to 90 percent today with the use of all available agents. The process of discovery often seems one of trial and error, but in fact the developments were orderly and had a cumulative beneficial effect, as shown by the results achieved in sequential studies (see Figure 2). These improvements in survival of afflicted children are im-

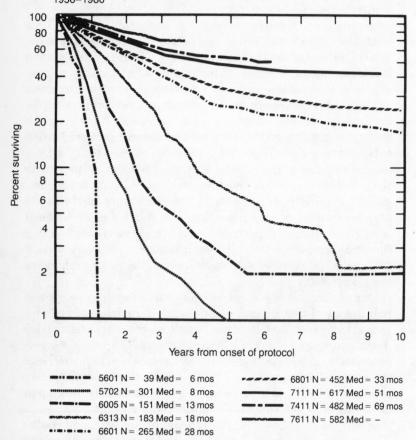

Cancer and leukemia group B
Acute lymphocytic leukemia survival in children under 20
1956–1980

▬‥▬‥▬ 5601 N = 39 Med = 6 mos		⁄⁄⁄⁄⁄ 6801 N = 452 Med = 33 mos
▪▪▪▪▪▪▪ 5702 N = 301 Med = 8 mos		▬▬▬ 7111 N = 617 Med = 51 mos
▬‥▬‥▬ 6005 N = 151 Med = 13 mos		▬‥▬ 7411 N = 482 Med = 69 mos
∿∿∿∿∿ 6313 N = 183 Med = 18 mos		▬▬▬ 7611 N = 582 Med = –
▪‥▪‥▪‥▪ 6601 N = 265 Med = 28 mos		

Figure 2 Results of sequential studies of leukemia patients, showing progressively improving survival rates. The first two numbers in the legend refer to the year the study was begun; the next two refer to the study number. "N" indicates the number of patients with leukemia in each study and "Med" means the median survival period of each group. For example, 5601, the first project, started in 1956 and studied thirty-nine patients. Their median survival period was six months. (With appreciation to the Cancer and Leukemia Group B and to Dr. James Holland; reproduced with permission from *Cancer Research* 45 [1985]: front cover)

pressive, and we believe that they will in time be achieved in other cancers as well.

Combination chemotherapy for leukemia was developed by selecting individual drugs that had both a different mechanism of action in killing leukemic cells and a different type of toxicity to normal cells, so that all the drugs could be combined and given at full doses without causing undue toxicity to the patient. The idea was to get convergent means of killing cancer cells but with different unwanted side effects, similar to the technique of giving radiation therapy from different directions to maximize tumor cell kill and minimize damage to normal tissue. For example, a drug whose primary side effect was to suppress normal blood cell formation could be given in combination with full doses of another drug whose primary side effects were on the nervous system or the lungs, but which did not affect the normal blood-forming cells. This seems obvious now, but at the time it was a major conceptual advance in cancer chemotherapy, and its rigorous proof was far from simple.

Once complete remissions were achieved by the use of combination chemotherapy, survival improved, but eventually all patients relapsed from their remission. We needed more information, new drugs, new ideas that would go further. Imagine the agonized frustration of seeing a child dying of leukemia restored to health for many months, able to go back to school looking perfectly healthy and with normal blood counts, only to have the disease return. Could it be that there was an underlying stimulus to turn normal cells into leukemic cells and that this persisted despite treatment? Or was it that not all of the leukemic cells had been killed or even that they could not be found for a time? Considerable insight into this problem was gained from the basic studies of Drs. Howard Skipper and Frank Schabel of the Southern Research Institute in Birmingham, Alabama, who developed quantitative cancer models in mice, inoculated them with mouse (L1210) leukemic cells, and then performed measurements to determine how many cells remained after treatment and how best to eliminate the remaining cells by retreatment with the same or different drugs. They recognized that a clinical remission during which the patient (the mouse in this case) looked perfectly normal still meant that millions of leuke-mic cells could remain undetected and these would eventually multiply to the point where the clinical evidence of disease would appear, although meanwhile the disease was unrecogniza-ble by the usual types of blood testing.

This discovery and others in mice led to a new treatment strat-egy in which patients received treatment during the time of clini-cal remission in order to eliminate the remaining microscopic areas of disease. It was found that the use of a second antileukemic agent could significantly prolong the length of a remission and that the effectiveness of the treatment during remission depended not only upon the drug but also upon the frequency with which it was given, and the dose. Intermittent treatment was more effective than daily treatment, and if the dose could be doubled, the remis-sions would last significantly longer. There were also some drugs that were more effective when given at first and not continued; other drugs, by contrast, were more effective with the patient in remission, and so on with other technical considerations. Further-more, as with the initial treatment to obtain a remission, the length of the remission could be improved by using combinations of chemotherapeutic drugs.

When *all* of this was done, and that took many years of work, many patients had lengthy remissions. However, in these patients the disease eventually recurred in the brain, caused by leukemic cells growing in the lining spaces (meninges) of the brain. This complication of leukemia takes time to develop and was not really appreciated until after we had some effective treatment to make it possible for children not to die early of other leukemia-related problems. Extensive additional studies showed that most of the antileukemic drugs that were given by mouth or by vein did *not* pass into the brain because of the blood-brain barrier, a physio-logical barrier to the free passage of materials back and forth between the bloodstream and the fluids bathing the brain. Radiat-ing the brain and/or giving chemotherapy directly into the spinal fluid had a definite effect in counteracting leukemia once it was detected in the brain, but that was rather late. It would be better to prevent this complication. So that same principle of treatment was applied earlier—as soon as the patients had been treated to the point of having a disease remission. This reduced the incidence of recurrence of leukemia in the brain from over 50 percent to less than 10 percent in patients who received this new type of central nervous system (CNS) prophylaxis therapy. Thus was born the use of combination chemotherapy to achieve a complete remission, followed by further combination chemotherapy using different drug programs to prolong the remission, and the concurrent use of CNS prophylaxis treatment: this resulted in long-term disease-free survivals, or cures, in 40 to 50 percent of patients. During the past decade additional drugs have improved the complete remission rate so that it now approaches 100 percent, and the use of these agents has made it possible to achieve an overall long-term cure rate of approximately 80 percent in children who are treated at the leading cancer centers. (See Figure 2 on page 58.)

That is largely the chemotherapy part of the story, but several other important innovations occurred along the way without which these advances could not have taken place. During the time of aggressive combination chemotherapy these patients are virtually devoid of normal white blood cells with which to fight infection, and of normal platelets to prevent them from having spontaneous bleeding or hemorrhage. Thus, in the past, patients with acute leukemia customarily died either of infection or bleeding if they did not quickly achieve a remission. Very meticulous work by many investigators documented the types of infections which these patients acquired, and vigorous pharmaceutical research on antibiotics led to very potent antibiotics that could destroy bacteria resistant to standard antibiotics, as well as fungi that frequently took the lives of leukemic children. Very recently it has become possible even to cure some potentially lethal viral infections. These major advances in the treatment of infection in immunodeficient leukemic patients have also benefited the entire field of infectious diseases, whether associated with cancer and leukemia or not.

Another major innovation, which originated from Dr. Emil Freireich and his colleagues while they were at the National Cancer Institute (NCI), was in new techniques of blood banking, so that fragile platelets could be obtained from normal blood donors and transfused into leukemic children, to provide them with sufficient numbers of platelet cells to prevent bleeding until they produced their own normal platelets in the weeks following chemotherapy. This revolutionized the entire field of transfusion of blood products and made an important impact on our ability to keep patients alive long enough for them to achieve a disease remission. The same research team also developed the technology to remove leukemic cells from the bloodstream of patients and replace them, for a short time, with white cells from normal donors. Interestingly, the techniques of continuous flow centrifugation, which permits platelets or white cells to be selectively removed, were developed by an engineer who left his regular job to work night and day on this while his child was being treated for leukemia. Unhappily, his own child did not respond, but his contributions have saved the lives of many patients since.

Other innovations helped to deal with new problems that could not be anticipated or appreciated until the time when there were long-term survivors. Some of the antileukemic treatments resulted in damage to the development of the brain in young children, and some led to the development of second cancers due to the mutagenicity and carcinogenicity of the particular drugs being employed. Again, these were not recognized problems until patients began to live long enough to experience them; but once they were found, other means of treatment had to be devised to minimize these risks. In addition, new immunological techniques were found to identify certain subgroups of patients who were at an unusually high risk for relapse of their leukemia, and special types of treatment had to be devised for them. In other words, the treatment that would cure the majority of patients could not cure the remainder, and since this could be largely predicted in advance, new treatments were devised for these patients that could be given them right from the start. This is very important in an aggressive disease like acute leukemia because if the first treatment fails, there may not be time to try another.

Treatment of acute lymphocytic leukemia in adults is not yet as successful as it is with children, but some of the same principles have now been successfully applied, and younger adult patients, particularly, have a possibility for cure that approaches that of children. The major type of adult leukemia, acute myelogenous leukemia, is only now at a point where a small fraction of patients are being cured; this is certainly a much tougher disease to treat. (In my next book will be more about the cure of leukemia.)

Many of the principles learned from treatment of childhood acute leukemia have also been successfully applied to treatment of other types of cancer. The cure of Hodgkin's disease is a good example of how we have capitalized on the extensive lessons learned from treatment of acute leukemia and of their application to a disease that primarily involves the lymph glands, rather than bone marrow as in leukemia. The thrust for a curative treatment of widespread Hodgkin's disease by Dr. Vincent DeVita, Dr. Emil Frei III and numerous other colleagues at NCI was based upon the use of multiple chemotherapeutic drugs that could be used in virtually full doses because they had differing toxicities—a direct extension of successful antileukemic therapy.

Certain types of cancer are better treated with different strategies than those used in acute leukemia. In some instances chemotherapy given prior to surgery is an effective means of both limiting the spread of disease and improving survival; an excellent example of that is preoperative chemotherapy for cancer of the bone (osteosarcoma), which enables more limited surgery to be done. The term recently proposed for this by Dr. Frei is "neoadjuvant chemotherapy," and this is also increasingly being used prior to surgery in patients who have cancers of the head and neck. The results in this group of people are very encouraging. Dr. Andrew T. Huang at Duke, a team of investigators at Wayne State University in Detroit and some other groups have used chemotherapy with great effectiveness following head and neck cancer surgery, and many long-term survivors are now being followed. In other instances, too, as described elsewhere for breast cancer, surgery is done first to determine whether the disease has spread outside the breast into lymph nodes, and following surgery chemotherapy is used as an adjuvant treatment in women who are likely to have disease recurrence. Sometimes surgery is used to remove large tumor masses to make the small remaining areas of disease more responsive to subsequent chemotherapy. This so-called cytoreductive or debulking surgery (described earlier in this chapter) is also performed in some patients with ovarian cancer and with recent success in rectal cancer.

Counteracting Side Effects of Chemotherapy The side effects of chemotherapy, by which is meant the degree of inconvenience and danger to the patient, depend upon the circumstances. Some of the major side effects come from depression of normal bone marrow function—meaning a decrease in blood counts and increased susceptibility to infection and to bleeding. There may also be loss of appetite, nausea and vomiting, with the nausea and vomiting sometimes being extremely troublesome; patients complain about them and dread to think about them if repeated treatments lie ahead. Sores may develop in the mouth and elsewhere in the gastrointestinal tract, leading to pain on swallowing or to diarrhea. There may be damage to the lungs, heart, kidneys or other normal tissues as well, but these are for the most part reversible, with some significant exceptions.

Over the years oncologists have learned to minimize the danger of some of these complications, and we are now learning how to minimize the discomforts as well. For example, because we know when the blood counts will reach their maximum degree of depression, we can monitor patients and look for early signs of infection and treat it aggressively with antibiotics. Similarly, when the number of platelets becomes too low, there is a tendency toward spontaneous bleeding—but we can monitor the blood counts and give platelet transfusions, thus virtually eliminating the danger. We also know how to adjust doses based on blood counts, to minimize the risk in subsequent courses of treatment. Many investigators had a hand in these advances, but Drs. Frei and Freireich, then of NCI, Holland from Roswell Park and the team of investigators from St. Jude's in Memphis were among the leaders in the pioneering studies that centered around the treatment of children with leukemia.

The problem of nausea and vomiting was extremely troublesome until recently because there were few preventive antivomiting drugs available, and our knowledge of how to use them was quite limited. Unfortunately, drugs that prevent the nausea and vomiting of motion sickness are relatively ineffective for the same problems when they are caused by chemotherapy. (Indeed, automobile and ocean sickness respond to drugs that are not nearly as effective as others in treating motion sickness in astronauts traveling in space.) Phenothiazines (Thorazine, Compazine, etc.) and sedatives such as barbiturates were somewhat helpful against chemotherapy-related nausea and vomiting, but only since about 1980 have there been significant further advances in combating nausea and vomiting by the use of drugs called antiemetics. Interestingly, the first major advance came when some young patients volunteered the information that when they were smoking pot (marijuana) they had less nausea and vomiting than if they took chemotherapy while not smoking. This led to the discovery by physician-scientists in Boston that the active ingredient in marijuana, tetrahydrocannabinol or THC, is a potent antiemetic and can often be effective when other drugs fail. (Further discussion of this is found in Chapter 10.)

Since then several new chemicals (metoclopramide, haloperidol, dexamethasone) have been found to be extremely useful in the management of this problem, and some are probably more potent even than THC. However, the drugs must be used in high doses and they often cause some side effects of their own, but these are usually trivial compared to the severe nausea and vomiting they counteract. For example, certain chemotherapeutic drugs, when given in high doses, cause nausea and vomiting in virtually 100 percent of patients, but with the use of the newer antiemetics the nausea and vomiting can be reduced in both frequency and severity. For a patient to have vomiting and retching every fifteen to twenty minutes for twenty-four to thirty-six hours following treatment is sheer misery, as you can imagine. However, it is only an occasional patient today who has severe and intractable nausea and vomiting for which we can provide no relief—that is how much progress has been made in about five years! Thus, patients who earlier would have dropped out of treatment programs because of these unpleasant side effects can now look forward to getting through the treatment without being incapacitated.

Curiously, certain conditioned reflex behaviors, which we call *anticipatory nausea and vomiting,* develop in some of these patients. Among patients who have had several courses of chemotherapy each of which is followed by severe nausea and vomiting, some 25 percent become "conditioned" to experience the same effects under the influence of an innocent stimulus or trigger—before they are even given the chemotherapy. We have seen patients drive into the hospital parking lot and promptly begin to vomit, or vomit when they smell the alcohol sponge used to clean off the arm prior to chemotherapy or even vomit when they see the nurse who administers the chemotherapy—even if that person is encountered out of uniform in a supermarket or elsewhere away from the hospital. Once this pattern is established, antiemetic drugs are not very effective, and the best strategy is to be aggressive in preventing it from occurring in the first place. This situation is reminiscent of that of the young hoodlum in *A Clockwork Orange* who is reprogrammed to behave serenely—the only problem being that he throws up whenever he hears Beethoven!

A new approach that we and colleagues at Memorial Sloan-Kettering have tried is to use drugs such as lorazepam that block short-term memory. It seems that patients who are treated with lorazepam often do not remember receiving their chemotherapy; even if they are uncomfortable and vomit, they do not remember it. We are very curious to know if blocking memory temporarily in this way will also block short-term learning and, if so, whether that will, in turn, prevent this conditioned behavior. Not much is known about conditioned responses in humans, but we have an opportunity to learn. Considerable efforts are being made to counteract this almost Pavlovian type of conditioned behavior by the use of relaxation techniques, hypnosis, desensitizing methods and the like. This does work exceptionally well in some patients, particularly children.

Effective new antiemetic drugs and other measures represent a marked improvement in the care of patients with cancer, and with the rapid dissemination of information through medical journals and meetings, most practicing oncologists are well aware of how to use them. (I have even edited a book called *Antiemetics and Cancer Chemotherapy* specifically for physicians.) Research on antiemetic programs may not be as glamorous as working with drugs that might cure cancer, but it makes it possible to use existing drugs that may have significant anticancer effects if only they can be used to their limit.

Thus, a whole new field of knowledge has arisen concerning the supportive care of cancer patients, the "high touch" if you will, in an effort to prevent or counteract the side effects of treatment, or "high tech." All of the side effects produced by the sizable number of anticancer drugs currently in use are now being examined to see how they can be minimized. For example, in the past we, and I include myself, thought we had learned that severe kidney toxicity precluded the use of what later turned out to be one of our most potent drugs against some cancers, a platinum derivative (cisplatin) of unusual structure. It is now known that simply providing vigorous fluid infusions before the drug is given intravenously is usually sufficient to prevent this complication. There are other drugs that can cause severe toxicity to the heart; now new chemical derivatives are being developed that we hope will have the same anticancer effect but without as much toxicity for that vital structure. The same is true for a number of other chemotherapies that have unique toxicities to normal organs. It has been found, for example, that even the drug that causes damage to the heart can be used more safely if it is given more frequently and in lower doses; that simple change in drug administration is increasingly being made to minimize the risk.

When chemotherapeutic drugs are used in combinations of threes and fours (and sometimes more), the complexity of the subject is quite formidable, and it is a real challenge to know when to use which antiemetic drugs and in what doses and frequencies. This field of chemotherapy is rapidly evolving, and only those physicians who stay current with it can take maximum advantage of discoveries as they occur—another reason to consider obtaining a second opinion.

Practical Illustrations of Chemotherapy Let us illustrate some of the practical aspects of chemotherapy by reviewing the situation of a forty-one-year-old schoolteacher and mother of two. Mrs. E. underwent a modified radical mastectomy in April 1982 for a 1.5 centimeter tumor in the upper outer portion of the left breast. Removal of fifteen lymph nodes under the arm revealed the presence of nests of tumor cells in six of the nodes, predicting the likelihood of disease being elsewhere in the body and of a later recurrence. Within ten days following the surgery she was started on a program of adjuvant chemotherapy with three standard drugs (cyclophosphamide, methotrexate and fluorouracil)—the so-called CMF regimen. Before she was given chemotherapy, her blood counts were retested and found to be normal. Full doses of drugs were given, both intravenously and orally, on the first day of treatment. When her blood counts were checked ten days later, the white count and platelet count were both depressed to the expected levels but not to the point of causing dangerous toxicity. At the end of three weeks she returned for reevaluation; the blood counts were found to be back to normal and she was given a second course of therapy. These cycles of chemotherapy were repeated every three to four weeks, depending upon whether the blood counts were sufficiently recovered to permit full doses of chemotherapy; if they were not, the treatment was delayed. The total period of treatment lasted over the course of one year (more recently adjuvant chemotherapy has often been shortened to six months). The major side effects that she experienced with her treatments were those of some nausea and vomiting for twenty-four to forty-eight hours following each course of treatment, and she received antiemetic therapy, which kept this from becoming severe.

Because of her work schedule the treatments were arranged to be given after morning classes on Fridays, so that every three to four weeks she would use the weekend to recover from the effects of chemotherapy and would not lose any time from work. The other side effect that she had been warned about in advance was that of alopecia, or loss of scalp hair. This developed gradually with thinning of the hair; she followed our advice and anticipated the problem by buying a wig and becoming accustomed to its use before the hair loss became severe. Toward the end of therapy, hair regrowth occurred and she was very pleased with her nice normal hair, actually a little curlier than before, as she recovered from the effects of chemotherapy. Although she had experienced intermittent episodes of gastrointestinal discomfort during which she would eat relatively little, she caught up on her nutrition at other times, and by the end of the course of chemotherapy she had even gained several pounds compared with her pretreatment weight.

Some women who receive chemotherapy for breast cancer have considerably more side effects than did Mrs. E., and sometimes this necessitates a reduction in dose or a decrease in the frequency with which the drugs can be given. However, the danger of recurrence of the breast cancer under these circumstances is so great that if the patient understands the issues and keeps in mind that the total period of chemotherapy is limited, the necessary motivation will usually be found to enable this program to be given. Chemotherapy of this type is given on an outpatient basis in the clinic, with most of the work done by nurses who are trained in the administration of chemotherapy—indeed, most chemotherapy can now be given in specially equipped treatment facilities in outpatient units, which is a considerable advantage to patients.

There are many special skills that are helpful in treating patients, and gaining access to the bloodstream to draw blood or give medicine to people who have hard-to-find veins is among the most important. We now have special catheters that can be left permanently in a vein if so desired, so that drawing blood samples or giving repeated intravenous treatments can be done as often as needed without discomfort. Another problem that this avoids is the danger of a toxic drug leaking out of the vein and oozing under the skin of the arm where it can cause a nasty wound, similar to that of a burn. Thus the techniques used by skilled chemotherapy nurses are extremely important for the care of patients who need repeated chemotherapy. Years ago the interns or senior physicians gave chemotherapy, and in some places they still do, but they are not nearly as skillful as a person who gives these kinds of treatments all day long. Often patients judge the competence of medical care by how often they have to be stuck when having blood drawn. Although we do not know of any relationship between being a good doctor and being good at drawing blood, there is no way to convince an uncomfortable patient of that! Patients also judge doctors on how well they relieve their pain—and that subject will be covered in Chapter 5.

Some of the procedures can be relatively unpleasant, such as repeated bone marrow tests and spinal taps for patients with leukemia. In these circumstances we have found it useful to use drugs that alleviate anxiety and that give temporary amnesia for the events in the clinic. As mentioned in the case of nausea and vomiting, we have reported the use on an experimental basis of a drug that blocks short-term memory and therefore prevents the sensitization of the patient to the unpleasant experiences in the clinic and immediately after treatment. Thus, even if these patients do have discomfort from the treatment, they may not remember anything about it and they will not be so anxious about returning for follow-up clinic visits. This is similar to the type of premedication that is frequently given before general anesthesia and that blocks the memory for events during the time in the operating room. We treated one elderly woman who had experienced severe side effects from treatments before we saw her and who had become quite wary and suspicious of doctors. She was treated in the hospital with our experimental drug in addition to the chemotherapy, and she did quite well although she did vomit once or twice. The next day she refused to go home, insisting that she had not yet received her chemotherapy nor even been seen by a doctor. She was pleased to learn from her family, since she would not believe it from us, that she had indeed been treated and had done well, and in the future she insisted on having the same type of treatment. There is still more work to be done with drugs of this general class. They are sorely needed, for many of the events that occur in the hospital or in the clinic setting are anxiety-provoking, setting up a vicious cycle of fear, anxiety and discomfort, which can become all-consuming if allowed to develop. This is an area of current research that seems quite promising. Also, relaxation and imagery techniques are very useful in such situations, when people who are trained in these methods are available to give the treatments.

INTERFERON AND OTHER TYPES OF IMMUNOTHERAPY The relatively new field of immunotherapy utilizes a number of different approaches that seek to eradicate cancer cells. One approach is to boost the normal immune response of patients by the use of natural substances such as interferons and interleukins. Interferons, for example, are thought to stimulate the immune system of the patient and make it more capable of eradicating cancer cells. Considerable research is going on in this area. Interferons were discovered in 1957 by Alick Isaacs and Jean Lindeman, who were delighted to find a natural substance produced by the body that interferes with viral infections, hence the name interferon. Indeed, skeptics of their work did not believe the discovery and dubbed their substance "imaginon." The discoverers had no inkling that interferon also had an anticancer effect, and so the substance was primarily of interest to virologists until fairly recently, when it was found to have anticancer properties in animals bearing tumors, and this lead was picked up for clinical trials.

Interferon was originally made in Finland through the efforts of Dr. Kari Cantell and the Finnish Red Cross, who obtained interferon as a by-product of routine blood donations for purposes of blood banking. The substance was used by Dr. Hans Strander of Stockholm, who treated children with bone cancer and thought that there were 50 percent fewer disease recurrences after surgery if patients were treated with interferon. He also found dramatic responses to interferon of a benign tumor of the throat caused by a virus-caused illness called juvenile laryngeal papillomatosis. While benign by the usual criteria in that they will not spread, these tumor masses cause obstruction of the air passage in affected children; fortunately these masses regress very substantially after interferon treatment and lives are thereby saved.

Interferon was exceedingly expensive and very scarce. (I used to joke that the reason that the Finns were so pale was because they were donating so much blood to the Red Cross.) The American Cancer Society, stimulated by that great supporter of cancer research, Mrs. Mary Lasker, and by Dr. Frank Rauscher, launched a major drive to purchase additional quantities of interferon for research in this country. The initial studies showed some anticancer effects in patients with breast cancer, lymphoma and multiple myeloma, and the media went absolutely wild with publicity about this new and miraculous treatment. The excitement did have some unfortunate effects, mainly in generating excessive expectations, but it also provided a great impetus for the development of various types of natural substances such as interferons (and later of insulin and growth hormone) by means of the new DNA recombinant technology, a major advance in the pharmaceutical development of complex biological substances. Sufficient interferon quickly became available to enable the conduct of large clinical studies all over the world.

Over the past five years many investigators have studied interferons, and the story is beginning to emerge, although it is still far from complete. One of the hopes was that since interferon is a natural product it would have few or no side effects and therefore be preferable to the use of chemotherapy. That turned out not to be the case; although most of the side effects are reversible, interferons do cause flu-like symptoms with fever, chills, malaise, loss of weight, loss of appetite, weakness, headache, muscle aches and depression. (It is my opinion that the flu symptoms are attributable to the interferon that the body produces naturally as a response to the viral infection.) We now know that interferon is not a magic bullet, but it does have significant anticancer effects in some diseases.

The most striking recent success story has been with a rare but fascinating form of leukemia, called hairy cell leukemia; close to 100 percent of patients given interferon have a very significant improvement in their clinical condition. Less impressive, but also important, are the anticancer effects in patients with malignant lymphoma, mycosis fungoides, Kaposi's sarcoma (in AIDS patients) and kidney cancers. Unfortunately, there is little by way of beneficial effect in some of the common cancers such as those originating from breast, colon and lung.

The next questions to be studied are whether interferon can profitably be combined with chemotherapy to enhance the effects against tumors, and whether mixtures of interferons are more effective than are single types of interferons alone (there are three major forms of interferon—alpha, beta and gamma). In addition to their usefulness for patients with cancer, interferons continue to be useful in conditions such as juvenile laryngeal papillomatosis, and in venereal warts (condyloma acuminata). The latter is a very distressing venereal disease that is unresponsive to most forms of treatment, but is remarkably responsive to interferon. There will be other uses for interferon in certain types of viral infections that are still being studied, including preventing or shortening the duration of the common cold, and possibly also in rheumatoid arthritis. It is comforting to those of us working in interferon research to know that this is a fundamentally important natural biological substance that the body uses regularly to limit viral infections, and so whatever we can learn about interferon in patients with cancer will ultimately be important also in understanding normal responses to viral disease. Naturally we are still eager to improve its effectiveness in patients with cancer, and we have not yet run out of ideas.

At present, work is progressing with other substances that, like interferons, are produced by normal blood lymphocytes. These substances are called lymphokines; a prominent one under investigation is interleukin-2 (IL-2). This has recently received a great deal of attention as a new approach (see Chapter 15). Another hope for the coming years lies in the use of monoclonal antibodies directed at specific antigens of the cancer cells; yet another lies in the use of chemicals to cause cancer cells to differentiate toward normal cells. The latter is entirely different from chemotherapy, which seeks to destroy malignant cells. There is also considerable interest in a tumor necrosis factor (TNF) that appears to destroy tumor cells to a greater extent than normal cells by mechanisms that are not entirely clear. (Further details of some of these approaches are given in Chapter 15). For the time being, however, immunotherapy is still in its experimental stages and cannot be considered as standard treatment. Indeed, other than interferon, there are no products of this type on the American market. Contrary to writings of some self-styled experts, we know of no way to produce superimmunity to cure cancer.

NUTRITION Before we discuss the nutritional needs of patients with cancer, it is worth reviewing some basic principles. So much has been written about diets and nutrition that the general subject has been made to appear far more complicated than it really is—a notion that also serves some who would advocate "special" diets for weight reduction, for example. Nutrition represents the sum of those processes that are involved in taking in and absorbing nutrients and of metabolizing or using them either for energy requirements or to lay down fat or enlarge muscles (or other tissues). If people eat and drink sufficient nutrients, that is, proteins, carbohydrates, fats, minerals, vitamins and water, and their expenditure of calories remains constant, they will stay in a steady state, neither gaining nor losing weight. If the caloric requirement or expenditure is greater than the intake, as it usually is in chronic illnesses such as cancer, then the calories will be spent at the expense of fat stores or muscle tissue. Of course, good nutrients are necessary for growth, for healing from illness and for providing a source of energy for those body functions concerned with immunity against infection and disease.

Although the nutritional needs of each individual are unique, and these vary for a given individual during different portions of the life cycle, everyone does require the same basic substances for calories (proteins, carbohydrates and fats). I will discuss the role of diet in cancer prevention in Chapter 7. Suffice it to say that *the normal U. S. diet contains sufficient vitamins that there is no need for vitamin supplementation, contrary to the misleading advertisements of many of the companies who make vitamins or cereals or who advocate some faddist diets.* Furthermore, the excessive intake of vitamins can even be harmful, and there are specific conditions associated with hypervitaminosis (too much) A, D, and others.

We all know that eating habits are established early in life and that they are very powerful and difficult to change. Although most healthy adults are concerned with curbing their appetites in order to lose weight, the cancer patient has quite the opposite problem, and now we want to focus on nutrition and give some practical advice for the patient who is being cared for at home. Chemotherapy not only causes nausea and vomiting, and a feeling of abdominal fullness, it also causes a loss of appetite and changes in taste. People with cancer often experience alterations in their taste sensation so that sweet foods may be more difficult to taste, whereas bitter foods may taste stronger than usual; this requires some change in the manner in which foods are prepared. Whatever can be done to make food taste better will help improve the appetite of the patient with cancer.

Protein-containing foods in particular may taste bitter, and since protein is an important nutritional component, one needs to find ways to make these foods more attractive. Some people can best accept proteins that are served cold or at room temperature, like cheese, cold cuts, tuna, chicken, eggs or egg salad, ice cream, milk shakes, puddings, custards and nuts. Meats can be cured, such as ham or bacon, or marinated; fresh fruits can be used to improve the taste of dairy products such as ice cream, milk and custards. Seasonings such as mint and lemon juice will also improve the taste and smell of food. *If you are cooking for the patient, the basic principle to follow is that whatever the individual desires is what should be used, rather than any particular formula. Vitamins should not be added to the diet without checking with the doctor, since in this case vitamins may precisely counteract the effect of antimetabolite drugs.*

It is true for all of us that food is more tempting when it is served in an attractive manner and in pleasant surroundings—unfortunately, that is difficult to achieve in a hospital environment, and this is one important reason why patients prefer to be at home during therapy. (Trays with plastic dishes and utensils will never raise consciousness for food, and rare hospitals do have proper dishes and silverware in their private VIP wards.) Varying the color of foods and using attractive dishes and silverware, nice place settings and background music are all simple and sensible means to make meals more attractive and appetizing. If, in addition, there is pleasant company to go with the surroundings, that reinforces the feeling that mealtime is enjoyable. Some find it helpful to take light exercise or have a glass of sherry before eating at night; most people who have health problems find that it is easier to eat their biggest meal of the day at breakfast. Again, there is no single formula for success—whatever suits the individual is what we want to encourage. And with patience and tolerance for some disappointments, sick people will appreciate and do well with specially prepared menus.

People who have nausea, vomiting and abdominal distress following chemotherapy will complain about difficulty in maintaining their weight, but this is not an invariable accompaniment of chemotherapy, as we have said. People who have nausea and vomiting for other reasons, such as in the first trimester of pregnancy, also complain of the same distress and yet they manage to gain weight. That is because *it is possible to compensate at times when the symptoms are not present,* and that is worth remembering for it also holds true between chemotherapy treatments. Thus, one should not be discouraged by temporary weight loss, because it can be made up for at a later time. However, when there is a feeling of fullness and nausea, foods that pass easily through the stomach, such as carbohydrate-containing foods, should be eaten; fattier fried foods, which take longer to leave the stomach, should be avoided. The volume of food in the stomach can also be reduced by reducing the volume of fluids taken at mealtime and then drinking them an hour or so later. Eating dry foods such as toast or crackers seems to relieve nausea, as does drinking cold carbonated beverages. Eating meals slowly and chewing food thoroughly and resting, even lying down, after meals can help to speed digestion. And there is a cookbook for patients who can't chew or have trouble swallowing (see bibliography). Often the smell of food may cause the person to have nausea, and if so, it is best for the person to stay out of the kitchen while meals are being prepared. *Most people find that eating smaller amounts of food more frequently and in a leisurely way is easier to manage than eating big meals at designated times when everyone else eats.*

If diarrhea is a problem, eating food when it is warm rather than hot can help, as can avoiding liquids while eating foods, and deferring the drinking of beverages until between meals. Lowering the roughage in the diet may also help to control diarrhea if that is a problem, since these fiber foods cannot be digested by humans and they help to speed the passage of stools through the bowel. Since roughage helps to make more regular and softer stools, fiber foods are recommended as part of our daily diet under normal circumstances; but they may be better omitted when the intestines are irritated, which means reducing the intake of raw fruits and vegetables, bran and other grain cereals and breads, and nuts.

Constipation is not a frequent problem in patients with cancer unless they are taking certain types of drugs or are bedridden, but if it is, high fiber foods and prune juice can act as laxatives. If the mouth is dry, liquids or soft foods are easier to swallow and if nausea is not a problem, butter, gravy, soups and syrups can be helpful as well. Many people dunk their foods in coffee, tea or milk, or swallow liquids along with bites of food.

If the mouth or throat is sore, soft cold foods such as ice cream, watermelon or grapes may be more acceptable, and swallowing may be more comfortable with the use of a straw. Under these conditions spices or highly acid foods such as citrus juices or tomatoes may have to be avoided temporarily. Finally, if all else fails, there are an abundance of food supplements available from pharmaceutical companies, which are also accompanied by attractive recipes. If sufficient calories cannot be taken by mouth, it may be necessary to use a feeding tube into the stomach or even, under special circumstances, to use intravenous feeding. Although it does not sound attractive, many patients who are having trouble eating sufficient calories to maintain their weight can learn to swallow a plastic stomach tube—like three swallows of a long piece of spaghetti. Once in, the tube can be used as a means of feeding them liquid nutritional supplements—and then the tube can be removed. A patient can often do this alone or with the help of another person. Again, there are a wide variety of excellent feeding preparations for this type of supplemental feeding.

The reason for discussing nutritional problems in such detail is that these are common, and too frequently the assumption is made that loss of weight is directly proportional to the rate at which the disease is progressing. This is not necessarily the case; patients with chronic illness often suffer from loss of interest in food, mental depression or other problems that are quite reversible if faced with a positive attitude and a willingness to experiment.

ATTITUDE AND IMAGERY Speaking of attitude, a great deal has been written about its importance in the causation of cancer and in the determination of outcome. Some of the ideas are very intriguing and sound intuitively plausible, but there is still little of substance that we can consider scientifically well-founded. For example, one commonly heard notion is that depression causes cancer, and this is based on the observation that patients who have cancer are more likely to be depressed than other people. While that is undoubtedly true, the conclusion is quite illogical because a person with any serious illness has more reason, and is certainly more likely, to be depressed than a well person—that tells us nothing at all about what they were like before they became ill, nor does it suggest cause and effect. However, more pertinent to this chapter on treatment is the claim that being active and aggressive about the illness, a "fighter," is more likely to cause a longer survival than being passive and quietly accepting of whatever comes along. There are some interesting experimental models that show that animals that struggle to survive will live longer than those who do not struggle against life-threatening circumstances. As physicians we also frequently observe individuals who have little interest in living who will often deteriorate rapidly and die. A positive attitude that permits a person to participate fully in medical decisions and in activities of daily living is tremendously important, and no one questions that. I recently cared for a young woman school administrator who had extensive kidney cancer and who not only lived about a year longer than anyone would have predicted but who spent virtually all of her time being active— right to the end. She had a remarkably strong will to live and her family was tremendously supportive of her. But notwithstanding this general phenomenologic background, a great superstructure is often erected that espouses the "willing" of outcome through imagery—and that is the part I call nonsense.

The Simonton program (see Chapter 14) is one prominent example that has attracted the fancy of the public because the idea of the individual's being in control of his or her body is attractive and positive—we want to control our destiny. Indeed, there is much that relaxation techniques, imagery and hypnosis can do to make patients feel better, to deal with pain or discomforts such as nausea and vomiting, and this is constructive. Not believable, however, are the derivative notions that people can "will" their immune cells to destroy the cancer in the body. Indeed, I have seen patients who have unfortunately delayed potentially curative treatment while engaging in this type of magical therapy at clinics. Like it or not, there simply is no basis to support the notion that we can cure cancer in this manner, although there is every reason to do careful studies on the role of attitudes and emotions in the entire process of coping with the disease. The field desperately needs good scientists who will devise and conduct the same type of careful clinical study with appropriate controls (i.e., not comparing sick people and well people but cancer patients with other patients who have life-threatening illnesses), such studies as are required in all other areas of medicine. There are no shortcuts to good scientific design. The clinics that claim to treat cancer with imagery are using fantasy to mislead the public, and for my part, they should be categorized along with other charlatans who prey on the victims of cancer. Not long ago I made this point to a group of hospice volunteers to whom I was teaching the fundamentals of caring for patients with cancer. Everything was going well until we came to this issue in response to a question. The audience became rather upset with my dismissal of imagery as having a primary role in cancer treatment, as suddenly they found their speaker to be a nonbeliever from the "traditional medical establishment." However, if wishing could make it so, we would have cured cancer a long time ago! But more about this subject later.

WHAT IS CANCER AND HOW DOES IT KILL?

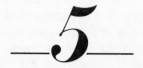

Cancer is classified by insurance companies as a "dread disease," and few would argue with that label. I once had to tell a young man that his symptoms were due to acute leukemia and he made the surprising reply, "Thank God, I thought it was cancer." In our country there are over nine hundred thousand new cases of cancer diagnosed annually and about half that many deaths. Looking at the positive side, however, more than three million Americans have survived cancer.

The name "cancer" is derived from the Greek word for crab, Karkinos, which is the term believed to have been used by Hippocrates when he named carcinos and carcinoma. His school attributed cancer to an excess of black bile, a notion that lasted for centuries. Not only was cancer described in the early writings of the Greeks and Romans, there is also excellent documentation of tumors' being present in Egyptian mummies dating back five thousand years. The disease goes back far before that, however, because there is pathologic evidence of bone tumors in dinosaurs and other prehistoric animals.

DEFINITIONS AND BIOLOGY OF CANCER It is difficult to give a single definition of cancer because almost any generality has its exceptions. Broadly speaking, any cancer is basically an abnormal growth of malignant cells. Two major types form solid tumors— *carcinoma* and *sarcoma.* Carcinoma is the term applied to malignant tumors derived from epithelial tissue (the outermost covering or lining of all free surfaces of the body), which may resemble normal tissue. Sarcoma is a malignant tumor, poorly differentiated, derived from connective tissue such as blood, bone and cartilage.

Three other major forms of malignancy include *leukemia,* sited in bone marrow and other blood-forming organs, causing them to cease their normal function and produce an overwhelming count of abnormal blood cells; *glioma,* sited in the nervous system and producing tumors of varying grades of malignancy; and *lymphoma,* originating in the lymph glands.

So in a practical sense cancer is a group of diseases, perhaps as many as one hundred, which originate from different parts of the body. Cancer has the property of growing uncontrollably and killing the individual by extending into the surrounding normal tissues and/or by spreading to distant parts of the body, a process known as metastasizing. Cancer cells arise from normal cells under the influence of cancer-causing (carcinogenic) stimuli, whether chemical or viral, as we will discuss in a later chapter.

We generally think of a tumor as a mass of rapidly growing malignant cancer cells, but there are also slow-growing tumors. Some, called benign tumors, generally will not kill the patient unless they happen to be in a critical part of the body, such as the brain. Rapid cell growth is not an invariable characteristic even of malignant tumors, for there are some cancers that grow more slowly even than certain normal tissues such as bone marrow or cells from the skin. When we speak of rapid growth of cancer cells we mean that the cells may double in number in a matter of a few days to a week, whereas slow-growing cancers (e.g., lung, bowel) may take one to three months to double in size. Slow-growing cancers produce tumor growths mainly because the cells accumulate and are not eliminated in a normal fashion.

The diagnosis of cancer is made by looking at cells under the microscope and seeing their characteristic abnormal features and abnormal pattern of growth. Cancer cells do have some resemblance to the tissue from which they originate, so a cancer of the liver (hepatoma) looks somewhat like a normal liver, and a malignancy of blood-forming cells (leukemia) has some resemblance to normal blood cells. At the same time these cancers also have abnormal features that are uncharacteristic of their normal counterpart cells. Cancer cells are often large and with irregular outlines; they have abnormal amounts of DNA and numerous cell divisions that are microscopically detectable signs of cells that are in the process of dividing. The frequency of these dividing cells within a tumor mass is roughly proportional to its rate of growth, as defined earlier. Sometimes the pattern of growth of cancer cells is so extremely abnormal and bizarre that it is difficult, if not impossible, to recognize the tissue of origin; then, when a tumor is found in an area of the body in which it did not originate, it may be a problem to find the organ from which it did originate.

Tumors are named after the embryonic cell from which they are derived. For example, we use the term *carcinoma* to refer to malignant tumors (or cancers) that are *epithelial* in origin. Epithelial cells are lining cells of skin, bronchial airways, glandular ducts and hollow organs such as the gastrointestinal or urinary tracts, so a cancer in one of these areas is called, for example, a lung, kidney or colon "carcinoma." Carcinomas are further subdivided into either *squamous* cell type or *adeno* cell type, depending upon whether they show features of skin or glandular formation; thus one might have an adeno *or* a squamous cell carcinoma of the lung depending on the cell type. *Sarcomas* are the other major form of cancer; these include tumors that originate from muscle, bone or fibrous tissues, like, for example, an osteosarcoma of the humerus (cancer of the upper arm bone). *Leukemias* are malignancies derived from blood cell elements that originate in the bone marrow (primitive white or red cell types), and *lymphomas* are from lymph glands and come in a number of different cell types also.

Tumors are further subclassified by pathologists by their appearance, mainly based on how closely they resemble the normal cell of origin. This has some predictive value in that well-differentiated tumor cells (i.e., those having clearly differing characteristics), which closely resemble the tissue of origin, are generally slow growing and may even be benign, whereas those that no longer have much resemblance to the cell of origin are called undifferentiated or poorly differentiated malignancies (carcinomas or sarcomas), and are generally more rapidly growing. Special stains, electron microscopic analysis or immunologic analyses may be necessary to properly classify the types of cancer, especially the leukemias and lymphomas.

Benign tumors are composed of cells that closely resemble the normal tissue, and their pattern of growth often produces a rounded mass; usually the tumor also has a surrounding fibrous tissue capsule that makes it easy to remove the entire tumor mass. Malignant tumors by contrast are more deviant in their cellular and organizational characteristics; the cells are likely to stick to one another and they readily outgrow their blood supply and become hemorrhagic (bloody). Cells from the edges of a malignant tumor tend to spread to surrounding normal areas and replace normal tissues and organs, and they also migrate *(metastasize)* to distant organs such as lungs, liver, bone marrow and lymph nodes. When they metastasize they generally resemble the tumor of origin, but at times the metastasis may be less differentiated than the original tumor, which may cause the pathologist to wonder whether a given metastasis represents a separate, primary tumor. This can be a diagnostic problem, as you can imagine, since we also know that a person who has had one type of cancer is more prone to develop a second, *independent* one, and such a person is more likely to develop a third one, and so on. Indeed, I have seen patients who, over the years, have had four to seven *different* types of cancers! "Them that has gits," as one stoic patient with a wry sense of humor said to me.

For cancer cells to metastasize to a distant organ, they have to break off from the main body of the tumor, migrate through surrounding tissues, erode normal blood vessels, be carried through the bloodstream to a distant area, pass out of the blood vessel and then be able to lodge successfully and grow into a new tumor in that distant site. That is a very improbable set of events for any one cell to manage; consequently, while many tumor cells may be shed from a primary cancer, few or none may survive the odds of this unlikely chain of events to cause a distant metastasis.

Nature habitually throws out billions of seeds or eggs or cells in order to perpetuate just one species. A fractional few find suitable conditions in which to germinate. This is true also for cancer cells. However, enough cells *shed over a longer period of time* will eventually give rise to one or more metastases. Some cancer cells have properties that enable them to grow better in the liver or in bone marrow, and some others in the lung or brain, for reasons that are not well understood. This same heterogeneity of cancer cells probably explains why resistant lines can survive chemotherapy, even when 99.99 percent of the tumor is killed; then, when these resistant cells grow back, they frequently are resistant not only to the original drug, but to other drugs as well. This is called "pleiotropic" drug resistance and it is a major problem that is now under intense study. Such cell lines are characterized by the presence of unique chemical glycoproteins in the outer membrane or cell wall.

Abnormalities in the genetic or *chromosomal structures* of cancers and leukemias are being documented by the use of new staining techniques. Some tumors have very characteristic changes of their chromosomes, so much so that a particular type of chromosome rearrangement, the Philadelphia chromosome, is almost diagnostic of one form of leukemia. We now can *see* many examples of chromosomal abnormalities, which is surprising in a way, since when a change in DNA is big enough to be seen by chromosomal analysis, it is a very gross change indeed. Much more subtle changes also occur regularly in cancers, but they require more sophisticated DNA mapping techniques to detect their presence. These techniques are possible through recent advances in DNA sequencing analysis, which offers the promise of teaching us much more about the nature of the malignant process.

If normal cells taken from animals are stimulated in tissue culture by a cancer-causing chemical or virus, they undergo a series of steps that results in *malignant transformation* and eventually become cells that look and act like cancer cells; they even acquire the ability to cause cancer in the animal from which they were originally taken. Up to a point the transformation process is reversible, that is, the cells can be persuaded to retrace their steps to normal activity. But beyond that certain point the cells have the capability to continue dividing indefinitely because they have now become permanently altered to a genetically stable condition. Grown in tissue culture, they become "immortal" in that they will divide indefinitely if they have sufficient nutrients.

Comparable events occur in the formation of tumors in humans, and some of these can be seen by looking at shed tissue cells in secretions taken from the cervix in the Pap test, or from the bronchial lining cells in tests of sputum cytology (cell analysis). Early changes in the cervix and in the bronchial lining cells are called *dysplasia,* and the cells are considered to be premalignant although they are not necessarily destined to become cancerous, particularly if the stimulus that caused them is removed. An excellent example of the capacity for reversal of dysplastic changes is seen in heavy smokers: after the smoker has quit, the cells gradually revert back toward normal. Unlike the inflammation that occurs in bronchial lining cells during bronchitis (infection in the tubes to the lungs), the changes of dysplasia in the lungs cause no symptoms by themselves, nor will they be likely to go away unless smoking ceases. Thus, for ex-smokers the risk of developing lung cancer slowly drops, as discussed elsewhere. By contrast, if the stimulus is not removed, the cells may gradually become more abnormal in appearance and begin to show microscopic invasion of the underlying normal cells; if they were biopsied, one could see a process called *carcinoma in situ.* This is a very localized cancer that is easily curable, particularly when it occurs in the cervix. If not discovered during this stage, the cells will invade the surrounding tissues more extensively and eventually give rise to the typical appearance of a malignant tumor.

It is thought that malignant transformation of cells may be more frequent than is clinically apparent, and that the development of true tumors or cancers is constantly being aborted by a process called immune surveillance in which the body's own defense system of normal immune cells recognizes transformed cells as "foreign" and destroys them. If this is true, then when immune surveillance is suppressed or becomes abnormal in some way, as may occur with aging, or with the use of drugs that suppress immunity, or in circumstances of impaired immunity such as the overall condition of ill health resulting from prolonged high stress or in specific conditions of attack such as AIDS, malignant transformation is unchecked and may lead to cancer (see Chapter 11).

Malignant transformation begins with the alteration of a single cell; that cell in turn gives rise to two daughter cells just like it, and so on. The time that it takes for one such cell "doubling" tends to be characteristic of particular tumors, and this changes as the tumor grows. An important concept is that by the time a tumor has grown to a size where it is clinically detectable, like, say, a lung mass one centimeter (0.4 inches) in diameter, which can be seen on a chest x-ray, it has already undergone approximately thirty doublings and reached 10^9 (one billion) cells. From that point on it takes only ten further doubling cycles to produce a tumor mass the size of approximately one kilogram (2.2 pounds), which is usually lethal. Thus, by the time a tumor is detected, it has already gone through the largest part of its biological life cycle. So when we speak of "early" cancers being curable by surgical removal, the reference to early is only a manner of speaking since even a small tumor already has more of its life history behind it than before it.

It happens that tumor cell growth is an irregular process. Furthermore, there is generally a long latent period, sometimes years, between the time when a stimulus occurs or is being applied and the evolution of a malignant clone of cells. For example, tumors that are produced by exposure to asbestos characteristically take fifteen to twenty years to become detectable, and those caused by radiation may take three to five years. Presumably they took some considerable time to get to the point where they began to grow at all. Once they begin to grow, they do so at a logarithmic rate until they get to a large size, when they begin to slow down; toward the end of their span, when tumors are very sizable, they actually grow much more slowly than they did at the beginning of their biological cycle.

Tumor growth curves are mathematically described by the Gompertz equation, first set forth by Benjamin Gompertz in 1825 to express his "law of human mortality." Since that time the Gompertz equation has also been useful in describing the growth of the human fetus, of individual organs and of tumors that grow in mice into which cancer cells are injected. Tumors, as described by the Gompertz curve, appear to grow exponentially over any short span of observation, say up to three or four doublings; long-term observation reveals a gradual slowing of the growth rate to an eventual plateau level at which the rate of new cell production equals the rate of cell loss. (For the mathematically minded reader the Gompertz curve and equation are given in Figure 3.) All of this is important because the sensitivity of cells to damage by chemotherapy or by radiation depends upon their rate of growth; curiously, slow-growing tumors are more resistant to killing than rapidly growing tumors.

Another important point about the growth of tumors is that the more rapidly they grow, the more likely they are to outgrow their blood supply and become dead or *necrotic* in the center—although cancer cells remain alive on the outer portion of the tumor, which derives part of its nutrients, including glucose and oxygen, from adjacent normal blood vessels. The main mass of tumor has its own blood supply, and this is the subject of considerable research at present. As the tumor mass begins to outgrow its blood supply, the oxygen supply becomes limited, a condition called hypoxia. This is a problem particularly when patients are being given radiation treatments, for the killing effects of radiation are less efficient under conditions of hypoxia. To alleviate this problem, radiation therapy has been given under experimental circumstances in which the patient is in a hyperbaric (high pressure) chamber, like a special diving chamber, in which the amount of oxygen supplied to the tissues can be increased; so far this approach has met with only limited success.

It turns out that cancer cells have the capacity for stimulating the growth of new blood vessels, which they subvert or parasitize, so to speak, for their own benefit. This so-called *tumor angiogenesis* is due to a factor produced by cancer cells, a process described in part by Dr. Judah Folkman of Harvard, which is essential to the survival of cancer cells within the body. One very exciting new approach to killing cancer cells is to try to inhibit this factor so that the cells cannot continue to survive and grow. It may ultimately become possible to inhibit angiogenesis by means that are very different from the usual drugs that kill cancer cells.

How do we know that cancers start from a single cell? We know that each cell carries certain characteristic markers specific for the normal tissue of origin, and this is dictated by inheritance from the parent cell. If cancer cells really originated from several cells at a time (rather than from a single cell), then they might express different markers in the different cells that make up a single tumor, but that is not the case. It is possible of course that multiple tumors might originate in a patient at the same time, but then each tumor would start with a single cell and would contain its own characteristic markers. Once a tumor develops, the cells within it show the capacity for variation and can mutate and develop new properties

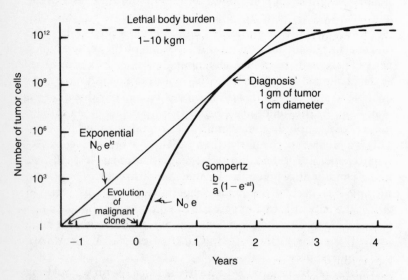

Figure 3 The Gompertz curve and equation, showing the tumor growth curve. Tumors appear to grow exponentially over a short span of observation, but long-term observation reveals a gradual slowing of the growth rate to an eventual plateau. (Kindly prepared by Dr. Edwin Cox and reproduced with permission from Cecil's *Textbook of Medicine*, ed. J. B. Wyngaarden and L. H. Smith, Philadelphia: W. B. Saunders Publishing, 1985)

while still retaining the original marker. This briefly summarizes a very large body of information.

HOW DOES CANCER KILL? How do cancers kill people or animals that are affected by them? Various mechanisms are responsible for fatal complications such as hemorrhage, but the major cause of death is that the cancer grows locally to involve a vital structure, or it spreads to a distant organ such as the brain or heart and does its principal damage there. Some tumors, such as liver and brain tumors, are prone to grow to a very large size locally and destroy the tissue in which they originate. Such a tumor either causes the vital organ to fail to function, or it obstructs or erodes blood vessels and thus causes fatal complications, or it ruptures an organ or exposes it to serious infection by destroying its normal protective barriers and causing ulcerations. Some tumors are prone to spread to distant organs *(metastasize)* even when they are still small—tumors of this kind are very difficult to cure by surgical removal because by the time they are first discovered they have already spread. A typical example of this is small cell cancer of the lung, one of the major types of lung cancer. Whether the tumors grow locally or at a distance from the site where they originated, they cause signs and symptoms due to expansion into vital areas— organs such as the liver, brain or heart, or bones, nerves or blood vessels.

The particular symptoms that a patient experiences depend upon the specific area in which the tumor is growing, and this can be unpredictable. I first learned this as a medical student when I examined a man who had a malignant melanoma that had metastasized right to the very tip of his forefinger. When I asked my instructor if this was not a very rare occurrence, he replied, with his customary acid wit, "Just think, if the cancer had gone another centimeter it would have missed him completely."

Anything is possible, and doctors have to be very alert to the many different manifestations of cancer. A headache in a previously healthy person is almost always due to an innocent cause, but an occasional patient will first come to the doctor with a problem of persistent headache and be found to have cancer. A cough can be due to many things, obviously, but occasionally it is due to cancer. Pain in the back is usually due to problems other than cancer, but it is not surprising if on evaluation a persistent pain in the back turns out to be due to malignancy. And so it goes, through virtually every organ in the body. (I remember when my medical school class first studied pathology, someone invariably thought they had the early symptoms of whatever it was we were studying—no matter how rare.) The opposite side of the coin is that *a patient with cancer can have signs or symptoms of any other disease as well—there is no law that prevents appendicitis or heart disease from occurring in patients with cancer. This is very important for doctors to remember because not every medical problem is due to cancer, and the treatment obviously depends on the cause.*

PAIN When people think about cancer they always think about pain, fearing that it will be an inevitable consequence of cancer. About 70 percent of patients with advanced cancer will have pain—this amounts to about twenty-five million worldwide. Fewer than one-third of these are not adequately controlled, an estimate that varies widely depending on availability of health care, ethnic background and personality. In this country, whereas pain is certainly a common problem, because of the pressure exerted by a growing tumor on nerve roots and the manner by which this is perceived by the brain, it is also one of the more manageable problems and *it is unusual when a patient's pain is so intractable that no satisfactory management can be found.* We hear much about these cases, which are certainly tragic, but they fortunately do not reflect the circumstances of most patients with cancer. We have an ever-increasing number of ways of combating pain, and doctors need to be comfortable in using the whole range of treatment options.

If pain is localized in one area, such as a bone, it is frequently possible to give radiation treatments to stop the pain or do a neurosurgical procedure, cutting or anesthetizing the pain fibers of that region so that pain is not perceived but the motor functions are not disturbed; then the patient can continue to use the body part, such as an arm or a leg. There are also new techniques of direct electrical counterstimulation of nerves to prevent the recognition of pain. It is possible to cut major pain pathways that transmit the signals from the source of the pain through the spinal cord and up to the brain where the pain is recognized, or even to inject areas of the brain that are involved in pain perception. If pain is more generalized, as it may be in a patient who has metastases to many bones, then we use whatever drugs are required to give pain relief. Sometimes simple aspirin or other anti-inflammatory drug serves to give relief, while at other times progressively bigger guns are required—up to narcotics such as morphine given orally if possible, by injection or, in extreme cases, by continuous intravenous drip. And some potent painkillers are now available in long-acting form, obviating frequent dosing and permitting sleep at night. By the way, heroin is no better than morphine for pain control. And then there are combinations of painkillers, such as aspirin and narcotics, that can work effectively when taken together. These and other means of obtaining relief from pain can greatly improve the quality of life for they permit the person to get on with a more normal set of activities. Indeed, if pain is allowed to get above a certain threshold, and this varies greatly for different patients, it reaches a point when it causes suffering.

I generally discuss the problem of pain early on with the patient, soon after the diagnosis is made, simply because it is such a prevalent fear that it probably has been a concern, whether the patient expresses it or not. It is rarely a problem when the patient has a curable cancer, and when the cancer is incurable, it is some comfort to patients to know that while pain is certainly a possible problem in the future, it will be handled by whatever means are necessary so that it will not be incapacitating. This is not to make light of the extreme difficulty of controlling cancer pain in some patients, and it certainly requires special expertise to do so at times. And pain can mean different things to different people. Basically it can best be described as whatever the patient says it is.

One of the more common problems is that patients are given medication that satisfactorily controls pain as long as they take it on a regular basis, but which may not be sufficient if they take it only when the pain becomes intense. It is necessary for the doctor to instruct the patient (and educate the family) to take the medication before the pain becomes severe, and to take it on a regular basis. This sometimes means setting the alarm clock for the middle of the night to have the patient awaken and take medication, so that he will not awaken several hours later with such severe pain that it is difficult to manage with the very drug that could have prevented it in the first place. This seems fairly obvious. Yet many patients fear "drugs" or dependency on drugs, and so prefer not to take them unless they "absolutely have to." Or they are afraid that if they take narcotics too soon, what will they do when they "really need it." The answer usually is "probably more of the same, and that's O.K." Many times, also, narcotics are perceived as illegal substances to be avoided if at all possible, and it is amazing, to me at least, to see patients with advanced cancer resist painkillers for fear that they may be habit-forming or that their friends and relatives will think less of them for using drugs. *In fact, it is important for the patient to know that drug addiction is rarely a problem under these circumstances and the error is more often of omission than commission.* This is in contrast to the situation that pertains with the recreational use of drugs. It is up to the doctor or nurse to explain this not only to the patient but also to family members. I have cared for numerous patients whose loved ones discourage them from taking "dope," to the great disservice of the patient.

NUTRITION Another problem that cancer often inflicts on its victim is to cause poor nutrition. Any patient who is chronically ill suffers a loss of appetite; but in addition, cancer often causes severe weight loss that may be all out of proportion to the size of the cancer. There is a peculiar syndrome known as cancer *cachexia,* in which the presence of cancer cells causes normal inflammatory cells to manufacture a polypeptide chemical that causes the breakdown of normal tissues such as muscle and fat. When this occurs, a patient who has a relatively small tumor can rapidly become debilitated as a result of severe weight loss or cachexia. If the tumor can be removed or controlled, the patient begins to gain weight again. It is difficult, however, to reverse weight loss in cancer patients, partly because they have a poor appetite and partly because the metabolic consequences of the cancer make it difficult to lay down new muscle and fat as would normally happen with the ingestion of a large intake of calories. Fat is mobilized, used up, at a more rapid rate in patients with cancer, and loss of high energy substances (adenosine triphosphate, ATP) also occurs. Although we are primarily interested in finding drugs that prevent or stop the growth of cancer cells, some researchers are also concentrating on medicines to break this cycle, which is destructive to the metabolism of the whole body. Hydrazine sulfate does this in rats that have experimental tumors, and Dr. Joseph Gold of Syracuse is advocating further research on this in patients with cancer. It seems to help prevent weight loss in patients and may extend life in lung cancer cases.

When a patient has a type of cancer that requires extensive surgery of the jaw, tongue, upper digestive tract, et cetera, it becomes particularly difficult for him to eat or to digest food. This poses additional problems with nutrition. As mentioned earlier, these can sometimes be counteracted by inserting thin stomach tubes and feeding the patient by pouring or dripping rich caloric liquids in through the tube, without the need for the patient to chew and swallow. If this is not feasible, as in the case of a patient who is in a postoperative state, or who has lost the portions of the bowel necessary for absorption of foodstuffs, then intravenous feeding can also be given to provide the patient with sufficient nourishment to sustain body weight. This is cumbersome and quite expensive, but it can sometimes be lifesaving as a temporary measure until bodily functions can be restored. We should also mention that there are many tasty recipes that can be prepared for people who cannot chew (see the bibliography).

The nutritional problems of the patient with cancer are further compounded by the treatments (chemotherapy, radiation therapy, surgery), which can decrease appetite and result in excessive loss of calories that cannot be replenished by normal means. Thus the effects of the cancer are compounded by those of the treatment. Malnutrition obviously weakens the patient and may make it impossible for him to tolerate treatments that could be given to well-nourished individuals. Occasionally a patient is so debilitated that he must be fed intravenously or by tube feedings to get him into a positive nitrogen balance and gaining weight *before* we dare give aggressive chemotherapy. Recognizing the severity of nutritional needs can make all the difference in allowing a patient the opportunity to respond to a course of treatment.

INFECTION Although it may seem surprising, probably more patients with cancer die of infection than from any other single cause. There are several reasons for this, but they generally boil down to the fact that a person who has had cancer for a long period of time is debilitated by loss of weight, compromised immune function and insufficient white blood cells from radiation and chemotherapy, and his normal defense mechanisms no longer protect him. In this condition the patient is highly susceptible to bacterial, fungal, viral and even parasitic types of infection that would not be a particular threat if he had not suffered these complications of cancer or of its treatment.

We have learned a great deal about infectious complications and how to prevent and/or treat them. This is important in improving the survival chances of all patients. With the advent of more potent antibiotics and of drugs that are effective against infectious diseases that were once untreatable, it is often possible to get patients through these complications. However, they are then prone to become infected by an organism that is resistant to the available antibiotics, because the extensive use of antibiotic treatment in itself creates resistant organisms, thus causing a kind of vicious cycle. Knowing when to use potent antibiotics and when to withhold antibiotics is part of the judgment that the cancer expert needs; sometimes consultants in infectious disease are particularly helpful with this question.

There are also complications unique to cancer treatment, which can be life threatening in themselves; these are discussed in Chapter 4, and in my new book on that subject written for professionals (see bibliography).

I hope that thus far I have managed to give you an overview of what cancer is and what its possible treatments might be. I will go on to describe in greater detail what else you need to know.

CANCER STATISTICS: THE BIG PICTURE

6

We are all at risk for cancer, whether male, female, black, white, rich or poor. The American Cancer Society estimates that seventy-four million Americans now living will eventually have cancer and the disease will strike approximately three out of every four American families. During the 1970s there were an estimated three and one-half million deaths from cancer, about twice that many new cases of cancer and about three times that many people who were receiving medical care or observation for a history of cancer. Cancer is difficult to deal with at any age, but it seems particularly tragic when it affects children—and it kills more children aged three to fourteen than any other disease. However, generally cancer strikes more frequently with advancing age, and so the risk rises steadily.

At the risk of being repetitive, I will say again that statistics are

95

a *guide* only, a clue to doctors and researchers as to where to watch out for trouble. In the final analysis, each person is unique, his or her own 100 percent statistic, not simply a point on a chart.

Yet it is important to know that there are over five million living Americans who have had cancer, three million of whom have had the diagnosis five or more years. Although the figures vary for different types of cancers, the risk of recurrence of cancer becomes less and less as the years go by. For example, a patient who had cancer of the bone more than five years ago and has had no recurrence is almost surely cured, and it is quite likely that a patient with breast cancer more than five years earlier is also cured, although with breast cancer it is not so unusual to have a recurrence later than that, as discussed previously. Still, to all intents and purposes one can consider that most of the three million people who had a diagnosis of cancer five or more years ago have been "cured"—they have no evidence of disease and should enjoy a life span similar to that of a comparable person who never had cancer. The definitions of cure were discussed in Chapter 4.

During the year 1987 about 965,000 people were diagnosed as having cancer; as far as their cancer is concerned about half of them can be expected to be alive five years after the diagnosis, unless they succumb to other factors such as heart disease or other diseases of old age. Looking at it another way (*not* considering other causes of death), some 385,000 Americans, or approximately 40 percent of patients who get cancer, will be alive five years after the diagnosis, which is a big gain over the past. In the 1930s fewer than one out of five patients was alive five years after diagnosis; in the 1940s this improved to one in four; and from the 1960s until recently one in three patients lived five years. Nonetheless, some 483,000 people diagnosed with cancer will die in 1987, which translates into 1,323 people a day. It is estimated that of those patients who will die of the disease, *about a third could have been saved by earlier diagnosis and treatment.* That makes it vitally important to concentrate on measures that could lead to earlier diagnosis.

A study of cancer rates shows an alarmingly high incidence of cancer among blacks, and blacks also have a higher death rate from cancer than do whites. In the last thirty years, cancer death rates in whites have increased by 10 percent, whereas in blacks they have increased by 40 percent. Thirty years ago, the rates were slightly lower in blacks than in whites. Blacks have a significantly higher incidence of cancers of the lung, large bowel (colorectal), prostate and esophagus. The incidence of invasive cancer of the cervix has dropped for both black and white women, but the incidence in blacks is still more than double that in whites. By curious contrast, the incidence of endometrial cancer, or cancer of the upper portion of the uterus, is twice as great in whites as it is in blacks.

Recent surveys have shown that black Americans tend to be less aware than whites about the warning signs of cancer and less likely to see a doctor if they do experience these symptoms. Thus, more whites than blacks have their cancer diagnosed when it is in the early, localized stage when the chances of a cure are greater. This may help to explain the higher death rate from cancer among blacks, but it is not entirely clear why blacks have a greater incidence of cancer than whites. Some cancers seem more related to socioeconomic status than to race, and since blacks tend to be at the lower end of the socioeconomic ladder in this country, that may be a partial explanation. In other cancers, however, socioeconomic status seems not to be a factor so this cannot account for what appear to be racial differences. This is a difficult subject to sort out, as are many other aspects of distinguishing the role of heredity and that of environment. A recent report by Dr. Harold Freeman shows that most of the poorer statistics for blacks, when they occur, are shared by other socioeconomically disadvantaged peoples, among whom whites are more numerous than blacks. The American Cancer Society is trying to change this picture.

The personal tragedy of cancer cannot of course be told in statistics, but the number of cases of different types of cancer and the number of deaths from these cancers represent a multiplication of these individual tragedies. Table 1 provides the figures on the more common types of cancer. The incidence and deaths from various cancers in different parts of the body are shown for males and females in Figure 4, page 99. To get a sense of what is happening in our country over time, we can also

Table 1 *Common Malignancies: Incidence, Signs, Recommendations*

Type	Annual Cases	Annual Deaths	Warning Signs	Recommendations*
Lung	150,000	136,000	Persistent cough, blood in sputum, chest pain	Most are cigarette-related. Screening not very effective
Breast	130,900	41,300	Lump, thickening, pain, swelling, change in nipple	Monthly breast self-examination. Show suspicious lesions to doctor. Baseline mammogram age 35–40, then every 2 years till 50, then annually
Uterus	48,000	6,800	Vaginal bleeding	Pap test every 2–3 years if perfectly normal on 3 annual exams
Colorectal	145,000	60,000	Rectal bleeding, change in bowel habits	Stools for blood yearly after 50; rectal exam yearly after 40; endoscopy every 3–5 years after 50
Skin	500,000	7,800	Unusual mole or skin change	Avoid strong sun or use sunscreen; show skin lesions to doctor
Prostate	96,000	27,000	None or blood in urine and difficulty voiding	Periodic rectal examinations—every 2 years over the age of 55

*Recommendations of American Cancer Society differ somewhat and are listed in Chapter 9.

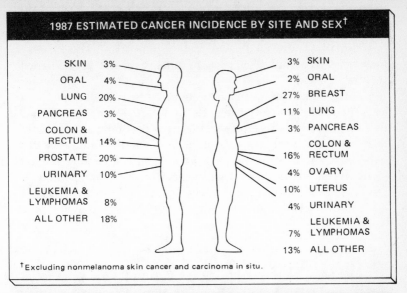

1987 ESTIMATED CANCER INCIDENCE BY SITE AND SEX†

SKIN	3%	3%	SKIN
ORAL	4%	2%	ORAL
LUNG	20%	27%	BREAST
PANCREAS	3%	11%	LUNG
COLON & RECTUM	14%	3%	PANCREAS
PROSTATE	20%	16%	COLON & RECTUM
URINARY	10%	4%	OVARY
LEUKEMIA & LYMPHOMAS	8%	10%	UTERUS
ALL OTHER	18%	4%	URINARY
		7%	LEUKEMIA & LYMPHOMAS
		13%	ALL OTHER

†Excluding nonmelanoma skin cancer and carcinoma in situ.

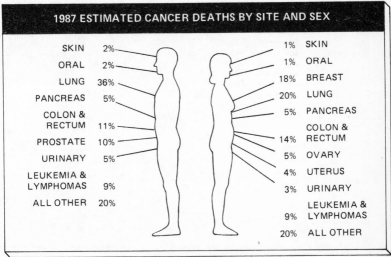

1987 ESTIMATED CANCER DEATHS BY SITE AND SEX

SKIN	2%	1%	SKIN
ORAL	2%	1%	ORAL
LUNG	36%	18%	BREAST
PANCREAS	5%	20%	LUNG
COLON & RECTUM	11%	5%	PANCREAS
PROSTATE	10%	14%	COLON & RECTUM
URINARY	5%	5%	OVARY
LEUKEMIA & LYMPHOMAS	9%	4%	UTERUS
ALL OTHER	20%	3%	URINARY
		9%	LEUKEMIA & LYMPHOMAS
		20%	ALL OTHER

Figure 4 Cancer incidence and deaths by site and sex—1987 estimates. The estimates of the incidence of cancer are based on data from the National Cancer Institute's Surveillance, Epidemiology and End Results (SEER) program (1981–83). Nonmelanoma skin cancer and carcinoma *in situ* have not been included in the statistics. The incidence of nonmelanoma skin cancer is estimated to be more than 500,000. (Source: Epidemiology and Statistics Department, American Cancer Society)

look at trends of individual types of cancer over a fifty-year period (Figures 5 and 6).

Clearly, some types of cancer are progressively declining as a cause of death, but it is not at all clear why. For example, we would like to think that cancer of the uterus is declining as a cause of death because of easier means of diagnosis, most notably the Pap test (see Chapter 9). However, there is no comparable test for stomach cancer, and not only is the death rate for stomach cancer falling, but the incidence is also falling. Presumably there has been a significant change in the national diet; something has been

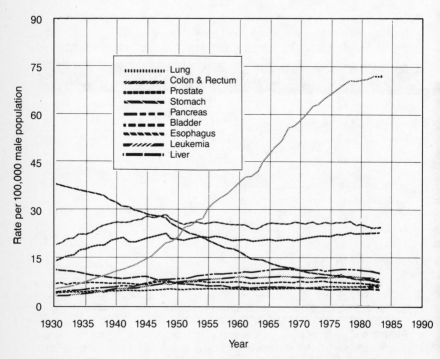

Figure 5 Male cancer death rates by site, United States, 1930–1983. The rate for male population is standardized for age on the 1970 U.S. population. (Source: Epidemiology and Statistics Department, American Cancer Society, 5-86)

removed that earlier was causing a high incidence of stomach cancer. (Stomach cancer is very common among the Japanese and we have some explanations for that in food preservation and dietary intake, as discussed in Chapter 7, but we have no comparable explanation for the change in incidence in our country.) At the other extreme is lung cancer, now the biggest killer among all cancers. The influence of cigarettes in causing this cancer is difficult to deny; this is discussed in much greater detail in Chapter 8. Other cancers are slowly creeping up as causes of death, while others are staying at the same rate. Not shown on the graphs is the

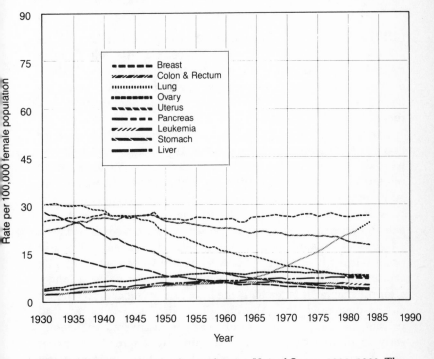

Figure 6 Female cancer death rates by site, United States, 1930–1983. The rate for female population is standardized on the 1970 U.S. population. (Source: Epidemiology and Statistics Department, American Cancer Society, 5-86)

decline in deaths of children from cancers. The most striking and gratifying achievements have been made with young patients with relatively uncommon tumors who, after successful treatment, have a full lifetime of normal health ahead of them. In contrast, the statistics on cancer of the prostate are not changing appreciably; when that is the cause of death, however, it generally affects people in the seventh and eighth decades of life. The affected individual is just as concerned, of course, regardless of age.

Let us now examine some of the facts and figures on certain of the more common types of cancer. Table 1, page 98, outlines some salient facts, warnings and recommendations about these problems.

LUNG CANCER An estimated 150,000 new cases of lung cancer occurred in 1987 and there were 136,000 deaths—talk about a tough bottom line! And this is only for the United States. Of these deaths, 44,000 were in women. Female deaths from lung cancer have been on a rising curve. They've "come a long way" to get there.

The relationship to cigarettes is discussed more fully in Chapter 8, but the Surgeon General's report of 1982 points out that those who smoke two packs of cigarettes per day have lung cancer mortality rates some twenty times higher than nonsmokers. In addition to heavy cigarette smoking, exposure to certain industrial substances such as asbestos may be related to an increased incidence of lung cancer, particularly when exposure is combined with a history of smoking. Lung cancer is difficult to detect sufficiently early to make it curable, and only some 5 to 10 percent of all lung cancer patients, whether white or black, live five years or longer after the diagnosis is made. If the lung cancer is localized when it is first diagnosed, then the overall survival rate is close to 40 percent, but only a minority of cases are discovered sufficiently early to fit that category. The warning signals for lung cancer include a persistent cough, blood in the sputum, chest pain and recurrent attacks of pneumonia or bronchitis.

BREAST CANCER An estimated 131,000 new cases were diagnosed in the United States in 1987, and there were 41,000 deaths.

Approximately 10 percent of women will develop breast cancer at some time during their lives; it has long been the major cause of death from cancer among women, although it is now being surpassed by lung cancer. The warning signals are a lump or thickening of the breast with swelling, skin irritation, distortion, irritation, retraction or discharge from the nipple, and pain or tenderness. The risk for breast cancer is greater for women over the age of fifty, as well as in those who have already had one breast cancer or who have a close relative who had it, and in women who have never had children or who bore their first child after the age of thirty.

The five-year survival rate for patients with localized breast cancer is close to 90 percent, but if the cancer has spread beyond the breast, the five-year survival rate drops to 60 percent, and worse if the cancer is widespread. There has been relatively little improvement in the survival of patients with breast cancer, although the types of surgery used now are much less radical than before and there has been great success in maintaining the cosmetic effect of the operated breast, either by means of reconstruction or by more limited surgical procedures, with or without the combined use of radiation therapy.

CANCER OF THE UTERUS It is estimated that there are 48,000 new cases of cancer of the uterus a year, which includes 13,000 cases of cancer of the cervix and 35,000 cases of cancer of the endometrium (upper portion of the uterus). Cancer of the cervix is most common in low socioeconomic groups and particularly among women with early sexual contacts and multiple sexual partners or whose partners have themselves had multiple sexual contacts (see also Chapter 7). Endometrial cancer tends to affect mature women, and the diagnosis is usually made during the sixth and seventh decades of life. It is estimated that there will be 6,800 deaths in 1987 from cervical cancer and 2,900 from endometrial cancer; but overall the death rate from uterine cancer has decreased by more than 70 percent during the past forty years, which is at least partly attributable to Pap tests and regular checkups.

The five-year survival rate for patients with cancer of the cervix is 68 percent overall. However, for patients who are diagnosed early, the five-year survival rate is close to 90 percent. If the cancer is truly early and involves only localized invasion (this is called cancer in situ), it is curable in virtually 100 percent of cases! Here is the best argument for the importance of early detection—it does make a big difference.

CANCER OF THE COLON AND RECTUM The illness of President Reagan in mid-1985 called public attention to cancer of the colon and rectum as a major health problem in the United States. The estimated 145,000 new cases in 1987 included 102,000 cases of colon cancer and 43,000 of cancer of the rectum; their combined incidence is second only to that of lung cancer. There were an estimated 60,000 deaths in 1987 from large bowel cancer, second again only to lung cancer. It is important to detect cancer of the colon and rectum early because there is a high cure rate with surgical removal of the tumor (this subject is discussed further under cancer screening). When colorectal cancer is detected in an early, localized stage, the five-year survival rate is around 80 percent, but it drops to about 45 percent if the cancer is first detected after it has spread to other parts of the body.

SKIN CANCER There are estimated to be more than 500,000 new cases of skin cancer per year, the vast majority of which are superficial and highly curable. In fact, these are so common that accurate statistics are not available, and skin cancer (other than malignant melanoma) is not listed in the cancer statistics. The incidence is far more common in individuals who have light complexions and who are regularly exposed to sunlight. The most serious type of skin cancer is malignant melanoma, which afflicts 26,000 people a year. There are an estimated 7,800 deaths per year from skin cancer, but 5,600 of these are attributable to malignant melanoma. For the more common types of skin cancer, survival is virtually assured when the cancer is detected early and treated by surgical removal. Malignant melanoma is the exception to this; the five-year survival rate is 83 percent, compared to over 95 percent for patients who have other forms of skin cancer.

ORAL CANCER There are an estimated 29,000 new cases of oral cancer per year, and they occur twice as often in males as in females; an estimated 9,400 deaths occurred in 1987. Cancer can affect any part of the oral cavity, from the lip to the tongue, the mouth and the throat. The five-year survival rates depend upon the location of the cancer in the mouth and vary from 31 percent for cancer of the pharynx to 92 percent for cancer of the lip, presumably because the latter is so much easier to detect early. The overall five-year survival rate for all patients with oral cancer is approximately 52 percent. I expect that the incidence of oral cancer and the deaths from oral cancer will rise substantially, after a waiting period, now that the use of chewing (smokeless) tobacco is on the rise in this country. Oral cancers are related to the use of tobacco and alcohol, and commonly to both together.

LEUKEMIA An estimated 26,400 new cases of leukemia occurred in 1987; half were acute forms of leukemia and half were so-called chronic leukemia. Although leukemia is generally considered to be a childhood disease, in fact it affects more adults (24,000 of the new cases were in adults, as compared to 2,000 cases in children) and it is far less curable in adults. There were an estimated 17,800 deaths from leukemia in 1987. The overall five-year survival rate for leukemia is, at 33 percent, still relatively poor, although that figure is out of date and will rise in the next few years. Rapidly changing trends in treatment are bringing clear improvement, as discussed earlier.

CHILDHOOD CANCER In 1987 there were an estimated 6,600 new cases of all kinds of childhood cancer and an estimated 2,200 deaths. About half of the deaths were from leukemia. Despite its rarity, cancer is still the major cause of death by disease in children between the ages of three and fourteen. There have been major new treatments for childhood cancer, not only leukemia, and the five-year survival rates in children are reflecting those improvements, although it takes time for these effects to be documented. The five-year survival rate for children with bone cancer is 47 percent, neuroblastoma 57 percent, brain tumors 53 percent, kidney tumors 81 percent, retinoblastoma (eye) 88 percent and Hodg-kin's disease 88 percent.

IF WE COULD CURE CANCER AND HEART DISEASE, THEN WOULD WE LIVE FOREVER? Cancer is a chronic disease that, together with heart disease, accounts for a majority of the deaths in this country. With the death rate from cardiovascular disease decreasing and the suggestion that the death rate from cancer will likewise decrease in the next two decades, what can we speculate about the life expectancy of the American population? Dr. James Fries wrote a fascinating article on this subject called "Aging, Natural Death, and the Compression of Morbidity." He pointed out that the average length of life has risen from forty-seven to seventy-three years during the twentieth century; but despite this phenomenal improvement the *maximum* life span has really not changed appreciably. Thus, for example, statistics on the number of centenarians have been available in England since 1837 and during this time, despite a tremendous change in average life expectancy, there has been no detectable change in the number of people living longer than one hundred years. In Sweden, where careful investigation of centenarians has been carried out, no one has yet exceeded 110 years of age, and the greatest documented age in the world was recorded in Japan, in a person 114 years old. Only approximately one in 10,000 persons lives beyond the age of one hundred in the developed countries of the world, and despite occasional sensational claims to the contrary from certain provinces in Russia where the record keeping is believed to be "creative," there is no documentation of any society that enjoys exceptional longevity.

Some 80 percent of the years of life that were lost to premature death for reasons other than trauma have been eliminated in the United States, and most of the premature deaths are now due to chronic diseases such as heart disease and cancer. Fries suggests that the ideal average life span is approximately eighty-five years of age and that if chronic diseases such as cancer are progressively eliminated, there will be more healthy people living out that ideal life span. That there is not a greater number of people living to be one hundred years of age now than there was in earlier times, despite improving overall survival of the populace, suggests that there must be death due to the process of aging and "natural causes," defined as death unrelated to specific illness. That is not yet a widely accepted view among geriatric specialists, but it has to be carefully considered. We are talking about a concept of an age "wall," to borrow a term from marathoners; that is, under ideal circumstances, when cancer and other chronic diseases are eliminated, more and more people will be living in a state of good health until they reach the "ideal age" somewhere between eighty and ninety, at which time they may be expected to die of "old age," presumably as the Lord intended. Meanwhile, other causes of premature death have been eliminated, particularly in children, and there are therefore more people at risk for developing diseases of the elderly, such as cancer. That is why there are so many cancer deaths in our society.

If you would like to think of an encouraging recent development, the average lifespan is now increasing because of improved longevity beyond childhood—presumably because of decreasing rates of death from certain diseases that affect adults. One epidemiologist characterized this dramatic change as equivalent to aging only 45 minutes out of every 60 minutes elapsed on the clock. Enjoy!

THE CAUSES AND PREVENTION OF CANCER

STUDIES OF CAUSATION—EPIDEMIOLOGY We all agree that an ounce of prevention is worth a pound of cure, but in order to prevent cancer we must know its causes. Unfortunately, our knowledge is incomplete; although we know some important causes, others have not yet been identified. In this chapter we will review the evidence on the causes, look at how that information has come into being and talk about how it can be used to prevent or reduce the incidence of cancer.

Several levels of information are needed to answer the question of what causes cancer. First we must recognize the common associations of cancer with certain occupational, environmental or genetic conditions. These insights often come from observant clinicians who note that an excessive number of patients have the same type of tumor and then trace it to a common association. This involves a kind of detective work that is called epidemiology—research in this area attempts to identify the environmental factors that are generally responsible for a large proportion of cancers in the population. *Remarkably, it has been estimated that as many as 80 to 90 percent of all cancers may be related to environmental influences, particularly those related to lifestyle,* as discussed below. Table 2 summarizes some of the more common environmental causes of cancer: these represent significant associations although they depend upon the level and duration of the exposure. By that we mean that one cigarette or one drink is not dangerous but years of intake are; by contrast, one high dose of radiation is enough to increase the risk of leukemia and other cancers. Once these associations are recognized, it is necessary to delve more deeply to discover whether these factors are real causes or whether they, in turn, are associated with some other, more critical factors such as age, race, sex or other simultaneous exposures. Finally, we must tackle the very difficult problem of finding the mechanism(s) by which the cancer is actually caused. The latter problem goes right to the genetic level because once a normal cell becomes transformed into a cancer cell, that change is self-reproductive and will be characteristic of all the "daughter" cells that make up the tumor.

The subject of cancer epidemiology (that is, the circumstances associated with the incidence of cancer) can be traced back to Ramazzini, who in 1770, in his book on occupational medicine, recorded the unusually high occurrence of cancer among nuns:

Experience proves that as a consequence of disturbances in the uterus, cancerous tumors are very often generated in the woman's breast, and tumors of this sort are found in nuns more often than in any other women. Now these are not caused by suppression of the menses but rather, in my opinion, by their celibate life. For I have known several cases of nuns who came to a pitiable end from terrible cancers of the breast. . . . Every city in Italy has several religious communities of nuns, and you seldom can find a convent that does not harbor this accursed pest, cancer, within its walls.

Calling our attention to the historical origins of cancer epidemiology, Dr. Michael Shimkin suggests that this may be the first

Table 2 *Environmental Causes of Cancer*

Agent	Method of Exposure	Site or Type of Cancer
Alcoholic beverages	Drinking	Mouth, pharynx, esophagus, larynx, liver
Androgen-anabolic steroids	Medication taken to build muscles or red blood cells	Liver
Aromatic amines (benzidine, 2-naphthylamine, 4-aminobiphenyl)	Manufacture of chemicals—used by industries and laboratories	Bladder
Arsenic (inorganic)	Mining and smelting of certain ores, pesticide manufacturing and application, medication and contaminated drinking water	Lung, skin, liver (angiosarcoma)
Asbestos	Manufacturing and application	Lung, pleura, peritoneum, kidney, gastrointestinal cancers
Benzene	Leather, petroleum and other industries	Leukemia
Cancer chemotherapy (melphalan, cyclophosphamide, chlorambucil, semustine)	Medication for cancer	Leukemia
Chromium compounds	Manufacturing	Lung
Estrogens Synthetic (DES)	Medication for menopausal symptoms, etc.	Vagina, cervix (?)

Table 2 *(Continued)*

Agent	Method of Exposure	Site or Type of Cancer
Steroid contraceptives	Birth control	Liver (benign), endometrium
Immunosuppressants (azathioprine, cyclosporin)	Medications for organ transplantation	Lymphoma (histiocytic), skin (squamous carcinoma), soft tissue sarcoma
Ionizing radiation	Atomic blasts, medical use, radium dial painting, uranium and metal mining	Nearly all sites
Nickel dust	Refining	Lung, nasal sinuses
Phenacetin-containing analgesics	Medication for pain	Kidney, bladder
Polycyclic hydrocarbons	Coal carbonization products and some mineral oils	Lung, skin
Tobacco chews and powder	Snuff dipping and chewing of tobacco, betel, lime	Mouth
Tobacco smoke	Smoking, especially cigarettes	Lung, larynx, mouth, pharynx, esophagus, bladder, pancreas, kidney
Ultraviolet radiation	Sunlight	Skin, including melanoma
Vinyl chloride	Manufacture of polyvinyl chloride	Liver (angiosarcoma)
Wood dusts	Furniture manufacturing	Nasal sinuses

Source: J. F. Fraumini, Jr., "Epidemiology of Cancer" in 17th edition of Cecil's *Textbook of Medicine,* ed. J. B. Wyngaarden and L. H. Smith (Philadelphia: W. B. Saunders Publishing, 1985)

recorded association of an occupation—in this case a nun, with a celibate way of life—with cancer of the breast, an association that has stood the test of many subsequent investigations. This is an especially curious occupational relationship because nuns, one might expect, would be far less cancer-prone than those who are exposed to chemicals that cause cancer, but in this case (breast cancer), it is, in fact, the normal physiology of pregnancy and nursing that decreases the risk of this form of cancer.

The subject of chemical carcinogenesis really began in 1775 when Dr. (later Sir) Percivall Pott, a noted surgeon at St. Bartholomew's Hospital in London, pointed out that cancer of the skin covering the testes, the scrotum, frequently developed among chimney sweeps and that it was caused by long-term exposure to soot. This was not an age when quantitation was in fashion so he had no firm statistical basis for his conclusions, but this cancer of the scrotum was certainly recognized by the chimney sweeps themselves since, as they said, "the trade call is the soot-wart." Sir Percivall made no mention of how to prevent this, either by avoiding soot or by proper hygiene of washing it off, but the cancer became rare in the following century as a result of appropriate regulatory action—and a decline in child labor.

In 1795 Dr. Samuel Thomas Von Soemmering pointed to pipe smoking as a cause of cancer when he wrote that "carcinoma of the lips occurs most frequently where men indulge in pipe smoking; the lower lip is particularly affected by cancer when it is compressed between the tobacco pipe and the teeth."

How does one come up with the notion that 80 to 90 percent of all cancers may be related to environmental influences? (This is a question I asked myself on first hearing this estimate—indeed, it still seems quite high to me.) The explanations are difficult, but let us go through it together. A great deal of importance is placed on the tremendous geographic variation in the incidence of different types of cancer. The rates in the low-risk countries are subtracted from the rates in the United States (or another high-risk country) and the resulting differences are thought to be due to environmental causes; the lowest rates are assumed to represent the baseline levels for spontaneous cancer that cannot be prevented and the difference between them and the rates in a high-risk country are presumed to be due to preventable environmental factors. The rates for certain types of cancer, such as those originating from the esophagus and liver, vary by as much as one hundred-fold in different parts of the world, and even the risk for common tumors in the Western world varies by ten- to forty-fold, depending on the country. Some of this variability may have a genetic basis. However, the data obtained from migrant populations provide strong evidence that environmental factors are involved. For example, for the Japanese who have moved to Hawaii or to the U. S. mainland the risk of developing various types of cancer changes from that which prevails in Japan to that of the United States. Their heredity remains the same, of course, but their environment has changed. Thus, although cancer of the breast is rare among Japanese living in Japan, it is much more common when they move to Hawaii or California; on the other hand, cancer of the stomach is common in Japan, but far less common among Japanese living in the United States. In these situations heredity is not a factor in causing the cancer. The best explanation for this type of environmental difference is that it is probably due to changes in diet, as discussed below, rather than changes of climate or work conditions.

Cancers in adults that are caused by environmental factors generally develop in the skin, in the upper respiratory and digestive tracts and in the bladder and prostate. Personal habits such as cigarette smoking, tobacco chewing, alcohol consumption and betel quid chewing are very important causative factors for cancer in different parts of the world; in fact, tobacco use accounts for 25 to 40 percent of all cancers (see Chapter 8). Smokeless tobacco products are also of great concern; oral cancer has been linked to dipping snuff, a very common practice in the southern United States. In parts of Asia, oral cancer is associated with chewing betel and other agents. Smaller proportions of cancers are due to occupational exposures, and many types of cancers may be linked to past exposure to certain viruses. We will discuss these below.

HAZARDS OF LIFESTYLE—DIET, OBESITY, ALCOHOL, RADIATION Current concern with smoking in public places, the popularity of dietary and vitamin programs that are claimed (rightly or wrongly) to prevent cancer, interest in breast self-examination and in other cancer-screening programs, intense interest in the control of pain and of nausea and vomiting, and the burst of new hospice programs that primarily serve terminally ill patients with cancer are all manifestations of the growing awareness of the prevalence of cancer and the need to "do something and not just stand there!" *There is a rekindled willingness to take charge of oneself and not be an object that only receives guidance and largesse from doctors and relatives.*

Now let us examine some of the hazards of the lifestyles of modern societies, with the term "lifestyle" referring to the total cultural, behavioral and dietary environment of the individual. We will discuss tobacco products in a separate chapter (8). Consumption of alcoholic beverages has also been found to be an important influence on cancers of the mouth, esophagus and larynx, and it multiplies the risk that tobacco smoking brings in these anatomic regions. *In other words, the risk of oral cancers for heavy drinkers who do not smoke is not nearly as great as for people who both drink and smoke.* Heavy alcohol consumption also markedly increases the risk of cancer of the liver and may increase the risk of breast cancer. The alcohol (ethanol) itself is not known to be a chemical carcinogen, but other additives in wines and beers have been implicated, along with nutritional deficiencies that are often associated with heavy drinking.

International studies suggest that Western diets are responsible for a large proportion of all cancers, although specific relationships are difficult to sort out. Obesity appears to be related to development of cancer; this is generally agreed among the experts. Diet is culturally conditioned, and is in turn related to hormonal status, behavior and cooking practices, which cover a broad panorama of possible relationships. Nevertheless, a diet that includes *a high intake of fat seems to increase the risk of colon cancer, breast cancer and uterine cancer; and of course, fat and caloric intake are also related to obesity, diabetes and hypertension.* That low intake of certain foods may also predispose to cancer has been well publicized recently; in particular, the *risk of colon cancer is increased by low consumption of fiber substances.* Intakes of vitamin A, carotene, and selenium that are well below that of the normal diet appear to be related to a higher incidence of lung cancer, while stomach cancer has been related to a deficiency of fruits and vitamins. *Although we know all these things, it is difficult to suggest other than a prudent (balanced) diet: avoid overeating, limit fat intake and consume two helpings a day of fruits and vegetables*—dark green vegetables, yellow-orange vegetables and yellow-orange fruits.* With this type of diet, added vitamins and other supplements are not necessary and can even be harmful.

A massive recent study from the People's Republic of China examining the relationships between dietary intake and cancer incidence concludes that a high cholesterol diet carries a very large risk of cancer, and a high protein diet also increases the risk over a low protein diet. Since cholesterol is in many fats and protein is ubiquitous in food (meat, fish, eggs, cereal, etc.), that leaves carbohydrates as the preferred source of calories in food. If the Chinese study is replicable in other societies, then the question is, how does one use such information—given that fats, proteins and carbohydrates comprise the nourishment in our foodstuffs? We are looking for more practical solutions. There are many other epidemiologic studies, but none is really solid enough for us to say that we know a safe diet; most, however, do agree that a high fat diet should be avoided and this, I believe, can be recommended to the American people as a way to minimize the risks of both cancer and heart disease. Specific recommendations from the National Cancer Institute are to decrease the average daily fat intake from 160 to 100 grams and to increase the average daily intake of fiber substances from whole grains, fruits and vegetables to 30 grams per day. Low fat and high fiber in the diet will lower the amount of estrogen (female hormone) in the blood, and this may explain why such a diet decreases the risk of breast cancer, since high estrogens are related to a higher incidence of breast cancer.

It is difficult to separate foods from the ways in which they are

---

*Because of the importance of the subject of nutrition and cancer and the controversy that surrounds it, I include as an appendix to this chapter an excerpt from a 1984 special report on the subject from the American Cancer Society, based on the work of a distinguished committee chaired by Dr. Sidney Weinhouse.

prepared. Stomach cancer is related to a high intake of dried, salted or smoked fish, pickled vegetables, and low intake of fresh fruit and vegetables (vitamins C, E, and A) according to Dr. John Weisburger of American Health Foundation. Food additives and contaminants have also been implicated in causing cancer, as in the eating of aflatoxin, a product of a fungus that can contaminate foodstuffs such as spoiled peanuts and that can cause liver cancer, as it frequently does in Africa.

Many suggested relationships between foods or food additives and cancer have turned out to be false, and some of these caused panic or near panic because of extensive, and often uncritical, media coverage. Some years ago there was the great cranberry scare when it was widely reported that cranberry juice and related products caused cancer; this devastated the cranberry industry for a number of years. It was found that there was no valid basis for the original claim, so fortunately for us all, but particularly for cranberry lovers, this proved to be a blind alley. More recently, artificial sweeteners such as saccharin and cyclamates have been said to have weak cancer-causing effects on the bladder of animals, but the risk in humans is very small, if any. Then coffee drinking was reported to be associated with a high incidence of cancer of the pancreas—that work has not been confirmed by subsequent studies and appears to be unfounded.

One interesting discovery that gives us hope for prevention is that certain foodstuffs, such as vitamin A, and retinoids in certain vegetables, can inhibit the development of particular types of cancer, such as those of the ovary and uterus. A great deal of work is now under way to try to use this information so that people who are at risk for developing cancer, such as smokers, can take an added substance every day to help reduce their risk. This research is only in the experimental stage, however; it may take years to find something that is both effective and nontoxic. (This subject is called chemoprevention, and it is discussed in a later chapter.) *Health stores that claim to sell products that prevent cancer are profiting from unsubstantiated hype—they have no independent knowledge or insights into this subject. Furthermore, there is a very real risk of toxicity from some of these substances, so there is possible danger without any certain benefit. Beware of this type of profiteering!* Remember that "cure" and possible, even probable, assistance in prevention are two very different things—and be guided accordingly.

Let me add a postscript to this section on diet since the scientific debate about the role of dietary constituents in causing cancer is quite vehement these days, fueled also by the economic interests of manufacturers of cereals and vitamins. Some experts rate dietary factors as responsible for only 2 percent of cancers, rather than the more often quoted figure of 35 percent. In a recently published letter to the journal *Science,* medical nutritionist Dr. Victor Herbert strongly objects to the advertising that promotes the intake of large amounts of high-fiber cereals to decrease the risk of colon cancer. Dr. Herbert cautions that Kellogg's All-Bran has not been shown to decrease risk and that intake of very large quantities of this food can produce deficiency of iron, zinc and calcium and may even cause intestinal obstruction. He has called for a study of these claims before they are allowed to be made publicly, and that seems quite appropriate to me.

The U.S. Department of Agriculture has been recommending that Americans eat adequate and varied amounts of fiber. By "adequate" they mean not less than 15 but not more than 35 grams of fiber from all plant sources—say half from the grain group (cereals, breads, pastas) and half from the fruit and vegetable group. In my view there is no good health reason to eat more than one bowl of cereal daily nor to subscribe to the use of the fiber pills that are widely advertised as protecting against cancer. The final chapter of this saga has not been written, so stay tuned. Meanwhile, eat a varied and balanced diet, minimize fat intake and avoid obesity—that's my considered opinion.

Radiation is another established cause of cancer, whether from solar or from ionizing sources. Solar radiation is the major cause of skin cancers; the evidence for that is based on the observation that skin cancers tend to arise on sun-exposed parts of the body and to occur among people who have outdoor occupations, such as sailors and farmers. There is also an inverse relationship between the incidence of skin cancer and the distance that one lives from the equator, as well as a strong relationship to the complexion of the skin. People with fair skin who sunburn easily such as those of Celtic origin (Irish, Australian) are very prone to develop skin cancer, while dark-skinned people rarely develop skin cancer.

Skin cancer is an important problem because of its frequency (40 percent of all cancers diagnosed). Skin cancer is curable in over 90 percent of cases, unless it is of the type called malignant melanoma, and even this can be cured if caught early. More young people in their twenties and thirties are developing skin cancer, presumably because they spend more time in the sun. Unfortunately, a tanned skin is considered by many to be a mark of beauty. Many people make it a goal to stay tanned for as much of the year as possible, not realizing that they are greatly increasing their chance of developing skin cancer. Tanning is now becoming somewhat less fashionable, curiously *not* because of the risk of skin cancer, but because of the widespread recognition that excessive sun exposure leads to premature aging (wrinkling) of the skin and therefore will diminish rather than enhance beauty. In this case vanity can be either harmful or useful depending upon whether one is seeking short-term or long-term benefit.

A number of points about the potential harmful effects of sun exposure are worth knowing. People at risk for skin cancer should apply sunscreens daily when they are exposed to the sun. In order to minimize sun exposure, it's useful to know that the sun is strongest between 10 A.M. and 2 P.M.; try to plan your outdoor activities for early in the morning or in the late afternoon. Covering yourself from the rays of the sun by wearing long-sleeved shirts, long pants and a hat when out in the sun will of course afford excellent protection. When sunning yourself on the beach, apply a sunscreen before exposing yourself to the sun and reapply it frequently and liberally—that means perhaps every two hours as long as you stay in the sun. If you go swimming or perspire heavily, reapply the sunscreen. The most effective sunscreens have a sun protection factor (SPF) of 15 or more printed on the label of the product. You should definitely use a sunscreen during high altitude activities such as mountain climbing and skiing, because at high altitudes there's less atmosphere to absorb the rays of the sun and the risk of sunburn is therefore greater. The sun is also stronger near the equator where the rays strike the earth most directly. Don't forget to use your sunscreen on cloudy days as well, because the sun's rays can be as damaging to your skin on a cloudy, hazy day as on a sunny day. If you develop an allergic reaction to one sunscreen, change to another—there are many products on the market from which you can choose.

There is a new cause for concern in that our atmosphere is losing its ozone layer and current and future generations will be more exposed to the harmful effects of the sun than our predecessors. This will predictably lead to hundreds of thousands of additional cases of skin cancer in the coming decade and thus a greater need than ever to take proper precautions. I would urge you certainly to avoid tanning parlors because the ultraviolet light from these not only causes sunburn and premature aging of skin but also greatly increases the risk of developing skin cancer. Keep infants out of the sun and teach older children to protect themselves from the sun at an early age so that they can develop good habits.

Ionizing radiation such as x- or gamma rays affects us all to some extent, although it is estimated that this radiation accounts for fewer than 5 percent of all cancers. It has been known for many years that people who have had x-ray treatments for arthritis of the spine or for a large thymus gland have a higher incidence of cancer and leukemia than the general population. Therefore, we no longer use those treatments. The old-time radiologists who received excessive radiation exposure because they were not aware of the need for proper shielding had a high incidence of leukemias, as well as skin cancers on their hands, with which they positioned patients in front of the roentgen tube. I knew an old-time radiotherapist who treated his own bursitis of the shoulder by radiation—once I found him sitting in front of the beam without so much as a technician in attendance. He told me that this was the best treatment for bursitis. Unfortunately, he later died of bone cancer. This behavior was downright self-destructive, but that was his choice.

Leukemia was also more common in radioactive radium dial watch workers who were unwittingly exposed at work because it was their habit to lick the brushes they used to paint the radium onto dials. Then, of course, after the atomic bombs were dropped came the dramatic revelation that many different types of cancer, particularly leukemia, follow in the wake of radiation exposure. Survivors of the bomb blasts had a high incidence of cancer beginning some two to four years after the exposure, peaking at about seven years and then returning normal in twenty to thirty years. It seems a particular tragedy that so many civilians who survived the trauma of being in Hiroshima or Nagasaki when the bombs struck subsequently had to bear and succumb to the late effects of radiation cancer years afterward. And now we can expect many hundreds or thousands of Russians to develop cancer if they were close to the nuclear accident at Chernobyl—*it is predictable and not preventable* after the exposure has occurred. It is also sad to think of the children and young people who were treated years ago with radiation for benign conditions like ringworm of the scalp or enlargement of the thymus in the neck, or who were exposed to frequent fluoroscopic monitoring of tuberculosis. The risks of doing these things were simply not known. When I was a child it was popular to frequent shoe stores that had fluoroscopic platforms for customers to stand on in order to look at the bones in their feet; now of course we know better than to incur such exposure. But it was such a fascinating temptation for children at the time.

One new potential problem is that of radon gas contamination of certain housing tracts, particularly in the Northeast. Radon is a naturally occurring, odorless, radioactive gas that, if the concentrations are high enough, may pose a risk of lung cancer equivalent to smoking. It is estimated by the Environmental Protection Agency that 5,000–20,000 cases of lung cancer per year may be caused by radon. There is not much known about this issue as yet, but fear, confusion and lawsuits of homebuilders are mounting. In Pennsylvania, New Jersey and parts of New York there is a geological formation known as the Reading Prong, which contains uranium that seeps naturally upward through the earth as the breakdown product radon gas. This poses no problem unless it is confined in a house without adequate ventilation pumps. It behooves federal and state governments to develop crash programs to investigate the risk, to encourage inexpensive technology to assess the levels of radon and to devise strategies for helping individual families and communities cope with this problem. We do not yet know enough to suggest firm recommendations other than these.

In a similar context, there have been many concerns expressed about formaldehyde contamination from certain types of building insulation. Although formaldehyde probably could cause cancers if it were in high enough concentration, there is no evidence that it is a cancer risk under any ordinary circumstances—not even for embalmers who work with this chemical substance regularly. The heavy odor of formaldehyde can cause uncomfortable symptoms to be sure, but fortunately it does not pose a practical risk for cancer as far as we can determine.

Unlike the inherent problem with radon, the potential exposure of people to nuclear waste is a predictable outcome associated with the technological uses of atomic energy for industrial and medical applications. The problems of safe handling, storage, transportation and disposal of radioactive wastes are very complex and beyond the scope of this book. Fortunately, many knowledgeable and concerned citizens, scientists and legislators are very busy trying to find some realistic answers to these man-made problems.

When I first moved to the South I was amazed at the number of patients who had had special x-ray tests of the liver made by the use of radioactive thorotrast, then very popular as a diagnostic test for amoebiasis, a parasitic infestation that produces diarrhea and liver abscesses. These abscesses could be seen on x-rays because the rest of the surrounding liver looked lighter. Unfortunately, the thorotrast remains in the liver virtually forever, so a seemingly innocent diagnostic procedure has the potential to cause cancer many years later. My first such experience as a medical resident was with a forty-year-old former professional baseball player in whom I diagnosed acute leukemia on the night of admission. The next day my attending professor, the famous Dr. Eugene A. Stead, Jr., was upset with me because I had been unable to find the medical records of this patient's only previous admission to Duke, which had consisted of only a two-day stay for diarrhea some twenty years earlier. To me there seemed no relevance of the leukemia to that episode, but Dr. Stead's cryptic attending note for the chart on that day was "Say for me—the present illness is related to the previous illness." Absurd? Imagine my surprise when a pathology resident came to the ward later that day to ask if my patient had ever been given thorotrast because he saw some typical thorotrast particles right in the midst of leukemic cells on the bone marrow specimen! We found that earlier chart, and the patient had in fact received a thorotrast study during the previous admission to rule out liver abscess formation; none had been found, but the damage was presumably done. While that did not prove that thorotrast had caused the leukemia, I learned something that day about taking a complete history from a patient and using all possible sources of information!

So if your doctor(s) seems to probe and ask questions ad infinitum, be glad—and respond. Better yet, check back in your own mind and records and build up a history, a profile of your health versus sicknesses, accidents, duration, when they happened, what physicians attended, what results were found, et cetera. And write it all down, along with every question *you* can think of. Certainly a job history would be useful too.

SEXUAL LIFESTYLE There are a number of factors related to sexual lifestyle that predispose to cancer. Perhaps the most important in terms of numbers of people affected is the relationship between sexual activity and cancer of the cervix, as mentioned elsewhere. We know that early sexual activity, say by adolescent girls; having multiple sexual partners as exemplified in the extreme by prostitutes; poor hygiene and not using barrier contraceptives such as a diaphragm are all associated with a higher than expected risk of cancer of the cervix. We know that women who are from traditionally monogamous groups, such as Mormons, Jews and Amish, and those whose religious convictions preclude sexual activity (nuns) have a much lower incidence of cervical cancer. Although low socioeconomic status is also related to a higher incidence of cancer, this is important only in that this is the group likely to demonstrate the other high-risk factor(s), such as sexual promiscuity.

It appears that there is also a "male factor," which relates to the high incidence of cancer of the cervix in women married to men who have multiple partners. This may explain the otherwise surprisingly high incidence of cervical cancer among Latin women, who tend to be "protected," while the men turn to prostitutes for their sexual experiences. It seems increasingly likely that cancer of the cervix is caused by human papilloma viruses, and that explains why sexual contact is relevant to its cause (see below).

Homosexual anal intercourse is associated with a particular type of cancer of the anus that is quite rare, and this cancer may also be related to virus transmission, although that is not yet certain. Male homosexuality also presents other risks for cancer. In the chapter on cancer and AIDS (Chapter 11), I describe the relationship between the virus that causes suppression of the immune system, which results in AIDS, and the susceptibility to some types of cancer. Here again we have an example of a sexual lifestyle that predisposes such individuals to particular types of cancer. More recently the disease has changed its clinical manifestations, such that heterosexual partners of infected people are also at increased risk. This is probably due to a greater prevalence of the disease in society as a whole, but it may also be associated with subtle changes in the characteristics of the virus itself.

Other unfavorable lifestyle situations, if they can be called that, insofar as cancer risk is concerned are *poverty* and *malnutrition*. As was mentioned in the case of cervical cancer, being in lower socioeconomic classes, whether black or white, predisposes individuals to greater risk of many forms of cancer than expected. Furthermore, once cancer develops, the length of survival seems to be shorter than average. It's difficult to sort out the possible factors that may be responsible for this, but malnutrition and the coexistence of other diseases that weaken the patient seem the most plausible.

It has been said that stress causes cancer, but the evidence supporting this is quite weak. The role of stress in causing cancer is discussed in Chapter 14.

OCCUPATIONAL AND ENVIRONMENTAL HAZARDS—ASBESTOS, VINYL CHLORIDE, AIR AND WATER Occupational hazards have been known since the time of scrotal cancer in chimney workers, as mentioned earlier. Asbestos workers are at present

a special problem because a great many people were involved in this important industry, and since the effects of asbestos were not recognized for twenty years, many people were exposed to it. Asbestos causes a peculiar type of lung cancer called mesothelioma; I have seen numerous individuals who were pipe-fitters, or welders, or who installed pipe insulation on submarines during World War II who came down with mesothelioma or other forms of lung cancer two decades later. (This problem has led to unique and enormous financial settlements from class-action suits against the manufacturers. Johns Manville was allowed to declare bankruptcy despite their huge assets, apparently because of the backlog of pending and projected suits against them.) Much more difficult to trace are the cases of mesothelioma that occur in people without any history of direct industrial exposure to asbestos, but in whose lungs asbestos particles are found. Careful examination, however, has shown that some of these occurred in people residing downwind from asbestos factories: it happens that the asbestos fiber travels very well in the wind and can easily spiral along for a mile or more and enter a residence through open windows. Asbestos is of major concern also because so much of this country's insulation was made with asbestos; when old buildings or schools are torn down, asbestos fittings are ripped out from pipes, in the process spraying the fibers into the air—this is now recognized as a dangerous practice. Thus, the cost of protecting workers who renovate buildings may make it impractical to do anything other than abandon certain buildings, unless better means of dealing with this peculiar mineral are found. How ironic that with our earlier lack of knowledge we could afford to construct buildings that now we may not be able to afford to destroy.

A few years back there was a great scare about vinyl chloride, which was discovered to be a probable cause of a peculiar type of liver cancer (angiosarcoma) among workers in the plastics industry, an observation made by an alert industry physician. Think about a world without plastics—can you imagine what it would be like to do away with vinyl polymers? There was concern about the welfare of workers, handlers of plastics, consumers of foods covered with plastics, et cetera. Fortunately, the problem exposure seemed to be limited to workers who had had unusually high exposures, such as those who scrubbed the vats used to make plastics. It has been possible to sharply reduce the exposure of workers and thus to save a major industry. There are similar concerns for people who work in the rubber industry, in coke and uranium mining, or those whose work forces them to be in dusty or smoke-filled environments, such as policemen in tunnels. There will probably never again be such a thing as an environment totally free of man-made carcinogens, but it is reasonable to work toward "safe" levels of exposure for our people, and most industries and workers share that goal. (The Delany Amendment seeks to reduce all carcinogen exposures in food to zero, regardless of whether the substance causes cancer in only one animal species out of ten and regardless of the intensity of the risk—clearly an unrealistic goal.) Realistic recent concerns have centered on contaminants in drinking water from rivers such as the Mississippi, or in water sources contaminated from waste storage dumps, or areas such as the now notorious Love Canal. The costs to society of finding safe storage areas are growing, and no one I know throughout the fifty states wants such a dump in his or her backyard! The ocean used to be the dumping ground, but hard lessons from toxicity to marine life have brought a realization of the folly of this solution. And what to do about the hazards of urban pollution? If it can kill the roadside shrubbery and animals in the city zoo and in the form of acid rain be swept off by winds to defoliate distant forests, what can it be doing to our risks for getting cancer?

Environmental hazards from the air that we breathe and the water we drink are often believed to cause cancers. We are concerned that air and water may become contaminated with carcinogens from industrial and atmospheric emission. Apart from the air in some workplaces (e.g., asbestos mines, waste dumps, manufacturing plants, coke ovens), the air that we breathe does not contain high levels of carcinogens. Take comfort!

Drinking water may contain mixtures of known or suspected carcinogens (e.g., asbestos, industrial chemicals, radioactive substances), and the process of treating water may generate small concentrations of chemicals thought to cause cancer. Fortunately the levels of our exposure are so low as not to pose a significant threat. Contamination of ground water by toxic wastes (chemicals, radioactivity) could become more widespread as older disposal sites begin to leak; although we are developing safer means of disposing of hazardous wastes, none is completely safe. Major water supplies are monitored for the presence of carcinogens by the Environmental Protection Agency, but even that cannot guarantee absolute safety in all regions. Unfortunately, for obvious reasons officials who are responsible for public safety do not always own up to their shortcomings, and public discomfort with environmental hazards is probably well founded and has good survival value.

We may yearn for the pure, simple pastoral life, but it may already be true that this is not to be found since even nature is not free of hazards from certain cancer-causing chemicals found in foods or soil—"nature is not benign," as one scientist observed. Nevertheless, that is no reason to stop looking for ways to improve our immediate environments, to prevent further contamination and to protect those areas that still contribute to the world's health, in terms of food, air and water resources.

DRUGS THAT MAY CAUSE CANCER Drugs are believed to account for fewer than 2 percent of all cancers. A number of medications have been discovered to cause cancer, and some others have been said to cause cancer, although on further analysis they probably do not. Some years ago it was discovered that synthetic estrogens taken during pregnancy produced cancers of the vagina in daughters who had been exposed to the estrogens while they were within the uterus—this was the first demonstration of the passage of a carcinogen across the placental barrier into the fetus, a very significant finding. There was controversy about evidence that estrogens increased the risk of uterine cancer, a particularly important issue because millions of women were taking oral estrogen contraceptives and estrogen following menopause. Further studies now suggest that there is no link between the use of oral contraceptives and uterine cancer, and that oral contraceptive use may even decrease the risk in young women, but the scare affected many people and the controversy regarding all of the risks of contraceptive hormones is probably not over yet. High doses of estrogens and long-term usage are still suspect as causes of uterine cancer in women beyond the age of menopause, and should be avoided. They have also been implicated in causation of breast cancer, but here the results are not conclusive. A combination of estrogen and progesterone may actually *decrease* the risk of cancer of the ovaries or endometrium (progesterone is the other major female hormone). Phenacetin used to be a common ingredient of various aspirin preparations and cold remedies, but now it has been removed because it is known to be a cause of bladder cancer. In this case, the identification of the cause led to the means to prevent the disease by removing the dangerous substances.

A more difficult problem, ironically, is that a number of potent chemotherapeutic drugs used to treat cancer may in some instances turn out to cause new cancers years later. A patient treated with certain types of drugs, such as the so-called alkylating agents, may be cured of the initial cancer only to develop a second cancer or leukemia three to ten years later. Recognizing this problem, we are trying to substitute equally effective chemotherapeutic drugs that are less likely to cause new cancers, but if a suitable substitute cannot be found, we have to admit that it is still preferable to be cured of the original cancer and have a 5 to 10 percent chance of developing a second cancer years later than not to survive the original cancer. This problem will be discussed further elsewhere.

Another peculiar problem caused by successful treatment of a disease is the cancer that is related to organ transplantation, or to some other condition in which there is a deliberate suppression of the immune response. Except in the special case of identical twins, it is possible to transplant an organ such as a kidney from a donor to a recipient person only because we are able to suppress the immune response of the individual who receives the donated organ; in order to do that we use drugs such as azathioprine, corticosteroids and cyclosporin A, which keep the donor graft from being rejected as a foreign tissue by the transplant recipient. Unfortunately, this makes the recipient far more susceptible to developing certain types of cancer, most notably the lymphomas, possibly because the normal ability to recognize a developing tumor cell is absent in people who have had their immune system partly or completely paralyzed. We have come to recognize this phenomenon more clearly in people who are immunosuppressed from a disease such as AIDS, for they have an extremely high incidence of cancer and, if they do not die of infectious complications, may die of cancer (see Chapter 11).

VIRUSES, CANCER AND ONCOGENES In our search for the causes of human cancer, the "hottest" area of investigation is the role of viruses. From an epidemiologic point of view, there is a very strong association between certain types of cancer and particular viruses. This current era of investigation of human cancer-causing viruses is based on the discovery by Dr. Denis Burkitt, a general surgeon working in Africa, that a form of lymphoma (later called Burkitt's lymphoma) was found in a particular geographic belt across central Africa. In this region there was also found to be a high incidence of Epstein-Barr virus (EBV). Burkitt's observation led to a productive collaboration with virologists and immunologists, among them the Henles of Philadelphia and the Kleins of Stockholm, who studied samples from people in this region of Africa and linked the virus to Burkitt's lymphoma. EBV has also been linked to nasopharyngeal cancers (nose and throat cancers), which occur in areas of the world such as Asia, where that disease predominates. It took years of work by many investigators to pin down these associations, as well as the discovery that hepatitis B infection is related to liver cancer, particularly in areas with high liver cancer rates, such as Africa and Asia. That means that people who have had hepatitis due to this virus are far more likely to develop cancer than those who have not. Indeed, there is evidence that the genetic material of the hepatitis B virus is actually in the cancer cells when they develop later. More recently, outbreaks of a peculiar type of leukemia (adult T cell leukemia) have been discovered in Japan and the Caribbean, and these have been strongly associated with a human T cell leukemia virus (HTLV-I), a strain very similar to the virus that is believed to cause AIDS (see

Chapter 11). Here again a malignancy, in this case leukemia, may develop years after the viral infection, for reasons not yet understood. The human papilloma virus is almost certainly involved in the causation of cancer of the cervix, possibly also in several other types of cancer.

Certain viruses are unquestionably related to cancer in humans, but some predisposing factors must also be involved, because not everyone exposed to these viruses develops cancer. What is there about the Chinese, Japanese or African populations that makes them susceptible to the cancers known to be associated with viruses? Is there some interaction between the viruses and the genetic background of the affected individuals, or between the viruses and cancer-causing chemicals such as aflatoxins that are also prevalent in the high cancer regions in Africa? The latter is a very likely possibility, and it would bring a linkage between chemical and viral causes of cancer.

The search for viral causes of cancer has been long, arduous and frustrating. It was relatively easy to show that viruses cause cancer in dogs, cats, chickens and birds and that under the microscope these cancers look for all the world like cancers in humans. Yet decades of searching for actual viruses in human cancer turned up only transient leads here and there, which generally could not be confirmed. The effort was very expensive and for a long time seemed always to lead to dead ends. Nonetheless, a tremendous amount was learned about the way in which viruses can cause cancers in animal cells and in tissue culture cells.

One of the most startling basic discoveries that put us on a new track was made by Dr. David Baltimore—who was awarded the Nobel Prize for his work. He found that RNA viruses carry into the mammalian cell a unique enzyme called reverse transcriptase that causes the cell to make a DNA copy of the RNA virus. After a series of intermediate steps, this new DNA product is then integrated into the chromosome of the host (mammalian) cell DNA, and thereafter the cell can, under the appropriate conditions, replicate itself, and express the genes from the virus. It is the replication of some of these normally suppressed genes that subverts the cell and transforms it into a cancerous growth. These cancer-causing genes are called proto-oncogenes when they exist in the cells, or oncogenes as they exist in viruses. It does appear now that the fifty or more known proto-oncogenes act as cancer-causing genes and that they can be activated by a variety of circumstances, including exposure to chemical carcinogens.

How does all this tie together? *It is fascinating to realize that for many years scientists who were studying chemical carcinogenesis and those studying viral carcinogenesis were working totally separately and in fact were constantly competing, because each thought his or her area was more important than the other in the search for causes of cancer. My guess is that it probably will turn out that both factors are necessary, and that neither alone is sufficient to cause cancer.* Thus, a proto-oncogene may be activated by a substance such as an aflatoxin, by ionizing radiation, by chemicals in tobacco, by hormonal influences or even by a second virus. If that proves to be the case, it will explain why when many people are exposed to a carcinogenic substance, only certain ones develop cancer. *We have known for many years from the work of Berenblum that cancer is (at least) a two-stage process and requires more than one transformation event in order to turn a normal cell into a cancer cell. The full complexity of this process is finally beginning to unfold.* Unfortunately, although the causes of cancer are being uncovered, we do not yet have any practical way to prevent it, but that will come later (see Chapter 15).

The first large attempt at a practical application of the latest information about viral causes of cancer will be a clinical trial conducted in Asia with a vaccine against hepatitis B virus. In that region of the world, hepatitis B infection is very common, and in the same population liver cancer arises years later. Indeed the liver cancer (but not the adjacent areas of normal liver) contains the DNA base sequences derived from the hepatitis B virus. The hope is that by preventing this type of virus infection in the first place, we will also be able to prevent the later occurrence of cancer. This is a very attractive approach because vaccination is so effective and inexpensive in preventing infections such as hepatitis B, but it will take years to know whether it is effective in preventing cancer. If it is, then further tests on EB virus and other suspected cancer-causing viruses can be performed.

In the case of animal tumors caused by viruses, we already know that immunization against the virus can prevent the cancer from occurring; this is quite clear in the case of the very common leukemia that occurs in cats and for which there now is an effective vaccine. If we can bring our knowledge of viruses in humans up to the point of our knowledge of viruses in animals, we will have made great progress; this is clearly happening from one day to the next. Every week the scientific journals report important new discoveries with oncogenes and new insights into the processes by which cells become cancerous.

From:

NUTRITION AND CANCER: CAUSE AND PREVENTION
An American Cancer Society Special Report

The following report was approved by the American Cancer Society's Medical and Scientific Committee and its Board of Directors in February 1984.

In most instances exposure to cancer-causing agents (carcinogens) takes place 20 to 30 years before a statistically significant increase in cancer can be detected. Only then can it be adduced that the increase in cancer may have been caused by exposure to specific carcinogens.

There is now good reason to suspect that dietary habits contribute to human cancer, but it is important to understand that the interpretation of both human population (epidemiologic) and laboratory data is very complex, and as yet does not allow clear-cut conclusions. Although associations of dietary patterns with various forms of cancer have been found, association does not necessarily imply causation. Causation in cancer is extremely difficult to establish.

In recent years a considerable number of dietary constituents have been found to protect against the occurrence of cancers in experimental animals. The diversity and widespread occurrence of these compounds in food suggest that it may be virtually impossible to consume a diet that does not contain substances that can inhibit carcinogenesis. Recognition of the range of inhibitors in the diet has led to two major lines of investigation that are currently being pursued. The first is directed toward understanding the impact that these inhibitors now play in preventing cancer and the second, how protective effects might be enhanced. Foods may have constituents that cause or promote cancer on the one hand or protect against it on the other.

No concrete dietary advice can be given that will guarantee prevention of any specific human cancer. The American Cancer Society nonetheless believes that there is sufficient inferential information to make a series of interim recommendations about nutrition that, in the judgment of experts, are likely to provide some measure of reducing cancer risk. These dietary recommendations are consistent in general with the maintenance of good

This report is based on a study by Sidney Weinhouse, Ph.D., Professor of Biochemistry of Fels Research Institute, Temple University School of Medicine in Philadelphia, Pennsylvania, and a Member of the Board of the American Cancer Society. He acknowledges with thanks the assistance of: David Kritchevsky, Ph.D., Associate Director of Wistar Institute in Philadelphia, Pennsylvania; Sushma Palmer, D.Sc., Project Director of the Committee on Diet, Nutrition and Cancer of the National Research Council, Commission on Life Sciences in Washington, D.C.; Michael J. Prival, Ph.D., of the Genetic Toxicology Branch of the Food and Drug Administration in Washington, D.C.; and Lee W. Wattenberg, M.D., of the Department of Pathology of the University of Minnesota School of Medicine in Minneapolis, Minnesota.

health. They are similar to and largely drawn from background statements previously issued by the American Cancer Society, the National Research Council of the National Academy of Sciences, and the National Cancer Institute. As new information is obtained from research, the Society's recommendations will be changed accordingly.

The first section of this report contains practical recommendations in areas where there are sufficient data. The second section includes comments on substances about which there is insufficient evidence to make specific recommendations at this time.

SECTION I
RECOMMENDATIONS

1. Avoid obesity.

That obese people are at increased risk of certain cancers has been demonstrated by the massive prospective study, Cancer Prevention Study I (CPS I), conducted by the American Cancer Society. This study, conducted over a 12-year period (1960–1972), found a markedly increased incidence of cancers of the uterus, gallbladder, kidney, stomach, colon and breast, associated with obesity. In this study, when data for obese men and women 40 percent or more overweight were reviewed, the women were found to have a 55 percent greater risk, and the men, a 33 percent greater risk of cancer than those of normal weight. Experiments in animals had indicated much earlier that the incidence of cancer is reduced and the life span is lengthened by providing nutritionally adequate diets that maintained animals at close to an ideal weight. For people who are obese, weight reduction may be one way to lower cancer risk.

2. Cut down on total fat intake.

Accumulating evidence from both human population and laboratory studies implies that excessive fat intake increases the chance of developing cancers of the breast, colon and prostate. Excessive intake of both saturated and unsaturated fats, whether from plant or animal sources, has been found to enhance human cancer growth in some studies. Numerous experimental studies have shown that high fat diets increase the incidence of breast and colon cancer in rats exposed to chemical carcinogens. Americans consume about 40 percent of total calories as fat. A decrease in the amount of fat we consume to 30 percent of total calories, on the average, has been suggested in the report of the National Academy of Sciences. For most people, this should mean a simple change in food habits, readily achieved by moderation in the consumption of fats, oils, and foods rich in fats—an effective way to reduce total calories.

3. Eat more high fiber foods, such as whole grain cereals, fruits and vegetables.

Fiber is a term used to cover many food components that are not readily digested in the human intestinal tract. These substances, abundant in whole grains, fruits and vegetables, consist largely of complex carbohydrates of diverse chemical composition. Agreement on fiber's role in cancer prevention is not universal. Proponents cite a large body of epidemiologic evidence that colon cancer is low in populations who live on a diet of largely unrefined food high in fiber. Other scientists point to epidemiologic data that do not support a preventive role of dietary fiber. They suggest that since refined diets low in fiber are likely to be high in fat, the latter factor may play a more prominent role in elevating cancer risk than low fiber intake. Even if fiber itself may not prove to have a protective effect against cancer, high fiber-containing fruits, vegetables and cereals can be recommended as a wholesome substitute for fatty foods.

4. Include foods rich in vitamins A and C in the daily diet.

a. Dark green and deep yellow vegetables and certain fruits are rich in carotene, a form of vitamin A. Many laboratory tests point to vitamin A (and certain synthetic chemicals related to vitamin A) as reducing the incidence of certain cancers in animals, and a number of human population studies indicate that foods rich in carotene or vitamin A may lower the risk of cancers of the larynx, esophagus and lung. Examples of foods rich in carotene are carrots, tomatoes, spinach, apricots, peaches and cantaloupes. Excessive vitamin A in the form of supplements (tablets or capsules) is not recommended because of possible toxicity.

b. Epidemiologic studies indicate that people whose diets are rich in ascorbic acid (vitamin C), i.e., those consuming diets high in fruits and vegetables, are less likely to get cancer, particularly of the stomach and esophagus. It is still uncertain whether it is vitamin C itself or other constituents of the vitamin C-containing fruits and vegetables that exert the protective effect. Vitamin C can inhibit the formation of carcinogenic nitrosamines in the stomach. The possible role of this inhibition of nitrosamine formation in modifying the incidence of human stomach and esophageal cancer is not known.

5. Include cruciferous vegetables, such as cabbage, broccoli, Brussels sprouts, kohlrabi and cauliflower in the diet.

Cruciferous vegetables belong to the mustard family, whose plants have flowers with four leaves in the pattern of a cross. Some epidemiologic studies have suggested that consumption of these vegetables may reduce the risk of cancer, particularly of the gastrointestinal and respiratory tracts. Tests in laboratory animals have revealed that the inclusion of cruciferous vegetables in the diet may be highly effective in the prevention of chemically induced cancer. A great deal of experimental work is in progress to determine what components of these foods are protective against cancer.

6. Be moderate in consumption of alcoholic beverages.

Heavy drinkers of alcohol, especially those who are also cigarette smokers, are at unusually high risk for cancers of the oral cavity, larynx and esophagus. Alcohol abuse can result in cirrhosis, which may sometimes lead to liver cancer. Epidemiologic studies in Africa, France and China have shown that the consumption of wine and other alcoholic beverages is associated with a high risk of esophageal cancer.

7. Be moderate in consumption of salt-cured, smoked and nitrite-cured foods.

Conventionally smoked foods such as hams, some varieties of sausage, fish and so forth, absorb some of the tars that arise from incomplete combustion. These tars contain numerous carcinogens that are similar chemically to the carcinogenic tars in tobacco smoke. The risks may apply primarily to conventionally smoked meats and fish. The food processing industry is now using a "liquid smoke" that is thought to be less hazardous.

There is limited inferential evidence that salt-cured or pickled foods may increase the risk of stomach and esophageal cancer. In parts of the world where nitrate and nitrite are prevalent in food and water, as in Colombia, or where cured and pickled foods are common in the diet, such as in Japan and China, stomach and esophageal cancers are common; and there is good chemical evidence that nitrate and nitrite can enhance nitrosamine formation, both in foods and in our digestive tracts. Many nitrosamines are potent carcinogens in animals and may be human carcinogens. Nitrite has been employed traditionally in meat preservation, where it acts as a preventive against botulism (food poisoning) and improves the color and flavor of meats. The U.S. Department of Agriculture and the American meat industry already have substantially decreased the amount of nitrite in prepared meats and are searching for improved methods of meat preservation.

SECTION II
TOPICS OF GENERAL INTEREST WITH
NO SPECIFIC RECOMMENDATIONS

The following substances or dietary practices have received much attention and therefore are reviewed, but no recommendations are made at this time. All are under investigation.

Food Additives

Various chemicals are added to foods to improve color and flavor, and to prevent spoilage. Some have been found to cause cancer in animals and have been banned. Several others are thought to be protective against carcinogens. Knowledge about the possible cancer risks or benefits of food additives is insufficient to warrant a recommendation for or against their use.

Vitamin E

There is no evidence that vitamin E prevents cancer in humans. While vitamin E is an antioxidant, and antioxidants may prevent some cancers in animals, more research is needed before the role of vitamin E in human cancer prevention can be assessed.

Selenium

Although there is evidence that selenium, a trace element, may offer protection against some cancers, this evidence is much too limited to justify a recommendation that selenium intake be increased. Because of the potential hazard of selenium poisoning, the *medically unsupervised* use of selenium as a food supplement cannot be recommended.

Artificial Sweeteners

At high levels, saccharin has been shown to cause bladder cancer in rats. Epidemiologic studies offer no clear evidence for an increase in risk of bladder cancer among people who are moderate users of this artificial sweetener. Of possible concern is the consumption of saccharin by children and pregnant women. The long-term consequences of this possible risk cannot be predicted from current epidemiologic data. New non-caloric sweeteners are now entering the market. Their long-term effects have not yet been studied in humans.

Coffee

Evidence about coffee as a risk factor in human cancer is inconclusive. Although some epidemiologic studies implicate high intake of coffee in bladder and pancreas cancer, others fail to make such a connection. Available information does not suggest a recommendation against its moderate use. There is no indication that caffeine, which is a natural component of both coffee and tea, is a risk factor in human cancer.

Meat and Fish Cooked at High Temperatures, such as by Frying or Broiling

Recent studies have demonstrated that the cooking of meat and fish at high temperatures such as by frying or broiling gives rise to a number of potent mutagens (agents that cause genetic changes) in bacteria, and some of them have induced cancers in animal tests. This subject is now being investigated in several laboratories.

Cholesterol

Although cholesterol is considered to be a risk factor for heart or blood vessel disease, there is little evidence that a high cholesterol intake or a high cholesterol level in the blood also poses the risk of cancer. Evidence relating low blood cholesterol to human cancer is inconclusive.

TOBACCO AND CANCER: THE BLIGHT AMONG US

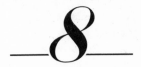

RELATIONSHIP TO SMOKING People often ask in all seriousness what they can do to protect themselves from getting cancer. This is a frustrating question for cancer experts, who are well aware that *lung cancer, the leading cause of cancer deaths, could be prevented in 80 to 90 percent of cases if only people would not smoke cigarettes. This change in habits on the part of smokers (or prevention of a habit in the case of potential smokers) could save over 100,000 lives annually.* But smoking not only causes lung cancer, it also causes or aggravates several other forms of cancer, heart disease, emphysema, bronchitis, sinusitis and premature aging of the skin. The carbon monoxide in tobacco smoke prevents oxygen from properly being transported by blood cells to your tissues and this causes a decrease in the capacity for exercise and potentially causes heart attacks. The American Medical Association estimates that at least thirty-four million Americans have lung conditions that are made worse by being around people who are smoking. This is a public health problem of staggering proportions, and we need to dissect the issues in scientific, economic, political, behavioral and emotional terms. The Surgeon General recently estimated that the number of tobacco-related deaths in one month is equivalent to all the deaths that have ever occurred from AIDS.

The tobacco industry spends some three billion dollars annually on advertising, far more than the entire budget of the National Cancer Institute. This is particularly impressive when one considers that these companies are not allowed to advertise on television—although it has been pointed out to me that when television covers baseball games the scoreboards are well decorated with cigarette ads, which we see almost every inning. *Such sums of money may be related to a conspiracy of silence by reporters on this subject,* which is not well covered even in magazine health columns. There is no greater educational need in magazines for young women than to discuss the health hazards of smoking, but the subject has for the most part been avoided. In talking to magazine editors about publishing articles to help their readers quit smoking, I find most unwilling even to consider such a piece for fear of losing advertising dollars from cigarette companies. This is why you see many articles in women's magazines on diet, exercise, mental health and beauty, but none on smoking. Leading women's magazines just don't publish articles on the harmful effects of smoking, and I find this irresponsible, and so does the Surgeon General. Recent advertising campaigns from the industry have hammered at the themes "let's review the facts" and "let's be calm and unemotional" about the question of smoking and lung cancer. The strong implication is that there is still a controversial issue that needs further study before any conclusions can be drawn. Well, let us review the facts indeed, and see how open the question really is.

In 1987 there were an estimated 136,000 deaths from lung cancer in the United States (92,000 in men and 44,000 in women); this type of cancer accounted for 36 percent of all cancer deaths in men and 20 percent of those among women. (At our local Veterans Administration Hospital, 226 patients died of lung cancer in a recent year; 225 were known smokers and one was questionable.)

The rate of increase in lung cancer deaths among American men appears to be leveling off and is possibly declining in men under age fifty, but the figures for women are far less encouraging. Age-adjusted rates have continued to show dramatic increases; *overall, lung cancer mortality for American women increased 337 percent between 1950 and 1980.*

A number of important relationships have been established between smoking and lung cancer. The first is between cigarette consumption and lung cancer, as illustrated in Figure 7. Several important relationships are apparent:

1   The records show that American males steadily increased their tobacco consumption between 1920 and the present.

2   Females began to increase their use of cigarettes after World War II, and since then the rate of increase has paralleled that of men.

3   After an interval of some twenty years following the increased consumption in males, the death rate from lung cancer began to increase steadily—in a line remarkably parallel to that of cigarette consumption. Earlier in this century lung cancer was a rare disease and medical professors would call their students' attention to it when they saw a case. For some years now it has been the most common cause of death from cancer among men and it has recently also become the most common cause of death from cancer among women—again, parallel to cigarette consumption among women.

4   Data shown in Figure 7 lead to the dire prediction of a continuing increase in lung cancer deaths among women, similar to that in men—a health problem of truly epidemic proportions. (We do not have the data for smoking prevalence in all other countries, but it is clearly on the rise in Asia and in Third World nations. On the positive side, the incidence of smoking in England is declining, and there has been a striking decrease among British and U.S. physicians.)

IS THERE ANY RELATIONSHIP BETWEEN THE AMOUNT A PERSON SMOKES AND THE RISK OF DEVELOPING LUNG CANCER? This is another important point in establishing the link between smoking and the risk of cancer. Figure 8 shows a steady increase in risk proportionate to cigarette consumption—the more one smokes, the greater the risk of contracting lung cancer.

What about the flip side of the question—*suppose smokers stop?* The data on this are summarized graphically in Figure 9. First, the risk for smokers taken as a whole is about thirty times that of nonsmokers (compare the bars at the extreme left and right). Curiously, for the first few years after ceasing to smoke the risk of being diagnosed as having lung cancer increases; thereafter it falls steadily, to approach the risk of nonsmokers. *Natural repair of the epithelial cells that line the air passages occurs over time—nature is remarkably forgiving!* What about the initial increase noted after smoking cessation? There is no firm evidence on this point, but the most plausible explanation seems to be that some people who stop smoking prob-

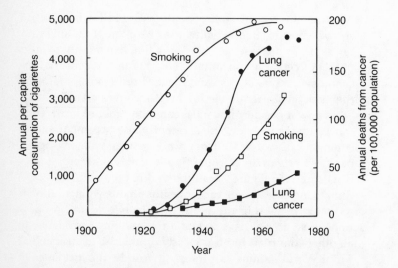

Figure 7 Trends in smoking prevalence and lung cancer among British males and females. The data for this chart are for England and Wales. In men, smoking (o) began to increase at the beginning of the twentieth century, but the corresponding trend in deaths from lung cancer (•) did not begin until after 1920. In women, smoking (□) began later, and the increase in lung cancer deaths in women (■) has appeared only recently. (Redrawn from the original by J. Cairns with permission from *Cancer Research* 44 [1984]: 5940)

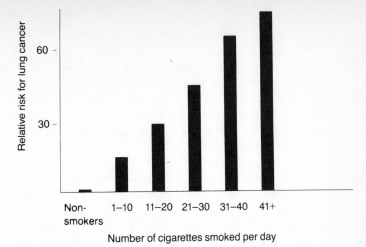

Figure 8 Relative risk of lung cancer by number of cigarettes smoked. (Redrawn with permission of Wynder and Stellman and *Cancer Research* 44 [1984]: 5940; data for smokers of filter and nonfilter cigarettes have been combined)

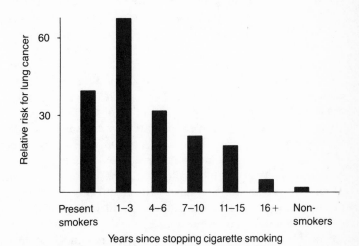

Figure 9 Relative risk of lung cancer after discontinuation of smoking. The relative risk for nonsmokers is shown in the short bar on the right; the relative risk for smokers is shown on the left. By sixteen years after cessation of smoking the risk falls almost to that of people who have never smoked. (Data published by Wynder and Stellman in *Cancer Research* 37 [1977]: 4608; reprinted with permission)

ably do so because they are already experiencing symptoms of ill health—coughing of blood, persistent cough, weight loss, chest pain, et cetera, which are due to a lung cancer that is already there but has simply not yet been diagnosed. Quite possibly the person senses there is something wrong and stops smoking before getting a chest x-ray or seeing a doctor.

ARE THERE REALLY CANCER-CAUSING CHEMICALS IN CIG-ARETTE SMOKE, OR ARE THE RELATIONSHIPS DESCRIBED ABOVE MERELY COINCIDENTAL? A review article by Drs. Loeb, Ernster, Warner, Abbotts and myself (1984) summarized the very extensive studies of this question performed by many investigators. The substances in tobacco—and there are hundreds of separate chemicals that have been identified—can be classified in two groups, those in the vapor phase and those made up of very tiny particles, or the particulate phase. It turns out that there are numerous potent carcinogens in both the vapor and the particulate phases. Some of the most potent of these known cancer-causing substances are listed in Table 3: *when these chemicals are given to animals they regularly cause cancer. The list of cancer-causing chemicals in tobacco includes a number of the most potent carcinogens known to man.* Anxiety about environmental hazards such as polluted air and water, asbestos, herbicides and radiation from nuclear power plants all relate to fears of developing cancer. Not all of the public concerns are well grounded, as we have seen, but how can someone who is not an expert know the difference between a silly scare about coffee or cranberry juice and a real risk from tobacco products? Even the publicity about tobacco risks emphasizes mainly the risk from smoking cigarettes, and takes little cognizance of the rapidly rising incidence of chewing of tobacco, which may pose health hazards of monumental proportions in the coming years. There is action to be taken that will help to safeguard our children and ourselves, and there are thoughtful legislators, insurance companies and health administrators who will listen.

Scientists are striving to find the causes of cancer, and progress is occurring at an amazing rate. But as we read about hazards of lifestyle, ask yourself how effective are we in translating this

Table 3 *Major Mutagens and Carcinogens and Related Substances in Tobacco Smoke*

	Amount in Smoke from One Cigarette
I. Particulate phase	
A. Natural fraction	
Benzo(a)pyrene	10–50 ng (nanogram)
Dibenz(a)anthracene	40 ng
5-Methylchrysene	0.6 ng
Benzofluoranthenes	90 ng
B. Basic fraction	
Nicotine	0.06–2.00 mg (milligram)
N-Nitrosonornicotine	0.2–3.7 μg (microgram)
C. Acidic fraction	
Catechol	40–280 μg
Unidentified tumor promoters	?
D. Residue	
Nickel	0–3 μg
Cadmium	80 ng
^{210}Po	0.03–1.00 pCi (picocurie)
II. Vapor phase	
Hydrazine	32 μg
Vinyl chloride	1–16 ng
Urethane	10–35 μg
Formaldehyde	20–90 μg
Nitrogen oxides	16–600 μg
Nitrosodiethylamine	0.1–28.0 ng

Source: United States Surgeon General, 1982.

information to nonscientists, and how effective are we in causing *changes in behavior* as a result of this knowledge? Not very effective, I would submit. Why are traditional quit-smoking programs so unsuccessful when *we know that we could prevent about one-third of cancer deaths (more than 135,000 people in the United States annually) plus perhaps another 200,000 others from heart and lung disease, if only people would act on the available information?* We should learn good health habits early in life, but what are the schools doing about this in our country? Not nearly enough!

If there are a large number of chemicals in tobacco that can cause cancer in animals when they are given singly, what can we infer about the likelihood that they may cause cancers in humans when they are all consumed together over twenty or more years? Very few scientists have much doubt about the cumulative risks caused by such exposure.

ARE THERE ANY BENEFICIAL EFFECTS OF SMOKING AS FAR AS CANCER IS CONCERNED? One has to look hard but there is one curious association that has been reported recently, which is that women who smoke have a 30 percent lesser risk of developing cancer of the upper portion of the uterus *(endometrium)* than do nonsmokers. However, the risk difference is present only for postmenopausal women and it is probably related to the association between estrogens and endometrial cancer in that higher estrogen levels increase the risk of developing this kind of cancer. Both the age at which menopause occurs and the bone density after menopause are related to the individual estrogen levels of women, and cigarette smoking opposes the effects of estrogen in both regards. Cigarette smoking changes normal metabolism of estrogen, a newly discovered and surprising effect. *Smokers experience menopause at an earlier age and their bones are less dense.* Presumably the lower risk of developing uterine cancer is also because smoking opposes the effects of estrogen in some manner that is not yet clear.

In commenting on the multi-institutional study of this issue reported by Dr. Samuel M. Lesko and associates, an editorial by Dr. Noel Wise in the same issue of the *New England Journal of Medicine* cautioned that even if some degree of protection is provided by cigarette smoking with respect to uterine cancer, this is not much comfort to a postmenopausal woman who smokes. The calculations go something like this. The yearly risk of developing uterine cancer among postmenopausal women (who have a uterus) is about 100 per 100,000 people; but only 70 per 100,000 for those who smoke. If approximately 20 percent of women who develop this kind of cancer will die from it, then the lives of approximately 30 of 100,000 times 20 percent, or 6 of 100,000 cigarette smokers, would be saved per year. This is more than counterbalanced by the annual number of lives that would be lost because of smoking, which is some thirty times higher than that, or 180 lives lost per year. Nevertheless, scientists are quite interested in finding out the precise mechanism by which cigarette smoking lowers the risk for developing this type of cancer. As far as we are aware, there is no other comparable case of a protective effect of smoking.

WHAT IS THE ROLE OF NICOTINE? It is now clear that nicotine is *the* substance to which smokers are physiologically addicted— and anyone who does not believe that smoking is an addiction has never been a chronic smoker and has never worked professionally with smokers. More people are habituated to cigarettes than to drugs or alcohol in this country because of those properties. Nicotine itself is not a carcinogen, but at the high temperatures that occur in the burning cigarette two derivatives of nicotine are formed that are themselves very potent carcinogens. (It is also quite likely that derivatives [metabolites] of some of the chemicals in tobacco, including nicotine, are carcinogens.)

WHAT ABOUT FILTER CIGARETTES? ARE THEY SAFE? You may wonder whether the advent of filter cigarettes has reduced these risks. Indeed, because they are perceived as safer, the market share of filter-tip cigarettes is now over 90 percent, and the consumption of low-tar cigarettes (less than 15 milligrams), has increased dramatically, particularly among women. In 1970 only 10 percent of women smoked low-tar cigarettes, but by 1979 this figure was up to 39 percent. This is a remarkable chapter in the larger tobacco story, and requires some explanation of the nature of filter cigarettes. First, the tobacco used is the same—it is not of higher grade than the tobacco in nonfilter cigarettes, and the tobacco is usually not even washed free of soil, dirt and insecticides. Thus, all of the cancer-causing chemicals that are present in (and on) tobacco are in filter cigarettes. (Remember the cigarette advertisement that bragged, "It's what's up front that counts"?) Second, the big selling point for filter cigarettes is that they have less tar and nicotine, and the brand that can lay claim to having the lowest content bases its advertising campaign on that. (The intense competition to have the lowest tar and nicotine is in itself ironic since the industry has never admitted that unfiltered cigarettes are harmful.)

In evaluating these advertising claims, we must bear in mind that the advertised amount of tar and nicotine in puffs of smoke is determined by the use of automatic smoking machines, whereas the amounts inhaled by the human smoker are determined by the very important factors of how hard he or she puffs, how the filter is held or squeezed, how close to the end the cigarette is smoked, and other factors that are in turn regulated by the blood nicotine levels that the smoker achieves by smoking. Now remember that nicotine is the chemical basis for the addiction. *The smoker unconsciously regulates his use of the product to provide the desired level of nicotine, and thereby a comparably increased amount of other harmful substances.* A recent study by Dr. Neal Benowitz and colleagues showed that when smokers cut down cigarette smoking from an average of thirty-seven cigarettes per day to five, the intake of tobacco toxins increased three-fold per cigarette and the daily exposure to tar and nicotine fell by only 50 percent. People are far more adaptable than the calibrated smoking machines that are meant to simulate the process of smoke inhalation.

Since the smoker of filter cigarettes has almost the same risk of developing lung cancer as the smoker of unfiltered cigarettes (actually it is about 20 percent less), it is a delusion to look for a "safe" cigarette that uses tobacco, and it is misleading to claim safety for filter cigarettes. In fact, all types of cigarettes are required to carry the same warning labels. A great deal of research has been aimed at developing a safe tobacco cigarette.

What about smoking cigars or pipes? As far as we know, the risk of inhaling smoke from either is as harmful as it is from cigarettes—and the hazard to others through passive smoking is probably comparable as well.

WARNING LABELS—EVERYONE'S FRIEND The American Cancer Society (ACS) has fought hard to establish and maintain taxes on cigarettes, because the cost of smoking far exceeds the revenue it provides, and because a higher price deters teenagers from smoking since they are dependent upon their parents for money to buy cigarettes, a point corroborated by a recently published study confirming this relationship between price and consumption. While the cigarette lobby has fought vigorously (and with considerable success) against greater taxation, they seem to have been more magnanimous about cigarette labeling. The cigarette label laws now require the use of four different types of warnings on a rotating basis. It was expected that the cigarette industry would fight these to the death, but they acquiesced and accepted these warning labels. What lies behind this acceptance, although it is surely not apparent to the public, is that the *tobacco industry needs these warning signs desperately for its own survival.* Most smokers have heard many times that smoking can be dangerous, and they are not paying attention to these warnings anyway; but the labels serve notice to the public, in a formal and legal sense, that there is a hazard that the smoker assumes in electing to smoke. In a recent lawsuit filed by the widow of a man who could not quit, the major basis for defense was that he knew the risks—they were plainly displayed on each package. The tobacco company won its case.

So far no one has won a suit against the tobacco industry, although a number of suits have been settled outside of court, and there is thus no legal record to serve as a precedent to support future suits. There are indications that the companies are prepared to pay up to five million dollars to defend each case, which means it is a hard, expensive and lengthy fight to win a lawsuit. A lawyer recently told me that he thought he had a winning case, but the cancer patient, himself a lawyer, decided not to file suit because he would be dead before the case was settled and the suit would be a great financial and emotional strain on his family. The climate for such suits is changing, however, with increasing public awareness of the danger, and it seems very likely that a longtime smoker, someone who can prove excessive exposure to passive smoking (see below) or someone who develops oral cancer from chewing tobacco will in time win a suit. That will predictably result in a great flurry of class-action suits, as happened in the asbestos industry when it was ruled that exposure to asbestos was the ultimate cause of mesothelioma.

The pro-tobacco people argue that smoking is a matter of free choice. *We scientists know that in choosing to smoke the smoker chooses to take some seven or eight years off his life expectancy* (from all causes of death), a fact that is now beginning to be taken into account in preferential premiums for nonsmoking holders of life insurance policies. What would be exceedingly detrimental to the tobacco industry is for a person with lung cancer, or his surviving family, to sue successfully on the basis that tobacco caused the cancer. There is certainly ample epidemiologic evidence for this, but one important counterargument is that the warning labels are clear and the individual knowingly ignored them as part of the freedom to choose. A counter to that argument is that once smoking is chosen, the smoker is not equally free to quit—because of the addiction problems mentioned earlier. Or, to put it another way, none of the "warning" labels baldly states that nicotine is addictive, a very significant omission. I am not a lawyer, but it seems to me that the freedom of choice applies only to adults, and it implies that they had freedom of choice to both start and stop use of this product. Those conditions are not being met.

ADVERTISING AND SOCIAL CONCERNS The social concern of the tobacco industry is inevitably called into question when one sees ten to twelve pages of glossy advertisements in magazines for teenage women (under legal age) showing an array of athletic, "cool" and sexy people in varying poses with their cigarettes. We are all exposed to such ads in print or on billboards. Another reminder of social irresponsibility is the fact that Third World nations are a major target for the expanding world markets of the cigarette industry and *these countries are sold U.S. cigarettes without warning labels in the language of the country.* As we sit in the comfort of America it is distressing to consider that tobacco companies are advertising vigorously even in Third World nations where food is scarce.

In a recent article in the *New York State Journal of Medicine,* and in a personal communication, Dr. David C. Sokal, an epidemiologist in West Africa, pointed out the impressive extent of cigarette advertising in countries such as Burkina Faso. He offered one young man who worked for him a 10 percent raise if he stopped smoking, but this was to no avail. During the course of discussing the dangers of smoking, this man remarked that the Marlboro man was really impressive. That caused Dr. Sokal to reevaluate the impact of cigarette advertising in that nation. A picture of a sun-bronzed American cowboy on a healthy horse rounding up fat cattle is a symbol of wealth and prosperity to a rural African child. In many villages if there is a horse at all, it is likely to belong to the village chief. Most of the herdsmen go on foot, and cattle are very thin. Nevertheless, tobacco companies promote cigarette smoking with billboards that are reaching more and more deeply into rural Africa. Also, news magazines such as *Jeune Afrique* (Young Africa), a French-language news magazine similar to *Newsweek* or *Time,* typically contain three to nine pages of full-color, glossy advertisements for cigarettes—sometimes constituting more than half the magazine's total advertising.

A particularly objectionable series of ads in Africa is those for Gauloises—their slogan is "A world to share." Figure 10 shows an advertisement taken from *Jeune Afrique* for Gauloises cigarettes, featuring motorbikes. Motorbikes in Africa are a much more relevant symbol of power than automobiles because Africans cannot relate to expensive cars whereas they can use either bicycles or inexpensive motorized bicycles. The motorbikes shown in the ad are a definite luxury item, but something that some educated Africans could dream about having, whereas a car would be totally out of reach. Recently, representatives of Peter Stuyvesant have

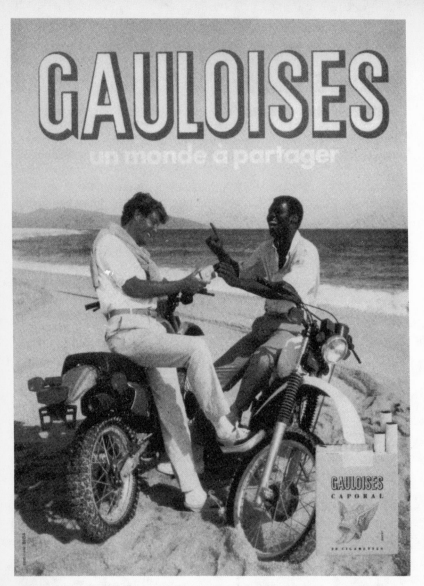

Figure 10 An advertisement for Gauloises cigarettes, reproduced from the magazine *Jeune Afrique*. The motorbikes pictured are a luxury item for Africans, but are something an educated person might dream of owning (whereas the American status symbol of the flashy automobile would be unattainable for most of this advertisement's readers).

aggressively been promoting their Ouagadougou cigarettes by hiring attractive young Burkinabe women to give away cigarettes. The women wear clothes made from cloth with the same pattern as the cigarette package, and they are driven around in a similarly colored, brand-new four-wheel-drive van.

Dr. Sokal points out that unlike the struggle against malaria, measles or famine, the control of health risks from cigarettes does not require enormous sums of money or resources, but rather wise cooperation among health workers and policymakers determined to discourage smoking in many countries. His article advocates revealing cigarette companies as the merchants of death that they are and outlawing the promotion of their products.

I have helped to care for some tobacco company executives stricken with smoking-related cancers. Often they have honestly believed that their products were safe and that it was statisticians who gave them a bad rap by "lying with figures." It is pathetic to watch reality begin to break through (if it does) when they discover that they are dying of lung cancer and that it may be related to their lifelong habit of smoking. It is really tough for them to accept because they have spent so many years believing (and wishing) the contrary—but nature is impartial and we all can be victims.

In a recent article in the *New York Times,* Stephen Klaidman, a senior research fellow at the Kennedy Institute of Ethics at Georgetown University, pointed out that passage of a bill banning all advertising of tobacco products would pose no threat to the First Amendment. Whereas both industry and some civil libertarians have argued that such legislation would ban a form of speech and be contrary to the original intent of the framers of the Constitution, there's no evidence that this would be inconsistent with the intentions of those who drew up the Constitution. Klaidman argues that James Madison and his colleagues would not have argued to protect the rights of purveyors of deadly products to send advertising messages to underprivileged children to move them to buy deadly drugs. Civil libertarians might argue that regulating advertising of a legal product is tantamount to censorship and could lead to the banning of automobiles or any other items that might be dangerous to the health of buyers. However, the Food and Drug Administration already regulates advertising of prescription drugs, and cigarette advertising is already banned from radio and television. In neither case have those limitations been applied to other areas. In "On Liberty," the classic essay by John Stuart Mill, Mill was as concerned with preventing harm as he was with assuring liberty and, indeed, he said that a person's liberty might be restricted if necessary to prevent harm to others. He felt that harm should be balanced against the value of protecting that liberty. Thus, given that about 350,000 Americans die annually from smoking-related illnesses, one should ask how much harm tobacco advertising does and how much harm banning such advertising would do.

Studies of smoking characteristics in this country show that there is an inverse relationship between socioeconomic status and lung cancer rates. For at least the last twenty years, college graduates have been much less likely to smoke than men with no more than a high school education, and professional men have lower smoking rates than blue-collar workers. The statistics are similar for women. Teenage girls are today the group for whom this country should feel the greatest concern: national surveys indicate that smoking has increased steadily among young women since the late 1960s. Young women of seventeen and eighteen are now smoking at a slightly higher rate than young men of the same age (26 percent vs. 19 percent). An additional concern is that *a high smoking rate among teenagers is associated with heavier smoking later and more difficulty in quitting than if smoking is initiated at a later age.*

Most habitual smoking begins during the teenage years, apparently influenced by peer pressure. Teenagers don't know the potential hazards to their health or to the fetus of a pregnant woman—and often they can't imagine anything pleasurable hurting them—ever. Describing the process of starting to smoke, continuing, stopping and resuming, Lichtenstein has pointed out that curiosity, rebelliousness, social pressure, confidence and availability of cigarettes are all recognizable factors. In the farmland of our tobacco-producing states, children often begin to smoke behind the barn when they are nine to eleven years old. More surprising to me is that parents, even in urban areas, will in many instances actually purchase cigarettes for their children.

Some success has been achieved in delaying the start of smoking by teaching children to resist peer pressures. Physicians are not often involved in these programs, so the opportunities for education lie with teachers, health educators and voluntary societies such as the American Cancer Society, the American Lung Association and the American Heart Association, which make effective use of the mass media. Not long ago I spoke to a group of eighth grade students and was pleased that not many had yet become smokers—at the same time, knowing the tragically ghastly results of lung cancer, it hurts me to see the many young people who congregate at shopping malls and smoke as they pass the time. Let me confess my dilemma—do I go over and make a friendly suggestion about the hazards of smoking, risking ridicule and rebuff, or do I walk away and miss an opportunity, just possibly, to do some real good? What would you do if you were in this position?

My colleague Dr. Arthur Holleb brought a bit of newspaper trivia to my attention. It seems that in Lonquor, a small English community, a nine-member committee was organized to preserve the right of the individual to smoke cigarettes, pipes and cigars. The chairman of this committee is the village undertaker.

QUIT-SMOKING PROGRAMS—THE HOW TO'S There are some 54 million people in the United States who smoke. Some nine out of every ten smokers say they want to quit. And 37 million people are actually ex-smokers. Some psychologists at Duke have been very interested in newer techniques of helping people to quit smoking, and they are convinced that giving up cigarettes depends more on skill than it does on will power. This is very positive, and very encouraging, because we can learn skills fairly readily—will power is more difficult to acquire. Successful strategies to quit smoking have to address both the addictive and the psychological aspects of smoking. Robert H. Shipley, Ph.D., author of a new book, *QuitSmart: A Guide to Freedom from Cigarettes,* says that 90 percent of America's fifty-three million smokers want to quit but don't know how, and that after a stressful day, for example, someone trying to quit may reason that "just one cigarette will help me relax, and after that I won't smoke anymore." Like the alcoholic, the reformed smoker is unable to stop with one cigarette—one generally leads to another. There may be certain times of day when smokers crave their cigarette, such as with the morning coffee. People come to believe that they can't get through a crisis without having a cigarette, that they will gain weight if they stop smoking or that they need a cigarette in order to concentrate and do their work. These psychological obstacles can be overcome, says Dr. Shipley, who also points out that about one-third of those people who give up smoking will gain weight while another one-third will actually lose weight.

Among other techniques, quit-smoking clinics often use aversive smoking procedures, such as asking a smoker who has quit for a day or more to hold cigarette smoke in the mouth for thirty-second periods without inhaling—this tastes foul, and burns the mouth. Furthermore, it produces muscle tension and headaches and makes such a negative impression on cigarette smokers that they are materially assisted to not want another cigarette. Other techniques used include self-hypnosis and relaxation training, as well as education about different types of techniques to decrease the dependence on nicotine.

Successful quitting involves skill, both in doing the right things and in thinking the "right" thoughts. One example of doing the right thing is to use brand switching; another is the use of nicotine "gum," to help soften the impact of nicotine withdrawal. In brand switching (the scientific term is "nicotine fading"), the smoker makes weekly switches to brands of cigarettes that contain progressively less nicotine, reducing the nicotine intake by about 40 percent each week. *After there has been adaptation to a cigarette brand that is very low in nicotine, the smoker quits cold turkey.* In his book Shipley describes the process in considerable detail, and he includes tables that permit smokers to find the nicotine content of their cigarettes and to plan progressive changes to fit in with the appropriate brand switching. For example, if you smoke Kent Golden Lights 100s, you are consuming 0.8 milligrams of nicotine in each cigarette, and you need to find a brand of cigarettes that provides about 40 percent less nicotine and switch to that brand for one week while keeping constant the number of cigarettes smoked. It is very important neither to increase the number of cigarettes nor to alter the manner of inhaling, in order to avoid compensating for the loss of nicotine. You should not smoke the cigarettes farther down to the end, nor should you cover up the air filter holes to crush the filter because these are also ways in which more nicotine can enter the bloodstream than would be the case otherwise. The following week, switch to another brand that contains about 40 percent less nicotine and repeat this process until you are finally smoking a brand that has 0.3 milligrams of nicotine or less per cigarette—this will take one to three weeks, depending upon your current brand. If you are already smoking cigarettes with 0.3 milligrams of nicotine or less, then you need not switch brands.

In another such example we might think of your smoking Benson and Hedges 100s, one pack per day, a brand that contains 1.0 milligram of nicotine. If you change to More Light 100s, that would reduce your consumption to 0.6 milligrams of nicotine per cigarette. If you then went to one of the lowest nicotine cigarettes, which contain 0.3 milligrams of nicotine per cigarette, such as Now 100 soft pack, you would have eliminated 70 percent of the nicotine as compared with what you were smoking two weeks earlier. *Now* when you quit cold turkey you will experience few of the physical symptoms associated with nicotine withdrawal.

When you use this brand-switching program, you will probably not enjoy the low nicotine brands as much as you did your regular brand; this is useful because it will be easier to give up smoking when you come to the point of quitting altogether. It is better to use this gradation system rather than to switch immediately to the brand lowest in nicotine because the latter course would be associated with more withdrawal symptoms and much frustration. Nicotine gum (Nicorettè) is another alternative to help smokers who are physically dependent on (addicted to) nicotine. This is a prescription drug that has only recently become available to U.S. physicians, but has been used for many years in Europe and Canada. Chewing nicotine gum helps because nicotine is absorbed through the membranes of the mouth and most people find that chewing ten to twelve pieces a day is sufficient to control the nicotine urge. The exact recommendation for the use of Nicorettè should follow your doctor's prescription. However, each piece of Nicorettè should be chewed very slowly until you taste it or feel a tingling sensation in your mouth—and this should be done only when you have the urge to smoke. Then, after you feel the sensation in your mouth, stop chewing and leave the gum in your cheek. In about a minute or so the taste or tingling will subside and then you can again chew slowly until you taste the gum and then leave the gum in your cheek again. Each piece is chewed slowly in this way for some twenty to thirty minutes to release most of the nicotine. Chewing too fast can produce light-headedness, nausea and vomiting, hiccups and upset stomach. It can also produce headaches and palpitations of the heart and excessive salivation. Some people should not use Nicorettè; for instance, it is not recommended for pregnant women or those women who may become pregnant while using this product, nor should patients use it who have heart trouble such as irregular heartbeats, angina or a recent heart attack. If you use the brand-switching method, you will probably need less Nicorettè than you would otherwise. The recommendation from Shipley is to begin using the gum on the day that you quit smoking and, after a few weeks, gradually week by week reduce the number by one piece of gum per day. After three or four months of this you can discontinue the gum entirely—except in response to the occasional urges that will probably arise.

Clearly the process of quitting smoking is more complicated than just eliminating nicotine withdrawal, since there is a strong psychological dependence or habit involved in smoking. Get rid of all cigarettes and ashtrays and other paraphernalia associated with smoking. We recommend a psychological coping strategy such as is found in professional clinics or is described in the *QuitSmart* book if you choose to "go it alone." (The *QuitSmart* book is available from J. B. Press, P. O. Box 4843-C, Duke Station, Durham, NC 27706.)

For another option, the American Cancer Society (ACS) has a FreshStart program designed to help you quit smoking and to stay off after having quit. The program consists of four one-hour small-group sessions led by a knowledgeable facilitator. The program tells you what you need to know and is presented in such a way that it can be a very positive and fulfilling experience. ACS has prepared a very readable Participant's Guide to give you valuable information about the program—it is available from your local chapter. In some ways I think avoiding the way back to smoking is more difficult than the stopping. Here are some helpful tips on this aspect of the problem from the Participant's Guide:

1   Make up a short list of small luxuries you have wanted, or items you would like to purchase as a gift for someone else. Next to each item write down the cost in terms of "packs of cigarettes." Use a special bank for the money you don't spend on cigarettes.

2   Visit your dentist after you quit and begin your "new life" with bright, white teeth. Try using lemon juice to remove tobacco stains from your fingers.

3   Begin a new sport or learn to dance. Be sure to consult your physician before making a major change in your physical activity, however; and always work your way up *gradually* in terms of time and intensity of exercise.

4   Get out of your old habits. Seek new activities or perform old activities in new ways. Don't rely on the old ways of solving problems. In short, don't be in a rut.

5   Stock up on light reading materials, crossword puzzles and vacation brochures you can read during your breaks from work.

6   Increase your time in places where you can't smoke, such as libraries, buses, theatres, swimming pools or department stores, during your first weeks off cigarettes.

7   Review your *FreshStart Guide* regularly. Make a list of the most important tips for you personally. Carry the list with you and review it often during your first month or so after stopping.

8   Finally, help a friend to stop smoking by sharing with him some of your experiences. Be certain, however, that your friend wants your help. Some individuals prefer to discuss their stopping, while others do not want to talk about it. Do, however, let others know the sense of pride and well-being you feel now that you have become a successful ex-smoker.

9   Enter the phone numbers of your *FreshStart* leaders and of a

buddy from that program in your regular telephone index or book.

10   Plan a major celebration for your six-month anniversary of being a nonsmoker!

The advice to pipe and cigar smokers is also to quit. As a heavy pipe smoker for twenty years who has recently reached a five-year "cure," I can tell you that it is hard to give it up, and as with the reformed alcoholic, there are certain times when the urge to smoke my pipe is very great. At those times I will chew on a swizzle stick (my assistant's bright idea), munch on a carrot, use relaxation techniques or change what I am doing altogether. Actually, like many ex-smokers, I am now very upset by smelling cigarette smoke and will move to another seat in an airport or restaurant. While I was a smoker I could not fully appreciate the discomfort that smoking can cause to nonsmokers. It is late now to apologize but I feel sad at having caused my family and other innocent people the discomfort and potential health hazard of being exposed to my pipe smoking, and I imagine even active smokers suffer these feelings. A great many physicians have quit smoking and this is very positive. Cigarette companies no longer advertise that "more doctors smoke _____ than any other brand" as they did for so many years.

We can also learn something from lung cancer patients who become ex-smokers. In a recent study of lung cancer patients, Nancy Knudsen, R.N., and colleagues discovered that many of them continued to smoke even after the diagnosis of lung cancer was made. The authors did, however, survey the smoking habits of all of their patient groups including former smokers who had smoked from one to four packs of cigarettes per day for a duration of fifteen to sixty-six years. Thirty-four of the fifty-one patients who quit smoking did so either at the time of their cancer diagnosis or immediately after their surgery, and the reasons were because they identified smoking with lung cancer or because of breathing complaints or other health worries, personal satisfaction of knowing that a person could quit, fear, acting upon the doctor's request, et cetera. The other seventeen patients who quit smoking did so before their lung cancer surgery. The suggestions that these patients made to help a person who is trying to quit smoking are summarized below:

Patient Suggestions to Help a Person Who Is Trying to Quit Smoking

(Source: Nancy Knudsen, et al., "Insights on How to Quit Smoking: A Survey of Patients with Lung Cancer," *Cancer Nursing* 8:3 [1985]: 148)

☐ A person has to make up his or her own mind and stick to it. He or she doesn't know it, but all smokers have a terrible odor emanating out of their lungs. I wonder if they ever think about this when they are making love!

☐ Avoid other smokers, visit an emphysema ward or talk with people suffering from it. Notice their inactivity.

☐ If you are the competitive type, get a friend or relative to quit too and try to outdo each other. I refused to let my husband say he had more will power than I had.

☐ Break your pattern. If you smoke right after meals at the table, get up and get busy. Chew gum instead. Do something different at the normal time. Break your pattern, be it sewing, reading, gardening, whatever. It worked for me.

☐ Try to realize the advantages of not smoking versus the pleasure and comfort while smoking.

☐ I sometimes suggest the possibility of lung cancer.

☐ If one can hold out for three or four weeks, they will find the smell of cigarettes obnoxious.

☐ Smoking is as much or more a habit of the hands as a craving desire. I found that after the third or fourth day, I'd forget about a cigarette; but whenever my hands stopped doing something, I automatically reached for my shirt pocket for periods up to three weeks. Most often I substituted a package of Life Savers or I would make up a package of carrot sticks, very effective substitutes. I ate a million.

Of course there are many patients with lung cancer who were heavy smokers and did not live long. Roswell Park Memorial Institute in Buffalo, New York, has a huge smokers "hall of fame," a sample of which is shown in Figure 11.

About one-third of the adults in the United States are regular

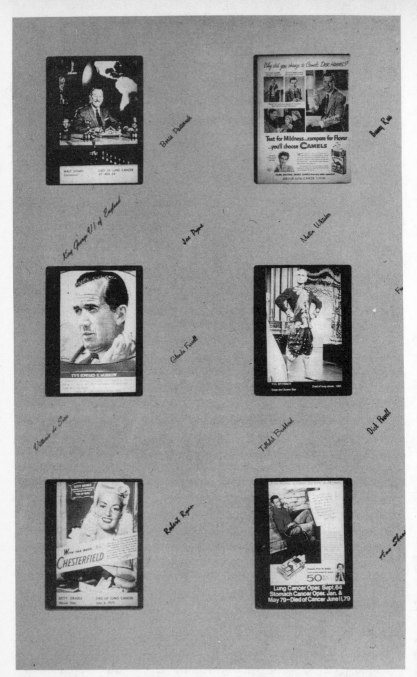

Figure 11 The Cigarette Hall of Fame at Roswell Park Memorial Institute, Buffalo, New York. (Photo kindly provided by Mr. Dante Terrana and Dr. E. Mirand)

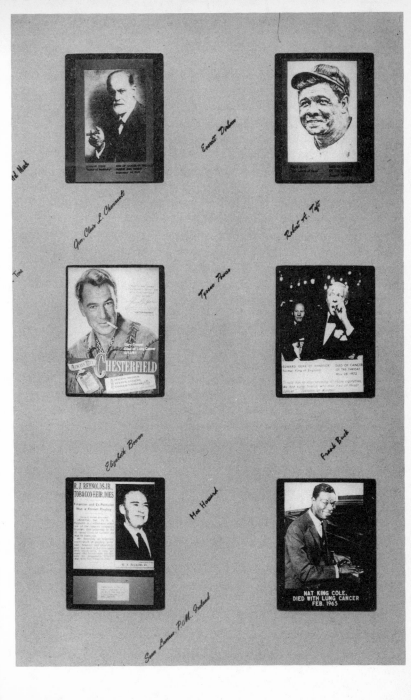

smokers, and there is a great need for more effective means to help people stop smoking, particularly since it can be stated that not only cancer, but also heart and lung disease risk factors are profoundly influenced by sustained abstinence from smoking. Despite the availability of quit-smoking clinics, most smokers who stop do so on their own and these intervention programs or clinics have not had a very high rate of success, the rates of dropout and recidivism (repeated relapse) being very high. Since most quit-smoking programs offer only six to twelve months of follow-up and rely on self-reporting, it is difficult to arrive at a meaningful figure for rate of success, but I estimate it overall to be about 20 percent in the traditional larger programs. Much more intense programs run by psychologists and comparable health professionals appear to be considerably more successful, but they are also more expensive and not yet suitable for large numbers of people. In reviewing the data from many different programs, C. S. Orleans, Ph.D., summarized all of this available information, as listed in Table 4.

Some transitional strategies have been conceived as adjuncts for smokers who wish to quit; for example, as described above, nicotine chewing gum has been recommended to lessen the degree of exposure to carcinogens and still deal directly with the physiological dependence on nicotine. Some 10 percent of heavy smokers may in turn become dependent on the gum. Furthermore, by itself the gum is not very effective in helping people to stop smoking, although it is perhaps useful in conjunction with other structured programs. From interview surveys we are aware that almost all physicians agree that it is their responsibility to set a good example for patients by not smoking cigarettes, and as a group physicians have had good success in stopping smoking. Yet two-thirds of smokers say that their personal physician has not advised them about the dangers of smoking: since physician advice can be quite effective when it is given, clearly there is much room for improvement in this department.

We shouldn't forget the Great American Smokeout, which celebrated its tenth anniversary in 1986. From humble beginnings in a small town in California, this ACS-sponsored program has gone

Table 4 *Smoking Cessation Methods: Initial and Long-Term Results*

Treatment Modality	Abstinence (%)	
	Initial	After 1 Year
Quitting on one's own		
Without any outside help	67	16–20
With self-help programs (mail, telephone)	20–40	16 (8–15 mo.)
Mass media and community programs		
Televised clinics	10	
Community media campaigns		5–9
Physician advice		
Pre-illness		5–10
Chronic respiratory illness or at risk for coronary heart disease		20–30
Postmyocardial infarct		50–60
Quit clinics		
Voluntary health organizations (5-day plans, American Cancer Society, American Lung Association, American Health Foundation)	60	16–22
Commercial quit clinics (Kaiser, Toronto Health Smokewatchers)	62	42
Majority psychological/behavioral treatment (hypnosis, behavior modification, psychotherapy)		
Abstinent participants		20–30
All participants		15–25
Promising behavioral approaches		
Rapid smoking plus	70–100	40 (6 mo.)
Normal-paced smoking plus	60	30 (6 mo.)
Smoke-holding/rapid puffing plus	70	50 (3–6 mo.)
Broad spectrum with smoke aversion	70–100	30–40 (6 mo.)

Source: Data published by C. S. Orleans and reproduced with permission from *Cancer Research* 44 (1984): 5940.

nationwide. Studies show that people who do pledge to stop on that occasion have a very favorable rate of success. They must be very well motivated.

PASSIVE SMOKING—A NEW PUBLIC CONTROVERSY Unfortunately, the subject of passive smoking has only recently come under study and so not all of the facts are in. However, a number of very important lines of evidence suggest that considerable caution is advisable, and it is not appropriate to assume that exposure to a smoke-filled environment is free of risk. Some of the evidence is as follows:

□ The harmful substances (carcinogens) that smokers inhale are the same as those that nonsmokers inhale when they are in a smoky environment. This is proven by analyses of the surrounding air.

□ We know that the nonsmoker who is exposed to passive smoking absorbs the substances because their presence can easily be detected in the urine. Perhaps the most telling test for these substances is the so-called mutagenicity or Ames test, which detects genetic mutations in bacteria when urine from exposed people is put into bacterial cultures. For example, airline hostesses who work in the smoking section can be distinguished from those who work in the nonsmoking section by the presence of mutagens in their urine. Volunteers who sit next to smokers, nonsmoking spouses of smokers and workers who work in smoky environments all have increased mutagens and nicotine metabolites in their urine.

□ Several studies, although not all, have shown that nonsmoking spouses of smokers have a higher incidence of lung cancer than nonsmoking spouses of nonsmokers; similarly, nonsmoking workers who work in a smoky environment have a higher incidence of lung cancer than nonsmoking workers who work in nonsmoky environments. The evidence continues to mount on this most important issue.

□ Changes in blood cell chromosomes are noted in people exposed to passive smoking. Furthermore, an important new finding is the presence of nicotine metabolites in the urine of infants cared for by mothers who smoke, a quiet form of child abuse.

As we said, the hazards of passive smoking are a relatively new area of concern and not all of the answers are in, by any means. The Surgeon General has recently come out with a very strong statement about the dangers of passive smoking. The tobacco industry would like us not to worry about this problem, and they suggest that nothing is known about any danger from passive smoking. However, until shown evidence to the contrary, I will continue to be worried about the risk of passive smoking for nonsmokers. I also subscribe to the 1984 recommendations of the American Association for Cancer Research, adopted unanimously by its members as follows.

RECOMMENDATIONS FOR PUBLIC POLICY "The American Association for Cancer Research accepts the evidence gathered by cancer scientists as establishing that cigarette smoking is the major preventable cause of human lung cancer. We therefore go on record as advocating that the greatest cancer prevention measure that might be undertaken would be for people not to smoke. As interim steps toward this goal, we recommend the following actions be taken by the government and members of our society to reduce cigarette smoking.

1   Take legislative action to reduce 'image advertising' and other types of promotional efforts designed to attract people to the practice of cigarette smoking.

2   Enact legislation designed to reduce the availability of cigarettes for children and young adults, particularly in school, military, and hospital settings. One measure would be to eliminate the tax-free status on cigarette sales in government installations.

3   Enact and enforce legislation that restricts smoking in public places.

4   Increase taxes on cigarettes and other tobacco products and

use the proceeds for research, education, and treatment of the diseases resulting from smoking.

5   Eliminate federal support for the production and distribution of tobacco products.

6   Increase the effectiveness of warning labels on tobacco products."

Lung cancer is grim in almost every respect. As mentioned in a separate chapter (9), screening tests seeking to detect lung cancer early enough that it can be cured have not brought any increase in the overall survival rate, presumably because when the cancer is discovered it is already too late to save the majority of patients. Furthermore, all the existing means of curative treatment are relatively ineffective except for surgical removal of a truly localized cancer, and this is possible to accomplish in only a minority of patients. A tremendous amount of work is being done to find more effective treatments for lung cancer, but nothing very promising is on the near horizon. How much better it would be to prevent this disease from occurring in the first place. On a positive note, the Defense Department deserves our praise for steps it has taken to discourage cigarette smoking in the armed forces. This courageous move will undoubtedly save lives and also reduce the health bills of our servicemen and women. And one major corporation, United States Gypsum, recently announced that all levels of workers at some of its plants must not smoke at work *or* at home. The legality of that action will be challenged and other companies will watch the outcome very closely. The action would certainly make an impact on their health care costs and on productivity.

SMOKELESS TOBACCO Snuff and chewing tobacco are two commonly used types of smokeless tobacco. Snuff is a cured, ground-up tobacco produced as dry, moist or fine-cut tobacco. Chewing tobacco also comes in several varieties—loose leaf, plug and chewing tobacco. Smokeless tobacco is usually placed between the cheek and gums or is chewed as the leaf or plug. The nicotine dissolves in saliva and is absorbed into the bloodstream.

At present, over twenty-two million Americans use smokeless

tobacco. I recently participated in a cancer symposium in West Virginia where a dentist reported on the situation in that state, in which it is estimated that as many as 75 percent of high school boys in one county are regular users of chewing tobacco and snuff. The typical user appears to begin chewing sometime during the fourth to the eighth grade, but many eight- and nine-year-olds already have suffered severe gum damage because they have been regular users since two to three years of age. Can you believe that? The risk of increased cancers is very great in users of these products, and a special problem is that of "snuff dipper's cancer," which has been known for years and almost always occurs at the point of contact of the gums with the chewing tobacco or snuff. A North Carolina study showed a fifty-fold increase in risk for cancer of certain parts of the mouth (cheek and gums) in women who habitually use snuff. A survey of 5,894 Oklahoma students showed that 13 percent of third-grade and 22 percent of fifth-grade males chew tobacco. Most students believe that dipping and chewing tobacco is less harmful to their health than smoking. And if you have seen baseball players chewing tobacco you know that significant role models are fostering this habit.

Connolly et al. recently reviewed the subject of the reemergence of smokeless tobacco (*New England Journal of Medicine,* April 17, 1986) and reviewed the overwhelming epidemiologic and experimental evidence that smokeless tobacco causes cancers in the mouth.

In addition to the risk for cancer, after some five years of use of smokeless tobacco a "pouch" results in the cheek at the site where the quid is kept. The muscles of the face are stretched and thin and the lining of the cheek becomes discolored. Another problem is that most people don't understand that smokeless tobacco is thought to be at least as strong an addiction as that of cigarettes, and we fear that the increasing use of these products in young people may lead to serious diseases when they reach middle age.

The Comprehensive Smokeless Health Education Act of 1986 bans radio and television advertising of chewing tobacco and snuff and requires that warning labels be printed on all smokeless tobacco packages and print advertisements.

The labels, required for the first time, will read:

WARNING   This product may cause mouth cancer.
WARNING   This product may cause gum disease and tooth loss.
WARNING   This product is not a safe alternative to cigarettes.

From an esthetic point of view I have the fantasy that an additional sign will appear that states: WARNING   This habit is disgusting!

ECONOMICS OF SMOKING AND LUNG CANCER When I speak to civic organizations in North Carolina about smoking and lung cancer, the importance of tobacco to the economy of the state is invariably brought up by someone in the audience. I get the feeling that my subject matter is about as popular as salmonella at a Fourth of July picnic. The entire tobacco industry obviously is of great economic importance in certain states, and it would be insensitive to ignore the needs of farmers, warehouse and factory workers and others in the industry, who are all good people. However, in recognizing the revenue side of the issue one must examine the costs. In this section we will pull together some figures that are very difficult to find, and then try to put them into perspective, drawing heavily upon analyses reported by Professor Kenneth E. Warner of the School of Public Health, University of Michigan.

In 1983 Americans spent well over $350 billion on health care, or in excess of $1,500 per man, woman and child. These costs do not reflect the loss of productivity associated with disease. It has been estimated that the total societal cost of smoking-related diseases (health care costs plus loss of productivity) is between $40 billion and $50 billion annually in 1980 dollars or around $60 billion in 1984 dollars. These figures do not include the value of human life nor do they measure the costs of pain and suffering to the victims and to their families and friends. One author (Abt) has pointed out that if such costs could be measured, they might exceed those that are more readily estimated for smoking-related diseases; he notes that the true social costs of cancer may be as much as ten times greater than the measurable costs.

Rice and Hodgson at the National Center for Health Statistics have analyzed the economic costs of smoking-related diseases. In

1980 the medical expenditures on all lung cancers in men totaled $1.003 billion, and in women, $595 million. Productivity losses attributed to smoking-caused lung cancer deaths were valued at $5.876 billion (in 1980 dollars). Thus, the total economic costs of smoking-induced lung cancer may be estimated at $7.47 billion in 1980 dollars, or approximately 17 percent of the entire cost of smoking-related illness. *In 1984 dollars, this cost would be approximately $10 billion!* Stark as these figures are, they may still substantially underestimate the true economic costs of smoking-induced lung cancer, particularly in women. The major reason for this is that the female share of the total is relatively small because many of the females who die are not in the work force, but are working in the household, for which they are not paid; another reason is that women's wages for labor are still less than men's in today's labor market.

In a recently released report prepared for the House Ways and Means Committee, the Office of Technology Assessment (OTA) estimated that the United States would spend between $12 and $35 billion to treat smoking-related diseases in 1985—the middle estimate in health care costs being about $22 billion, or 6 percent of all U.S. health care spending. "This amounts to about 72 cents for each pack of cigarettes sold in the U.S.," OTA says in its report on smoking. Estimated medical care costs are $1.7 billion to $5.4 billion, while Medicaid costs amount to $0.3–1.1 billion. After subtracting out the state share of Medicaid and adding in other federal programs that provide health care to the elderly, it is estimated that the federal government pays between $2.1 and $6.6 billion for treating smoking-related disease. OTA estimated that the federal costs would amount to about $4.2 billion in 1985 or about 14 cents for each pack of cigarettes. Their most recent estimate on the loss of productivity from smoking-related diseases ranges between $26 and $61 billion with a middle estimate of $43 billion. According to that report, "the middle estimate amounts to about $1.45 for each pack of cigarettes sold." The total for smoking-related health care costs and lost productivity amounts to between $39 and $96 billion with a middle estimate of $65 billion. The middle estimate equals $2.17 per pack of cigarettes.

It is also difficult to calculate the individual costs of smoking-induced lung cancer. The most obvious cost of smoking is the direct outlay of some $15,000 that the average smoker can expect to spend buying cigarettes over a lifetime of smoking. This is a concern that all smokers share, but this may pale when insurance companies begin putting a premium on smokers, and when employers do preferential hiring of nonsmokers. These tangible pocketbook costs of smoking are far more meaningful to the individual smoker than the potential costs of lung cancer that may occur in the indefinite future. Nonetheless, *it is estimated that the average economic burden of lung cancer is $60,000 per case,* a figure arrived at by dividing the total social cost due to loss of productivity and medical expenditures by the number of cases.

Does the revenue generated from cigarette sales offset the costs of smoking-related lung cancer? The answer is clearly no. If one looks at these figures, as we did in an article in *Cancer Research* (December 1984), one cannot avoid the conclusion that nonsmokers are subsidizing the ill health and loss of productivity of smokers—there is a very substantial gap between the taxation of tobacco at 16 cents per pack and the much larger cost to society. Nonetheless, the industry is constantly lobbying to reduce or eliminate the tax. You and I need to express our views on this to our elected representatives—you can be sure that the powerful tobacco lobby will continue working to lower or eliminate the tax. Furthermore, it might be preferable to place the tax on each cigarette rather than on the pack since companies are now moving toward having twenty-five cigarettes per pack rather than twenty.

Let me also mention a more cynical view of the economics of smoking that is based on the notion that smokers tend to live some seven to eight years less than nonsmokers, which lowers their average life expectancy down to about the time of their retirement. Thus, their premature death prevents tens of thousands of people from entering the dependent geriatric population and spares society the cost of social support programs such as Social Security, Medicare benefits, et cetera. (Tobacco industry advertising campaigns have obviously not yet seized upon the cost-saving features of premature death due to tobacco-related diseases as an argument for smoking!) A recent analysis of the "macroeconomics" of disease prevention in the United States by Gori and Ritcher discusses this issue; and another paper, by Leu and Schaub, analyzes the national health care costs of the Swiss economy since the late 1800s and compares them to what would have occurred in the absence of smoking. Leu and Schaub arrive at the conclusion that total health care costs in the nonsmoking society are not very different from those of the smoking society. However, *there is one critical difference between the two societies: more people live longer and healthier lives in the nonsmoking society.* Thus, whereas the total effect of nonsmoking may not be cost-saving, it may be a very cost-effective way to improve the nation's health.

The American Cancer Society has a target of a smoke-free young America by the year 2000. Make sure your children belong to that graduating class.

CANCER SCREENING AND DETECTION: HOW USEFUL ARE PERIODIC EXAMINATIONS?

9

Often patients who find they have cancer ask me what they might have done sooner to prevent it from occurring or to find it earlier. And what should other members of their family do to check themselves? Cancer prevention issues are extremely important and are dealt with elsewhere. This, however, is the place to answer the question about *early* diagnosis. The importance of screening and early detection was exemplified by President Reagan and Mrs. Reagan, who were probably cured of cancers of colon, skin and breast. Although it can make a critical difference to find cancer early, there are instances when early discovery is of no advantage because the treatments are not too different—or, unhappily, not too satisfactory whether the cancer is found early or late. The result of a brain tumor in a critical area or chronic leukemia would probably not be very different if found two months earlier or later, whereas the result of cervical, breast or colon cancer might be very different. Considerations such as these (and even they change as new treatments become available) influence my recommendations to you regarding what tests to take and how often.

Naturally the first step is the hardest one to take, and that is to face the possibility of developing cancer as we would face other significant hazards of living. We check our cars for safety and use seat belts, have our blood pressure and blood sugar tested periodically—particularly if there is hypertension and diabetes in our family, and so on. *We have to recognize that there are special terrors, irrational fears that sometimes interfere with our ability to function sensibly, and it is here that knowledge can be so important in overcoming inertia or paralysis.*

So let us get down to the substantive business of describing what we know and what we can do to find cancer early.

PRINCIPLES OF SCREENING FOR CANCER Cancer screening involves the use of cost-effective tests to find early stage cancer when it is still curable with local treatment (like surgery or radiation). These tests are designed to discover specific forms of cancer among large groups of people who have absolutely no symptoms of disease but who may be "at risk" because of their age, occupation or personal habits. Although the idea sounds rather straightforward, it is full of controversy because of changing technology, costs and societal expectations. Frankly, many of us in this field are uncertain about what advice we should be giving to the public with respect to screening for more than a few types of cancer. Here we will discuss the issues surrounding cancer screening and distinguish between cancer *screening* and cancer *detection,* which involves a more individual approach with fewer cost-benefit considerations.

If the tests available to us were reliable, inexpensive and capable of finding a tiny cancer in literally any part of the body, we would want to use them for everyone. *Since there is no single test that detects all cancers, the focus of screening is on those signs that are abnormal in some of the more common cancers such as those of the cervix, skin, bowel, breast, prostate and lung, with particular emphasis on those cancers in which curability depends upon early detection. The problem is finding a reliable test for a reasonable cost that will be used by the people at highest risk for developing a particular cancer.* When we speak of reliable, we mean a test that can detect the great majority (greater than 85 percent) of cancers if they are indeed present and not pick up many so-called false-positive findings, which incorrectly suggest the presence of a cancer when none is there. This can be a major logistical problem. Consider for a moment that most women have some lumps in the breast during the course of their menstruating years, but only a very small fraction of these ever turn out to be cancerous. A test that could not distinguish between benign and malignant lumps would not be of any use, since we would either not use it at all or end up with an unacceptable cost because it would involve so much unnecessary surgery. Table 5 lists the well-considered recommendations of the American Cancer Society; my own vary slightly from those for practical reasons of cost, availability and discomfort of some tests. It is important to recognize that screening is not an exact science; but like statistics, it can be a great help in drawing attention to patients who are in high-risk groups.

PAP TEST The classic example of a screening test that is good, i.e., cheap, efficient, usually reliable, effective and having positive long-term results, is the Pap test, named after the father of cytologic diagnosis, Dr. Papanicolaou. In this test a few drops of vaginal fluid are taken by a doctor or nurse and placed on a glass slide, which is then stained and examined by expert technicians and pathologists. So much work has been done with this test that we can be satisfied about its accuracy. (I am referring to the test that is taken in the doctor's examining room and performed by reputable laboratories, not the so-called home Pap test.) Another factor that makes this test particularly important is that early cancer of the cervix is regularly cured with simple and inexpensive treatment, whereas if the cancer grows large before it is detected it may not be curable or may require very extensive surgery. The death rate from cancer of the cervix has been declining steadily; this trend admittedly began even before Pap tests became widespread, but the test is believed to be a very important factor in the continuing decline in mortality. Women who are screened regularly

Table 5 *Summary of American Cancer Society Recommendations for the Early Detection of Cancer in Asymptomatic People*

Test or Procedure	Population		Frequency
	Sex	Age	
Sigmoidoscopy	M & F	Over 50	After 2 negative exams 1 year apart, perform every 3–5 years
Stool guaiac slide test	M & F	Over 50	Every year
Digital rectal examination	M & F	Over 40	Every year
Pap test	F	20–65; under 20 if sexually active	After 3 negative exams 1 year apart, perform as directed thereafter
Pelvic examination	F	20–40	Every 3 years
		Over 40	Every year
Endometrial tissue sample	F	At menopause, women at high risk*	At menopause
Breast self-examination	F	Over 20	Every month
Breast physical examination	F	20–40	Every 3 years
		Over 40	Every year
Mammography	F	Between 35–40	Baseline
		40–49	Every 1–2 years
		Over 50	Every year
Chest x-ray			Not recommended
Sputum cytology			Not recommended
Health counseling	M & F	Over 20	Every 3 years
and cancer checkup†	M & F	Over 40	Every year

*History of infertility, obesity, failure to ovulate, abnormal uterine bleeding, or estrogen therapy
†To include examination for cancers of the thyroid, testicles, prostate, ovaries, lymph nodes, oral region and skin

Source: Reprinted with permission from *CA-A Cancer Journal for Clinicians* 35 (1985): 199. © 1985, American Cancer Society, Inc., and updated in 1987.

are much less likely to die of cancer of the cervix. Indeed, *the use of the Pap smear is said by recent studies to reduce the risk of mortality from invasive cervical cancer by 75 percent. Yet surveys show that at most 80 percent of women between ages 20 and 39, and 57 percent between 40 and 70 follow the recommended guidelines on screening for cervical cancer. And this represents our best case for cancer screening.* The use of the Pap smear in the recommended way could further reduce mortality (see Chapter 16). The social problems associated with screening are important to recognize because this particular cancer is most common in lower socioeconomic groups, the very people who are hardest to reach with public health measures. We need better community organization to get people to a screening clinic, involving active church groups, use of buses—whatever it takes!

Today the only major questions about cervical cytology screening (or Pap tests) are about at what age the test should first be done and how often it needs to be repeated. As we have pointed out, cervical cancer is more common among women with multiple sexual partners, and since social mores have become more permissive in recent years, it is wise for sexually active women to have a Pap test in their early twenties, say at age twenty-one, and then repeat the test approximately every three years (this figure is quite debatable—some experts suggest more frequent testing). The decision of how often to have a Pap test should be based on the results of the most recent test, and the medical advice for one individual may differ from that for another. We know that cervical cancer never arises out of the blue without a previous period of a precancerous or dysplastic phase, and this can also be detected microscopically with the Pap test. Any cytology that shows a significant abnormality calls for ordering another test in perhaps six to twelve months, to be followed by another decision as to when the test should be repeated. *An abnormal test is not a cause to panic but should be an incentive to follow through with periodic testing as advised by the physician.* In my opinion a cytology that shows no abnormalities whatever need not be followed so frequently since that appears to be a waste of resources.

BREAST CANCER SCREENING The technique of breast self-examination (BSE) was recently introduced as a screening test for

177

9: Cancer Screening and Detection: How Useful Are Periodic Examinations?

breast cancer, and it is rapidly growing in popularity. It can be taught in schools by nurse volunteers or physicians, costs nothing to use, gives women responsibility for this aspect of their health and familiarizes them with changes in breast tissue that occur during the menstrual cycle. *BSE is best performed monthly on the same day of the cycle, preferably just after the menstrual period. It can detect suspicious lumps or call attention to fibrocystic breast tissue* (notice I use the word tissue and not disease, since such tissue is not abnormal and does not lead to cancer), *which can be quite lumpy, painful and tender.* Since breast cancer is one of the two most common causes of death from cancer in women (lung cancer is the other), and early breast cancer is curable in the majority of patients, this exam offers a real opportunity for minimizing the danger. Obviously it is important to learn the proper technique, to follow up on any questions and to show any suspicious lump to a doctor. BSE's limitations are that it is very difficult to find a cancer that is less than one inch in diameter, nor has it yet been proven that BSE actually saves lives, although we hope that it does.

Figure 12 on pages 178–79 illustrates the American Cancer Society recommendations for breast self-examination and describes the technique.

What about mammography as a screening procedure? Mammography is a kind of soft tissue x-ray developed specifically for breast examination. It can give major evidence that a lump felt by the patient and/or doctor has characteristics of cancer. It can never completely exclude the possibility of cancer, but certain features are so typical as to simplify the decision about whether or not to operate. The cost of the mammography procedure is not trivial (the average is about $150 per study), which alone makes it inaccessible for many low-income people. There are clinics that are bringing the price down to the range of $30–$50, a major advance. It also requires an expert radiologist to make the interpretation since we are looking for very tiny areas of cancer—and there are still not enough people well trained in this technique to handle the workload if 50 percent of the women followed the recommendations for screening. For women who have a mammography done and are found to have a spot that looks suspicious to the radiologist, surgical biopsy or removal of the lump is usual. When the

Figure 12   HOW TO EXAMINE YOUR BREASTS Monthly self-examination of the female breasts is recommended by the American Cancer Society as a safeguard against breast cancer. This simple three-step procedure could save lives by finding breast cancer early, when it is most curable.

STEP 1   In the shower: Examine your breasts during bath or shower; hands glide easier over wet skin. Fingers flat, move gently over every part of each breast. Use right hand to examine left breast, left hand for right breast. Check for any lump, hard knot or thickening.

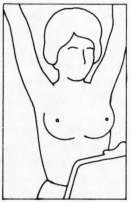

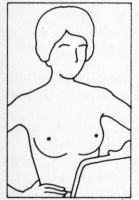

STEP 2   Before a mirror: Inspect your breasts with arms at your sides. Next, raise your arms high overhead. Look for any changes in contour of each breast, a swelling, dimpling of skin or changes in the nipple.

Then, rest palms on hips and press down firmly to flex your chest muscles. Left and right breast will not exactly match—few women's breasts do.

Regular inspection shows what is normal for you and will give you confidence in your examination.

STEP 3   Lying down: To examine your right breast, put a pillow or folded towel under your right shoulder. Place right hand behind your

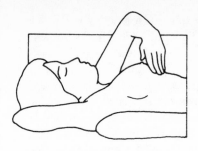

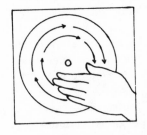

head—this distributes breast tissue more evenly on the chest. With left hand, fingers flat, press gently in small circular motions around an imaginary clock face. Begin at outermost top of your right breast for 12 o'clock, then move to 1 o'clock, and so on around the circle back to 12. A ridge of firm tissue in the lower curve of each breast is normal. Then move in an inch, toward the nipple, keep circling to examine *every part of your breast,* including nipple. This requires at least three more circles. Now slowly repeat procedure on your left breast with a pillow under your left shoulder and left hand behind head. Notice how your breast structure feels.

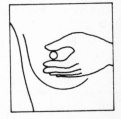

Finally, squeeze the nipple of each breast gently between thumb and index finger. Any discharge, clear or bloody, should be reported to your doctor immediately.

Why you should examine your breasts monthly Most breast cancers are first discovered by women themselves. Since breast cancers found early and treated promptly have excellent chances for cure, learning how to examine your breasts properly can help save your life. Use the simple 3-step breast self-examination (BSE) procedure shown here.

For the best time to examine your breasts: Follow the same procedure once a month about a week after your period, when breasts are usually not tender or swollen. After menopause, check breasts on the first day of each month. After hysterectomy, check your doctor or clinic for an appropriate time of the month. Doing BSE will give you monthly peace of mind. And have a physician examine your breasts every 3 years from age 20 to 40, and every year after 40.

What you should do if you find a lump or thickening If a lump or dimple or discharge is discovered during BSE, it is important to see your doctor as soon as possible. Don't be frightened. Most breast lumps or changes are not cancer, but only your doctor can make the diagnosis.

radiologist finds the mammogram suspicious for cancer when the lump cannot be felt, only one or two out of ten biopsies will determine that it is cancer. ("Let's just watch it a while and see" is nevertheless usually unwise advice.) The finding that leads to surgical biopsy and pathology study is far more expensive than the mammography ($750–$1,000 or more), but if it is an early cancer then a life has been saved. If the lump turns out to be benign, it is a great relief, but it has been expensive, uncomfortable and worrisome—that's the trade-off. A very small amount of radiation is used in performing mammograms, but the benefit seems to far outweigh the risks.

But let us suppose the mammography test is negative; how often should it be repeated? On this point the advice varies somewhat, as with the Pap test. A negative test does not exclude with certainty the possibility that a cancer was missed because it was too small to be detected or lacked the typical features; also, a negative test obviously does not guarantee that the person will not develop cancer of the breast in the future. A baseline mammogram is recommended for all women between age thirty-five and forty. The consensus is that routine mammography screening is appropriately performed every one to two years after the age of forty and annually after age fifty, unless a person finds a new lump during the course of monthly self-examination. While that may be ideal, such a degree of frequency is probably unrealistic for most women. Also, women who have a greater than normal risk of cancer—strong family history (mother, sister, aunt)—or who have had a prior breast cancer should be screened more often than average, and should start screening at an earlier age.

I have seen women who turned out to have breast cancer although their mammography testing did not suggest cancer. This is very unfortunate but it can happen with every test that we use in medicine. But mammography also finds cancers earlier than other tests, as with Nancy Reagan, and thus saves lives. It has been estimated that fewer than 5 percent of American women above the age of fifty have annual mammograms and that probably fewer than one-third of eligible women have ever had a mammogram. A large study of more than 60,000 women done by the Health

Insurance Plan of New York found that the mortality from breast cancer is reduced by 30 percent in women over age fifty who are screened for breast cancer by mammography and physical examination. A recent American Cancer Society report confirms that important finding. *However, the lack of improvement in survival figures for breast cancer on a nationwide basis indicates that screening is not taking place with sufficient frequency.* It would be very helpful if improvements in technology could reduce the costs of mammography, and such advances are coming. We must remember that mammography is still a new procedure and its full advantages and limitations have yet to be realized. It is not a final answer at this stage, but it is very important for women to know about and to use it.

TESTICULAR CANCER Although testicular cancer is relatively uncommon, unlike breast cancer, we are trying to introduce testicular self-examination into school health programs. Since this is a cancer that occurs predominantly in young men and it is now highly curable, this simple screening test is extremely useful. The American Cancer Society provides educational programs about cancer screening free of charge for interested groups who contact their local chapter. In our local ACS chapter in Durham, a practicing urologist has volunteered his time to give excellent sessions to high school students while women nurses provide demonstrations of the techniques of BSE to the female half of the class. Almost more important, such high school training can be used to stimulate curiosity about the larger problems of cancer and thus serve to better equip a rising generation with the capability to cope more effectively.

LUNG AND BOWEL CANCER—THE "TOUGH" PROBLEMS Screening tests for two common types of cancer are far more controversial, and of less certain benefit. In an effort to detect lung cancer early, periodic chest x-rays (at six- or twelve-month intervals) and sputum cytology similar to a Pap test have been tried in large groups of people. Although these means will detect cancers earlier than they might be found if a person waited until there were symptoms to see the doctor, so far the tests have not been shown to make much difference in the outcome. Unfortunately, most patients still succumb to their lung cancer even if they have participated in a screening program, and such programs are expensive if continued over the years. Large research studies that are now in progress may lead to new recommendations, but on the basis of present evidence it appears that we need to develop less expensive tests and tests that will detect lung cancer earlier than do the existing techniques. *The best insurance against dying from lung cancer is not to get it in the first place, a policy that is the most cost-effective of all* (see Chapter 12).

Cancers of the "bowel"—which includes cancers of the esophagus, stomach, colon and rectum—are among the leading causes of death from cancer. Because these cancers tend to bleed into the bowel before they give rise to symptoms, screening for blood in the stools has been widely advocated as a useful test for early detection. The idea is to test the stool for the presence of blood by reacting a small specimen with guaiac, a special chemical that is impregnated onto paper and that causes a visible color change (blue) in the presence of blood. People can be taught to check their own bowel movements or they can be screened at a doctor's office. *However, large studies have not confirmed the usefulness of the test in cancer screening and its ultimate place is still controversial:* the major problem is that there are many false positives and false negatives. For example, eating red meat will cause a person to test positive; therefore people must go on a meat-free diet for perhaps five days before the stool is tested—and that is usually not practical in a screening situation. False-negative stool tests also occur because these tumors may bleed only intermittently; thus a single negative specimen does not exclude the diagnosis of cancer. I remember one woman in whom we suspected intestinal blood loss and in whom I performed eleven consecutive negative stool examinations before she had three positives in a row. Conversely, more innocent blood loss may come from bleeding hemorrhoids, which are far more common than cancers—yet finding hemorrhoids does not necessarily preclude the presence of cancer elsewhere in the bowel. So the problem is a difficult one to resolve.

The problems that surround the testing of the stool for blood can be illustrated by the experience of President Ronald Reagan, as reported by the media. In March 1985 he had a routine examination, as part of which four stool samples were tested for blood—two of the tests were negative and two were positive. Because of the knowledge that meats can cause false-positive tests, the President was advised to change his diet, and the stool was retested. At this time he had six tests, *all* of which were negative—even though at that time he had a malignant tumor growing in his colon near the appendix. Dr. Charles Moertel from the Mayo Clinic is quite experienced in this area and he believes that in some 20–30 percent of cases a false-negative test such as happened with the President will occur. The test (Hemoccult) also gives far too many false-positive results. The most common causes of false-positive reactions are meat and other substances in the diet that react with the guaiac reagent; these include fresh fruits, fish and vitamin C tablets. False-positive tests are so common, in fact, that only 5–10 percent of people whose Hemoccult test is positive actually turn out to have colon cancer, but obviously a person whose test is positive needs further evaluation. And this requires a great deal of uncomfortable and expensive testing, as described below.

Opinions as to the value of the Hemoccult test vary widely among the experts—indicating that we simply do not have the answer. Various independent study groups, including one convened by the National Cancer Institute (NCI) in 1978, have concluded that the weaknesses of the test for screening purposes outweigh its benefits. Dr. David Eddy, who advises the American Cancer Society and the NCI about screening tests, argues that for people over the age of fifty, annual Hemoccult tests and sigmoidoscope or colonoscope examinations every few years make sense since colon cancer is such a major killer and yet so curable if caught early. Dr. Eddy has put together a mathematical model to evaluate the costs and benefits of screening. He concludes that if you are over the age of forty, having an annual stool test for blood will decrease by 15 percent your chances of ever getting colon cancer, and decrease by 30 percent the chances that you will die from this cancer. That type of effect is comparable to the benefit that women receive from mammography over the age of fifty, yet the tests can be done at only a fraction of those costs. Other experts, such as Dr. John Bailar, a statistician and physician from Harvard, disagree and feel that the model does not tell the full story. There clearly is now a great increase in awareness of the problem of colon cancer among the American public, and this will undoubtedly result in more screening tests being performed. Perhaps after some additional period of years we will have answers to these questions.

Meanwhile, recent surveys indicate that many (although not all) experts believe that testing for blood in the stool is not a cost-effective way to reduce deaths from that disease, yet in the final analysis it is still advocated as a place to start. The illness of President Reagan has made everyone aware of the more sophisticated tests for colon cancer, and most hospitals certainly experienced a greater demand for testing for colon cancer immediately after the President's illness. However, it is extremely costly and uncomfortable to follow up on positive stool examinations by doing these. Colonoscopy (passing a flexible tube into the bowel) or taking x-rays of the large bowel (barium enema) do not lend themselves to large-scale screening, nor will they ever be popular with those for whom they are recommended. Parenthetically, the tests are sufficiently uncomfortable that I do not know of many doctors who, with no symptoms, have these performed routinely on themselves or their families. Nonetheless, periodic colonoscopy is still recommended by ACS as a screening test to detect early colon cancer. The shortage of experienced examiners would make that impractical if everyone followed the advice, but apparently that takes care of itself since most will not. I agree that it is desirable to have colonoscopy done and would recommend it, particularly for those in high-risk groups (older people, and those with previous colon cancer, previous polyposis or ulcerative colitis). Examination of the colon with the flexible colonoscope is much more efficient than with the rigid sigmoidoscope, which only visualizes part of the large bowel (colon). A periodic rectal examination is certainly a more practical test since a surprisingly large number of colon cancers can be detected by means of such an examination. In fact, it used to be said that one-half to two-thirds of colon cancers could be felt by an experienced observer.

Unfortunately, relatively fewer of them now occur so close to the anus and the odds are not nearly that good. We do not know why the distribution of cancers appears to have changed so that a greater proportion are now located higher up in the colon.

MOUTH AND SKIN—THE "EASY" PROBLEMS One simple technique that is not used nearly enough in cancer screening is examination of the mouth for oral cancers. An experienced dental technician or dentist can quickly examine the tissues in the mouth for cancer or for a suspicious precancerous lesion. Ask your dentist to check you each time you go for a dental check-up. As discussed further in Chapter 8, *I predict that the growing use of chewing tobacco among young people will lead to an epidemic of oral cancers in coming years, and therefore screening programs must be made available to them.* (It would make sense to me if an added tax on tobacco went to pay for such health programs.) What is crucial is to pinpoint the target population of people who are especially at risk; in the case of oral cancers these are tobacco users (including smokers), heavy consumers of alcohol and those with poor oral hygiene. Unfortunately, some of these groups are characteristically difficult to reach with medical or educational programs—a problem very familiar to those conducting all other kinds of public health programs.

Careful self-examination of the skin for nonhealing sores or suspicious moles is something an individual can do to facilitate early diagnosis. This is particularly important for persons who have a fair complexion and who get considerable sun exposure (farmers, sailors, sun-worshipers, etc.). Ronald Reagan is a well-known survivor of skin cancer from this high-risk group.

There are three major types of skin cancer: basal cell carcinoma, squamous cell carcinoma and malignant melanoma. Basal cell carcinomas tend to be raised, clear growths on the skin, which may crust, ulcerate and sometimes bleed. They occur most often on the face and other exposed areas of the body. Squamous cell carcinomas are usually raised, pink growths just under the skin. They most often appear on sun-exposed areas of the body but, like basal cell carcinomas, may also appear elsewhere. Malignant melanomas are usually small brownish or black patches or lumps having an irregular outline. They may crust on the surface of the skin or bleed. Many of these melanomas may arise on preexisting moles such as on the hands, feet or face and back. The American Cancer Society has publications available that show some of these disorders in color, and of course a dermatologist is the one who is most familiar with the appearance of these types of conditions.

Screening for skin cancer is relatively new but it is eminently sensible. There are almost a half-million new cases reported annually in the United States, the vast majority (over 90 percent) of which are curable. The American Association of Dermatology and its 7,500 members have recently instituted free annual skin cancer screening for the public in hundreds of locations throughout the country. The first year of operation included 23,000 people and found one hundred malignant cases of skin cancers that were not previously treated.

CANCER DETECTION Cancer screening programs are sometimes called cancer "detection" programs. However, I prefer to think of cancer screening as widespread, relatively low-cost tests applicable to large populations, in which the specificity and cost-effectiveness of tests are the key ingredients, and of "detection" more in terms of direct physician-patient contact, in which case everything "reasonable" is done to find *all* kinds of cancer, more or less regardless of cost. Although the goals are similar, individualization of the approach is different. (This is not a standard definition, for many people use "screening" and "detection" interchangeably.) For example, a well-to-do executive can afford to pay for tests that cannot be justified on a public health cost-effectiveness basis. The concern of a particular individual may be so great that periodic colonoscopy is in order; in fact, it is advisable after a certain age. It might seem odd that someone would want to have such an uncomfortable and expensive procedure, yet if close relatives have had colon cancer, periodic colonoscopy would be reasonable to do, especially since this cancer is far more curable when detected early. Interestingly, President Reagan's brother had surgery for colon cancer just weeks before the President's illness.

Relatively new procedures such as mammography are still expensive for use in mass screening programs. But they are an important part of cancer *detection* for women who are in high-risk groups (i.e., over forty, family history of breast cancer, nonchildbearing). In our view mammography and other such cancer detection tests are part of good comprehensive health care, but they do involve more thought and planning by the doctor than a Pap test screening program, which is very inexpensive and cost-effective. Pelvic and rectal exams should be part of a regular checkup, as scheduled by you and your doctor, and a test of the stool should also be done on each such visit, because a positive test will be given follow-up attention and a negative test can be repeated at a later time. Also, a self-administered stool exam can then be followed up by laboratory tests or x-rays if necessary.

I strongly advocate that everyone have a thorough baseline evaluation by an internist or generalist who is particularly cognizant of preventive measures that can be taken for cancer and heart disease, and who will do a reasonable series of baseline tests including blood counts, urinalysis, chest x-ray and EKG. Then, if problems arise in the future, the physician can refer back to the norm for that individual. Such an evaluation also provides a fine opportunity to give cancer education about smoking, self-examination and other tips regarding health maintenance and stress avoidance. At the same time the evaluation can be used to detect other common ailments such as hypertension, diabetes, et cetera, at little added cost.

Thus, cancer prevention and early detection should ideally be part of a comprehensive medical program that first establishes the baseline for the individual young adult (age twenty to twenty-five) and follows with future workups that emphasize those areas that require attention—whether through periodic screening or more in-depth evaluation to follow up on specific problems (e.g., coughing up blood, blood in the stool, finding of a tumor mass). In this broad context I favor regular medical evaluations every year or two. Unfortunately, the cancer aspect of a general workup, as outlined above, is often given inadequate attention. Indeed, there is some merit in having a physician with a special interest in oncology as the person in charge of the evaluation, provided that the individual is also competent in comparable issues that affect the cardiovascular system.

Some may object to the distinction drawn here between tests suitable for mass screening and those specifically and selectively ordered by a thorough doctor for a concerned patient. Clearly the issue involves economics—what a person is willing to pay to detect disease at an earlier and presumably more curable stage. This economic distinction is made not because I advocate any such thing—indeed, it is unfortunate and unjust—but because I think it describes reality. And it may be only when such issues are made clear that a public, better informed and willing to express what it wants, will demand the earlier screening and insist on more equitable and affordable arrangements for the later, specialized detection. Nothing is free. There is no "free" comprehensive cancer detection program, any more than there is a free lunch. It seems timely to think through these medical-societal issues and see if we could do better with our resources in finding early cancers—I think we can. Certainly it is true that screening and subsequent early detection would save literally millions of dollars currently spent on prolonged treatments for "late" cancers.

The American Cancer Society has also publicized some of the major warning signals associated with cancer, and these are appropriately arranged to spell the word CAUTION.

Change in bowel or bladder habits.
A sore that does not heal.
Unusual bleeding or discharge.
Thickening or lump in breast or elsewhere.
Indigestion or difficulty in swallowing.
Obvious change in wart or mole.
Nagging cough or hoarseness.

I have covered some of these items in other ways, but they bear repeating, perhaps in a more personal way. A change in bowel habits usually means that if you are used to having a regular bowel movement almost daily and now begin to have problems with constipation for no known reason, or if the stools become narrower, say the width of a pencil, or if there is blood or black tarry-looking material in the stools without your having recently eaten beets or similar substance, then you should become suspicious. This is also true if you have a symptom called tenesmus, which means that having just finished having a bowel movement, you feel the urge to go again immediately. With respect to bladder habits, the reference is primarily to the presence of blood in the urine, which definitely needs to be checked if it occurs. Similarly, you need to pay attention to a sore that does not heal somewhere on the skin, such as on the face or hands, or a mole that ulcerates and bleeds anywhere on the body, including the scalp, genitalia, hands and feet. If a wart or mole begins to grow, change color or ulcerate, that also should cause you to see a physician. Unusual bleeding from any source is a caution, such as from bowels and bladder as already mentioned, but also from the sputum (not a simple nosebleed) or discharge from the nipple. A thickening or lump in the breast or elsewhere is self-explanatory, but to notice it implies that you have an awareness of how the area felt previously, and that is why regular breast or testicular self-examination is so important. Indigestion or difficulty in swallowing may be a sign of disease of the tube leading from the mouth to the stomach (esophagus) or anywhere in the upper gastrointestinal tract. A nagging or persistent cough or hoarseness is often due to bronchitis or to a benign disease, but bears checking, for it could be a warning signal that calls for a chest x-ray or other evaluation.

SUMMARY In summary, screening for and early detection of cancer are related but somewhat different issues because, as I use the terms, screening programs need to be justifiable for large population groups based on the cost of finding a curable cancer. *If the cost of a particular screening test is low, if the results are reliable, if the tumor it tests for is common and if the cure rate is high, then screening programs are ideal.* However, if a test is expensive, if the kind of cancer being tested for is rare (e.g., choriocarcinoma) or the kind of cancer is common but to find it early makes little difference to survival (e.g., lung cancer), then the test is unsuitable for screening large populations. Nevertheless, if an individual has the means (with or without insurance) and the desire to pursue even low-yield procedures for the sake of finding something useful, or if the person is in a high-risk group because of a strong family history, then I'm in favor of it and it should be arranged between the person and the doctor. Ideally this interaction should be part of the larger goal of health maintenance. The current status of screening tests for cancer is haphazard in this country, and there is a great deal of room for improvement if we wish to provide our citizens with the advantages of present-day medical science. We need to pull our health leaders, cancer experts, insurance people and legislators together and see what we should be doing for our people and how it can be paid for—bearing in mind the tremendous societal implications of failure to make early diagnosis.

MARIJUANA AND THC: FROM POT TO PRESCRIPTION

"Let the jury consider the verdict," the King said, for about the twentieth time that day. "No, no!" said the Queen. "Sentence first—verdict afterwards."
—LEWIS CARROLL, *Alice's Adventures in Wonderland*

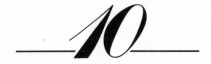

I used a similar title for an editorial written for the *Annals of Internal Medicine* to call attention to the peculiar problems of bringing tetrahydrocannabinol (THC) into the practice of medicine as an antiemetic drug to counteract the nausea and vomiting often caused by cancer chemotherapy. I was very much involved with research on THC, the active ingredient of marijuana, and it is of some interest to highlight the development of this substance, not because it is currently a major problem, but because it illustrates some of the peculiar (perhaps unique) circumstances that can arise in drug development. Marijuana itself comes from the Indian hemp plant, *Cannabis sativa.* The first record of its use was in 2737 B.C. by the Chinese Emperor Shen Nung; he termed the substance a "liberator of sin" and "delight giver." It was later used in the Middle East, where its acute toxic effects of loss of equilibrium and mental detachment were discovered—some think these may have given rise to the notion of "flying carpets" from the *Arabian Nights*. The first marijuana use in Western civilization appears to have been documented by Napoleon's generals (the relationship of that usage to the events at Waterloo is not a matter of record, however).

It is interesting that marijuana was listed as an approved medicinal in the U.S. pharmacopeia from 1850 until 1942, when it was removed as an approved agent; it has only very recently been resurrected, after it was discovered to have potent antiemetic effects. Research with this agent was greatly facilitated by the discovery and synthesis of its active ingredient, THC, in 1964 by an Israeli scientist, Dr. Mechoulam. Ironically, the son of another scientist (whom I will not identify), who specialized in studies on the effects of marijuana, was being treated with chemotherapy for cancer and he noticed that when he smoked pot he had much less nausea and vomiting, an observation not lost on his father. This was followed by a critical study by Drs. Sallan, Zinberg and Frei in Boston, who found that indeed THC reduced nausea and vomiting after chemotherapy. Shortly thereafter, we wrote a protocol to study this substance, not so much because we wanted to do research on this subject, but largely because it was only under research conditions that we could get THC for our patients who were suffering from severe nausea and vomiting—it was a serious medical problem for our patients and it required a solution. We were not aware at the time that the study of the connections between the vomiting center in the brain and the stomach and the musculature involved in vomiting would be as complicated and as interesting as it is, but that is another story.

Getting the approval and supplies of THC for our research program took eighteen months. We have a thick file of correspondence with various government agencies, each of which had to give its approval—literally a paper mountain. Indeed, the same obstacles had to be faced by any investigator in this country who wanted to study THC at that time or, for that matter, any other Schedule I drug—classified as such because they are alleged to be habituating and dangerous—such as an investigator studying heroin for relief of pain. The process of obtaining permission or licensing is almost prohibitively costly in effort and time. It is not comforting to realize that there never was a scientific reason to justify classifying marijuana or THC as a Schedule I drug. There was certainly no need to regulate its medicinal trials so tightly. A child could have obtained the drug illegally on any day in most schoolyards, but cancer patients could not get it until investigators went through this lengthy application process. Many potential investigators told me that they simply gave up because of the amount of time and effort involved. Nonetheless, we found THC quite successful in two-thirds of those patients who had failed to respond to other antiemetics—this was most worthwhile. This beneficial effect often made the difference between whether a patient would come back to receive potentially lifesaving chemotherapy, drop out of treatment entirely or, more commonly, delay chemotherapy treatments because of anxiety about their unpleasant effects. Occasional patients did experience temporary troublesome side effects from THC, typical of marijuana overdosage, and for them the THC was not an improvement even if it controlled their vomiting.

After publication of the initial reports from several institutions, including the National Cancer Institute, a blue-ribbon scientific panel of experts was asked for its opinion by the Department of Health, Education and Welfare (HEW). The experts agreed that THC was promising in the management of nausea and vomiting in patients with cancer and recommended its approval, but we understand that the then Secretary of HEW, Joseph Califano, overruled them, and this essentially stalled the treatment's development for a number of years. It is my conjecture that the government had so much invested in talking about the harmful effects of marijuana that it wanted to suppress *anything* that might give the opposite impression, regardless of the circumstances. Ultimately, several factors helped get approval in 1986 to market THC in this country. The first was that a growing number of investigators felt, as I did, that it was worth the effort to obtain this drug for their patients, and they managed to get approval for research protocols. Second, when the National Cancer Institute became convinced that this was an important addition to the supportive care of patients with cancer, they introduced a unique government-approved program in which they became the distributors of THC and provided it free to specially licensed pharmacies and individual physicians. This was an (unpublicized) act of kindness that cost the National Cancer Institute many millions of dollars that might have been spent for other purposes, but at least it provided an avenue for cancer patients to obtain THC legally. Still, the program probably reached only a fraction of the patients who might have benefited from use of THC.

Many patients of course obtained THC illegally. However, I learned from patients that some concerned law enforcement officers, such as local sheriffs in small communities in the South, were considerate enough to provide confiscated marijuana for medicinal use to cancer patients in their communities. To me this is a remarkable story in its own right, although not one that I could easily investigate—for obvious reasons. In contrast is the case of an idealistic but seriously misguided young general practitioner from the Outer Banks of North Carolina who was arrested at gunpoint by a platoon of state troopers dressed in camouflage while he was cultivating marijuana plants in his garden—he claimed he was planning to use the marijuana to treat nausea and vomiting in his cancer patients. He was prosecuted and sentenced by a judge in Manteo, North Carolina, which greatly damaged the career of this young man. Although he had shown rather poor judgment, he nevertheless argued pointedly through his attorney that the law had no right to interfere in the practice of medicine, given that the patient was in need of (and agreed to) the use of a substance that had been shown to be effective under research conditions. This was a really interesting constitutional issue, but it was never dealt with by the judge who, on a technicality, disallowed most of the expert testimony for the defense dealing with the effectiveness of marijuana or THC for this problem, and the physician was convicted based on the undisputed fact that he had broken the law. Having spent all of his money on his defense, and thoroughly disenchanted with the legal system in his case, the doctor decided not to appeal to a higher court, against the advice of his attorney.

10: Marijuana and THC: From Pot to Prescription

As studies of the efficacy of THC in preventing or minimizing nausea and vomiting continued to mount, the pressure grew to make this drug available to patients. At the same time, the National Cancer Institute did not want to remain responsible for providing the drug indefinitely. Pharmaceutical companies were invited to consider applying to license THC and to initiate the formal process that would lead to its marketing, if the tests of safety could be met. Since there was no competitive drug in the marketplace at that time, one might have expected that pharmaceutical companies would be eager to stand in line to be the first to offer such a product, but that was not at all the case. Indeed, no major U.S. pharmaceutical company was interested in taking on this product. Only a company based outside the United States, Unimed, made an effort to become a licensee at that time. The clinical development of the drug had already been completed, and Duke and several other institutions turned research records over to Unimed, without of course revealing patient identity. But even with the work largely accomplished, there were numerous legal, Food and Drug Administration (FDA), patent rights and manufacturing problems that delayed the marketing of the drug for many years after it should have been ready to prescribe to cancer patients. Our governmental procedures protected the cancer patient population all too well in this instance in a horrendous and mindless abuse of power; the system is in need of overhaul.

Why was no other pharmaceutical company interested in sponsoring this drug? There are several possible reasons. The most likely is that the drug was then classified as a Schedule I drug, which meant that unless it was reclassified as Schedule II (and that could not be predicted), its use would always be so restricted that even if it were commercially marketable, the number of physicians who would be eligible to use it would be few. Further, the precautions required of a pharmacy that handles a Schedule I drug make it necessary to invest in major capital equipment: all drugs must be locked in safes that are bolted to the floor to prevent theft, and accountability procedures are complex and carefully monitored by both state and federal drug enforcement agencies. Another factor may have been that the stigma of taking an illegal "drug" worries many patients to the point where they prefer to have the discomfort of nausea and vomiting, thus affecting sales. Finally, I have good reason to believe that some pharmaceutical companies avoided the matter altogether because they feared the government was so strongly opposed to marijuana that it would resist its licensing, resent its eventual licensing for medical uses and recall that resentment when the sponsoring company had other, unrelated dealings with the FDA.

Several pharmaceutical companies prepared synthetic derivatives of THC and entered them into clinical trials. One of these, Nabilone, is approved in Europe and Canada and its approval for marketing in the United States is supposedly imminent. I say "supposedly" because the approval situation has not changed in over two years and at this writing Nabilone is still not available except on a research basis. Nonetheless, these preparations seemed to have a far better chance of approval than THC because they were not initially treated as Schedule I drugs, although they have very similar results, so their eventual prescription use would be handled in the same way as are narcotics. THC was eventually handled the same way as well, but first it had to be "declassified" from Schedule I to Schedule II, which is a much harder road for a drug to travel than classifying it Schedule II from the beginning. There is surely no good reason to be more concerned about the safety, security and abuse of THC and its derivatives than there is about narcotics that physicians use for pain control, which are Schedule II—indeed, the reverse is true.

There are several curious little side chapters to this drama. An organization called NORML, the National Organization for Reform of Marijuana Laws, has waged a long and vigorous lobbying campaign to legalize marijuana because of its purported medicinal effects; NORML claims it helps not only nausea and vomiting, but also relieves pressure in the eyes of glaucoma patients. The organization fought hard for legalization of marijuana, yet its members seemed to oppose the licensing of THC, probably because they feared that once the FDA had approved a pure marijuana derivative (marijuana being exceedingly impure) there would be no reason for governmental agencies to respond to their petition to license raw marijuana—their drug of preference. The debate about whether marijuana has useful properties over and above those of THC has not been resolved, nor has the role of either of these drugs in management of glaucoma, although a number of patients are quite certain that marijuana has helped them when other drugs have failed. One would think that these controversies would be resolved by proper clinical experimentation and not by courts of law or regulatory agencies—it is part of the Alice in Wonderland aspect of the story of THC that debate rather than experiment is used to deal with these questions.

Ironically, now that THC has recently been marketed by Roxane Laboratories, who purchased rights to it as an antiemetic medication from Unimed, the many years of delay have provided time for development of numerous antiemetics that may be equally (or even more) effective for certain chemotherapy drugs, thus making THC less important to us today than when no alternative drugs existed. This was a sad chapter in our history, in which the very federal agencies that were designed to protect us were in fact interfering with access to the best medical care. I hope such a series of events never occurs again, but nothing fundamental has changed, and this is one of the things that drives patients out of the United States or outside of the law to obtain certain medications. We need a careful and dispassionate review of such problems to determine how the public need and trust can best be served and then to instruct the regulatory agencies accordingly. That is how I would interpret the description of government of the people, by the people and for the people.

CANCER AND AIDS: A DOUBLE WHAMMY

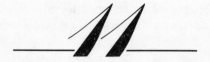

THE CLINICAL SYNDROME AND ITS CAUSES In the cartoon strip "Li'l Abner," Al Capp created the character of Mr. Bfystyk, a little man who walks through life with a black cloud perpetually over his head, symbolizing the misfortune that follows him everywhere. That image comes to mind when I think of the unfortunate people who have both cancer and acquired immunodeficiency syndrome (AIDS). Unlike cancer, which was known in antiquity, AIDS is a newly discovered syndrome, and its incidence is rising in epidemic proportions. As of July 1987 the Centers for Disease Control (CDC) in Atlanta had records of 45,000 U.S. cases of AIDS and 26,000 deaths. Still these are small numbers compared to cancer. What is more alarming, the number of cases continues to increase rapidly. One staggering estimate is that even if there were no more new infections as of 1987 there would be about 200,000

11: Cancer and AIDS: A Double Whammy

AIDS cases and over 50,000 deaths in 1991, based on the number of people (1.5 million) who are currently infected with the virus.

In a study published in *Science,* Dr. James Curran and coworkers point out that for single men aged twenty-five to forty-four living in Manhattan and San Francisco, AIDS is the leading cause of premature mortality as measured by years of potential life lost. Figure 13 illustrates the incidence of cases as projected through 1986; and the geometric increase has not yet begun to plateau. Other estimates corroborate this view: 35,000 cases were diagnosed in the first five years of the AIDS epidemic, and the Public Health Service estimates that 235,000 new cases will occur in the next five years. Within five years the cost of medical care alone for these patients will be in the neighborhood of $15 *billion.* Furthermore, the disease is worldwide. In the United States, AIDS was originally described as occurring predominantly in three groups of people, characterized as the H's—*h*omosexual men (73 percent), intravenous *h*eroin drug users (17 percent) and *h*emophiliacs (1

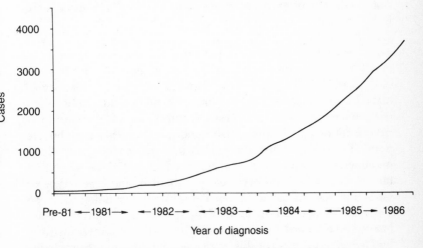

Figure 13 The incidence of AIDS in the United States, with projections through 1986. Note that the curve continues to rise and has not yet reached its plateau, or peak incidence. (Adapted from J. W. Curran, et al., *Science* 229 [1985]: 1352; copyright 1985 by the AAAS)

percent). It also occurs frequently among *H*aitians, possibly because many of the afflicted men had served as prostitutes for gay men. Now the shadow of the disease is extending outward to include heterosexual contacts of bisexual men, heterosexual and homosexual partners of I.V. drug users, female prostitutes, offspring of affected mothers, occasional transfusion recipients and, very recently, even a group of cancer patients who received a very dubious remedy in which the serum was apparently contaminated with both hepatitis B and the virus associated with AIDS. (It is a grim irony that some patients who were being treated in this way for cancer were infected with AIDS and/or hepatitis B virus—the black cloud again!) I know of a hemophiliac who acquired AIDS virus from a contaminated batch of clotting factor and then passed it to his wife who passed it on to their infant son, presumably by intrauterine exposure. And now we have to face the reality that the risk for getting AIDS is present in heterosexual contact with a partner infected with the virus—there is heterosexual as well as homosexual transmission, in other words. A new study has shown that if either partner in a marriage contracts the AIDS virus, there is a 50 percent chance of the other partner's acquiring it also. This is of great concern among servicemen in Germany and Italy who get infected from prostitutes and bring the infection home.

AIDS is a profound and devastating disease of the immune system in which certain key elements of blood lymphocytes (called T-lymphocytes) are qualitatively and quantitatively defective, which renders the person susceptible to so-called opportunistic infections (see below). Also abnormal are other lymphocyte populations (called B-cells and natural killer cells) and blood monocytes. During the few years in which AIDS has spread its terror, a great deal has been learned about it, and a new type of virus that appears to be responsible for its transmission has been isolated. Discovered both at the Pasteur Institute in Paris by a team headed by Dr. Luc Montanier and at the National Cancer Institute by Dr. Robert Gallo and his associates, this strain of human immunodeficiency virus (HIV-III) is closely related to another HIV strain (I) that is known to cause an unusual form of leukemia arising from the T-lymphocyte population of cells. Actually there are now at least three strains of virus known to cause AIDS and another one that infects people in Africa but seems not to cause this disease. What is most remarkable is that some of the most important research on AIDS has been performed by cancer researchers, probably because they discovered a viral cause for T-cell leukemia, seemingly another new disease, which is caused by a novel virus closely related to the one that causes AIDS. Thus these investigators were all primed for discovery due to the convergent causes of these conditions.

Are these really new diseases or are we just learning to identify them? As far as AIDS is concerned, it may have existed in Africa for a time but it is clearly a new disease in the rest of the world. The AIDS-causing virus is very similar to the green monkey virus in Africa, which has crossed the species lines to infect people, often prostitutes, although it does not cause AIDS. A virulent change (mutation) in the virus is probably what has triggered the AIDS epidemic, the latest plague to affect the human race. Curiously, this became a political problem in that African nations, such as Uganda, Zambia, Zaire and Rwanda, were denying that they had a problem with this disease, fearing that it would discourage tourism and hurt their economies. One can consider this a form of genocide, regardless of their motives. Previously they had withdrawn their participation in international scientific meetings, presumably for these political reasons. This was unfortunate for many reasons but especially because African AIDS differs in significant ways from the disease with which we have become all too familiar. It seems to affect men and women in equal numbers and is predominantly spread by heterosexual transmission. It is now clear that exposure to the AIDS virus has occurred throughout Africa, with estimates in prostitutes varying from 27 percent (Zaire) to 88 percent (Rwanda). Very recently the embargo on information seems to have been lifted, and this is a welcome development. They once again join the community of nations concerned with problems of world health.

Once a person is infected, the virus circulates throughout the body and infects the lymphocytes; now the patient has a condition that is called pre-AIDS, in which he has minimal or no symptoms but is infectious to others. Then there is AIDS-related complex (ARC), in which the diagnosis can be made by testing the blood, but the patient has only a mild version of immune suppression with loss of energy, weight loss, swollen lymph glands and fever. At any given time there are many more people who are in the waiting-pattern of pre-AIDS (perhaps 1.5 million people at present), than there are with ARC (about 100,000) or who have the frank manifestations of AIDS (13,000 cases as of this writing). How long the disease remains in the pre-AIDS or ARC state is not known at this time. Nor do we know whether the progression to the clinical manifestations of AIDS is inevitable. Fortunately, there is now a blood-screening test that can eliminate the risk of transfusing infected blood products, at least from licensed blood banks. However, serious blood shortages have resulted because of fear and confusion—some people even have the erroneous notion that one can contract AIDS by giving blood. It continues to be important for us to give blood to the Red Cross as often as possible to help our friends and neighbors, and ourselves in turn.

The peculiarity of this viral infection, which is transmitted (as far as we know) only by close sexual contact or by blood contamination, is that it paralyzes the immune system and renders the individual vulnerable to infections of all kinds, including some that almost never affect healthy individuals and may be found to infect only animals or are bacteria or fungi ordinarily found only in soil. The organisms that lead to "opportunistic infections" that endanger AIDS patients include parasites, fungi, bacteria and viruses—often more than one at a time. It also infects the brain and can cause major brain damage in its later stages. (AIDS can also socially paralyze communities with fear, as with parents' boycotts of schools in New York City and elsewhere when young AIDS victims are permitted to remain in school.) Many AIDS patients also have a tendency to develop various forms of cancer; particularly common among them is an otherwise rare form of cancer called Kaposi's sarcoma, which is a cancer of blood vessel tissues. It is noticeable in numerous areas of the skin, but it also affects internal organs such as the liver. Kaposi's sarcoma is generally a rapidly growing malignancy in these patients—if they do not succumb to infection, they will succumb to widespread malignancy. Malignant lymphoma is another form of cancer that is seen frequently in AIDS patients.

TREATMENT Neither AIDS nor Kaposi's sarcoma is particularly susceptible to treatments available today, but Kaposi's sarcoma will, at least temporarily, respond to a variety of chemotherapeutic drugs as well as to interferon. Interferon is particularly interesting in that it is not only an anticancer substance, but also an antiviral substance. If the HIV-III virus is causing the cancer, or at least causing such a profound deficiency in the immune system that the cancer can spread rapidly, an antiviral drug, at least theoretically, might slow or prevent the growth of the cancer. And indeed, the work at a number of institutions indicates that some 20 to 40 percent of patients with Kaposi's sarcoma and AIDS will respond temporarily to interferon, but then the disease returns and the interferon is no longer effective. Also, it is disappointing that interferon has not helped these patients to become resistant to either the AIDS virus or the other viruses to which they are susceptible. Clearly AIDS patients are missing more in their antiviral resistance than just interferon. And, indeed, a number of missing factors have been described, and these will shortly be tested in AIDS patients. Chemotherapy used for other cancers is also used for Kaposi's sarcoma patients, with about the same response rate as for interferon, but again the disease will return. There have been no permanent cures.

A small number of other drugs are also being tested in AIDS patients. Among these are antiviral drugs such as HPA-23, which inhibits an enzyme important to the virus; Suramin; Ribavirin; Foscornet and other drugs that may stimulate the immune response, such as interleukin-2 and several others. Azidothymidine (called AZT) is the most promising of the new drugs. It is of considerable interest because it is so effective in inhibiting the virus in tissue culture and, most importantly, it is the first drug that improves the survival of treated AIDS patients. It was recently approved for marketing for certain types of AIDS patients. We still have much to learn about its use.

We recognize that the homosexual community is in a state of panic over this situation, and rumors of miracle drugs are spreading through the grapevine. The heterosexual community's panic is rapidly spreading. There may be insidious social effects if blood screening for jobs, for instance, becomes required. However, we may be quite certain that anyone who finds a cure will not keep it a secret. Efforts at disease prevention, by "safe sex" methods and education about dirty needles, are being expedited in the gay community, and these are most important of course.

Ideally we would like to find a vaccine against this virus, and many excellent scientists are working hard toward that goal.

IMMUNITY AND CANCER The convergence of cancer and AIDS is terrible for the patient but from a scientific point of view we stand to learn a great deal from it about how a normal state of immunity serves to impede the growth of common cancers. Some years ago Sir MacFarlane Burnett speculated that some cells, even in healthy people, constantly undergo malignant transformation and that this process becomes more frequent as people age. However, normal defense mechanisms recognize a transformed cell as a "foreign" cell and destroy it before it begins dividing into a tumor. This theory has been neither proven nor disproven, but clearly our experience with patients who are immunodeficient shows that their tumors grow rapidly. This also happens in people who take chemotherapy to suppress the immune response so that they will not reject transplanted organs such as kidney grafts from relatives (other than identical twins). Earlier we were puzzled to find that patients who had been given transplanted kidneys would develop unusual kinds of cancers, such as lymphomas, at a rate far in excess of what would be expected in the normal population. We know now that the drugs used to suppress the ability of the patient to reject the transplanted kidney will also depress the immune response, in a manner somewhat like AIDS.

These discoveries remind me of some experiments we did thirty years ago when Dr. Dean Burk and I injected mice first with tumor cells and then with chemotherapeutic drugs and showed that the drugs killed the tumor cells. If, however, we injected the chemotherapeutic drugs shortly before injecting the tumor cells, the tumors grew more rapidly than they would if no drugs were given at all—demonstrating that potent drugs could reduce the animal's natural resistance if the timing was inappropriate. As discussed elsewhere, chemotherapeutic drugs used to cure certain types of cancers or to suppress immunity for purposes of organ transplantation may predispose patients to a higher incidence of cancers such as leukemias or lymphomas, again indicating that a partial paralysis of the normal defense mechanism could be a contributing factor in the development of cancer.

The virus that causes leukemia in cats also inhibits their immunity, much as does the AIDS virus. The ability to paralyze the central lymphocytes involved in the immune process may be a common property of such viruses.

Now that the HIV-III virus has been found, a great deal of work is being done to develop a vaccine, like that for cat leukemia virus, that will prevent AIDS and presumably also the cancers that are found in AIDS patients. Whether the efforts will be successful or not is unknown at present. For some viruses it is possible to make an effective vaccine, but other viruses are much more adaptable and can change their surface characteristics so much that they are not destroyed by viral antibodies. Unfortunately there are reasons to believe that the AIDS virus may fall into the latter category; still, the prospect of having one or more vaccines for these strains of viruses is very exciting, because they might work to prevent the disease.

Indeed, at this time we know of sixteen different strains of the HIV-III virus that have been isolated from patients who have AIDS. This is very reminiscent of the situation with influenza, where there are many different strains of flu virus. This poses a serious problem because it is possible to develop a vaccine against only one strain at a time, and not against all the different types within that virus family. Nonetheless, there may well be a common chemical region that is shared by all of these AIDS-causing viruses, and if that is the case, it may be possible to develop a vaccine. Dr. Gallo has found some common components on the envelope proteins of all these strains and it is against these that vaccines will be attempted for the purpose of causing immunity.

SERENDIPITY—PREPARING FOR LUCK It is amazing how much has been learned in such a short time about this (presumably) new disease. As mentioned earlier, the discoveries have come largely from cancer researchers from the National Cancer Institute who were working on other problems that turned out to be relevant to AIDS as well. This is an excellent illustration of the universal nature of science, and it also shows the beneficial effects of cancer research in other areas. This is a very important point to understand. There are many other examples of this—cancer researchers at Burroughs Wellcome developed drugs that were intended to suppress cancer but turned out also to be very effective in preventing graft rejection of kidneys, enabling the field of organ transplantation to proceed. Now they have developed chemotherapy against viruses—acyclovir against herpes and AZT against AIDS. They also developed a drug for leukemia that also lowered the level of uric acid in the blood; my former chief and colleague Dr. R. Wayne Rundles found this to be the most effective treatment known for gout, because the abnormal deposits of uric acid in the joints (tophi) could be melted away during weeks and months of treatment.

Much of what is known in the field of immunology was an outgrowth of work by many cancer researchers, and that knowledge is now being applied to many types of allergic diseases. By the same token, many of the advances that have proven useful in cancer research were made by people working primarily in other areas, such as biochemistry, genetics, anatomy, endocrinology, et cetera.

In reflecting on this fact some years ago, Dr. Howard Skipper, in his address to the American Association for Cancer Research, poked good-natured fun at the narrow way in which many scientists are trained and pointed out that it takes all kinds of different talents to make the great unexpected discoveries, because "nature is not trained as we are." This universality of science is also worth remembering because at times there is bickering over whether too much money is being spent in one area of science or another; it is more important to support excellent science than to be concerned about what it is called. The cure of AIDS, if and when it comes, will be testimony to that principle.

ON REDUCING THE ENORMOUS
ECONOMIC BURDEN OF CANCER:
PERSONAL AND NATIONAL

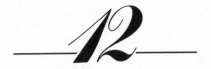

OVERVIEW It is hard enough for the individual afflicted with it to face the physical and emotional impact of cancer. But how can we deal with the additional staggering financial burden that often goes with this illness? *And what can you do* as a potential patient, family member or friend of a patient, or as a responsible member of a society that likes to think of itself as a caring social network? In this chapter I will give you information and some suggestions and options that I hope will help you decide soon—and not after the fact. And for practical purposes we had best assume that at some time, like it or not, you may well have to be involved.

In 1983 this nation spent over $350 billion on health care, in excess of $1,500 for every man, woman and child. By 1987 health care expenditures had risen to $511 billion or 11.4% of the gross national product. More than a month of work is required to pay for health care in one way or another; cancer ranks third behind circulatory diseases and injuries as a contributor of these staggering costs. The costs of cancer in our country are difficult to measure and difficult to define, and estimates vary widely depending upon which factors are considered. The most obvious costs are the out-of-pocket expenses for hospitalization and outpatient treatment, nursing home care, doctor bills, drug costs, rehabilitation care (including prosthetic devices), rental of home care equipment such as hospital beds and oxygen, et cetera.

In addition to these direct medical expenditures, there are indirect costs of cancer to the patient and family, such as travel expenses to and from medical care facilities, having to arrange for family members to accompany the patient during hospitalizations or for clinic visits, child care and the like. Another huge cost is the loss of earnings due to those illnesses we collectively call cancer—earnings that are lost because of the premature death or medical disability of the wage earner. The total figure is estimated at some $26 billion in 1977 dollars—much more in today's dollars. The majority (92 percent) of the earning losses are due to premature death.

Sometimes the losses are far out of proportion to the frequency of the disease. For example, although cancer of the respiratory organs (predominantly the lung) is of course the largest cause of lost earnings, cancers of the lymph glands and blood-forming tissues, such as lymphomas and leukemias, represent approximately half as much in lost earnings even though their frequency is considerably less. The reason is that the patients afflicted are much younger and would therefore have a longer earning capacity had they lived as wage earners.

Another way of looking at the cost of cancer is to compare its impact to that of heart disease, stroke or accidents, by checking the number of deaths, the years of life that are lost per death and the lost earnings per death. Cancer is a close second to heart disease in the number of deaths, second to accidents in years of life lost, and second to accidents in earnings lost per death.

WHAT CAN WE DO TO HELP REDUCE COSTS? Before we analyze further the national problem of these staggering costs, let

12: On Reducing the Enormous Economic Burden of Cancer

us look at what patients and their physicians can do to minimize the financial drain on the afflicted person and family.

Clearly it is expensive to have cancer, and some cancers are far more expensive than others. Costs vary widely depending on where the patient lives, whether the patient is cared for in a community hospital or a university hospital and whether or not the physician believes in treating cancer aggressively at all costs. Very few people can "afford" to have acute leukemia, although obviously we have no choice in the matter; the cost of care for an adult with leukemia is in the neighborhood of $100,000 over the course of one or two years. At the other extreme are skin cancer—a noninvasive melanoma—or cervical cancer. These can be relatively inexpensive to remove.

Health insurance is another variable. Some policies pay most of the bills while others have a cutoff figure beyond which the patient receives no further coverage; still others may limit coverage to a particular amount in any given year. Because the costs of our illnesses do not necessarily correspond with the benefits of any particular insurance policy, more and more people are buying policies specifically designed for expensive diseases such as cancer. Is that necessary or desirable? Although I am not an expert on these business matters, here are some practical suggestions that you might wish to consider concerning your insurance policy. These have been learned by the experience of other patients and our hospital business office. As with all such matters, it is best to plan well in advance, because once cancer strikes it is too late to make a change.

1   The most important point about any type of insurance contract is to be sure to read the "fine print" and find out what the policy will and will not cover. Most people (and I include myself) rarely check this out for any type of contract that we sign—so you must make a conscious decision not to put it off any longer. Do it now!—and ask yourself questions about hypothetical situations that could happen to you and see if you can find the answer. If you cannot, either you missed seeing it or that situation is not covered. Find out which it is by asking your insurance agent or employee benefits officer.

2   *Be sure that your insurance policy has major medical coverage.* It is not important for the policy to cover every small health bill, but it is obviously important that it cover major medical illnesses such as cancer, in which the bills can be extremely high. To help reduce the costs of coverage it is often useful to have a substantial deductible so that the costs of smaller bills are not passed on to the insurance company. Remember that it costs the company about the same amount of work to process a small claim as it does a large one, and your premium pays for the company's costs plus profit. The same principles apply to automobile insurance—it is less expensive for you to have a higher deductible and to pay the $50 charge for repair of a dent than to have all expenses covered and have the company pay. I'll say more about this later.

3   Be sure that you have a supplemental policy that has a feature that will also cover drugs and other expenses that you may have at home. Many insurance companies do not routinely cover these kinds of expenses.

4   Once you are eligible for Medicare you will still need a supplemental policy to help defray those costs that Medicare doesn't cover, particularly professional fees. It is advisable to buy a supplemental policy under a large group plan or to continue on the policy that you have when you retire. You do not need a series of supplemental policies; one good one will usually suffice. I know of elderly people who can barely afford to buy their groceries who own six or more supplemental insurance policies because they were frightened by some (questionable) television advertising. (Those who work for the federal government don't need Medicare, but the rest of us do.)

5   Medicare and other insurance policies have a statement to the effect that *they cover a certain percentage of "usual and customary charges."* Most people do not understand that insurance companies establish these charges by looking at the financial records of several institutions and determining a usual fee for a particular service; then they will pay only their required percentage of that average *no matter what the actual charge.* It is

a little like trading in your beautifully kept ten-year-old car and finding that the dealer looks in a well-worn little black book and tells you that it is almost worthless. With respect to professional bills, for example, if your doctor bill is $600 but the usual and customary charge for that service according to your insurer's version of the "little black book" is $400, then the insurance company will pay only the percentage, say 80 percent of the $400 ($320) and not of the $600, and you are out the difference ($280). In most cases the supplement will pay only the 20 percent of $400 and not the difference between the $400 and $600. Thus, if different doctors have different charges for the same service, the amount you will be reimbursed by the insurance company depends not on the amount of the bill that you receive, but rather on *what the company has determined is a usual and customary charge.* This is also true for Medicare insurance. The implications of this are quite profound because insurance companies are very democratic—they consider all doctors who render a given service to be equal! I happen to think that it is appropriate for an expert in a field to charge more than a recent medical graduate, just as a top music teacher charges more for lessons than does the average one in a community. However, the patient will have to pay extra for that luxury, if you call it that. More and more often, such financial issues are governing the practice of medicine—but more on that later. There are special cancer policies, which are understandably quite popular, but of course they do not cover you for other diseases that can be just as expensive. By and large, however, a major medical insurance policy will offer equal coverage if you have taken care to purchase a supplemental policy. If you do have a cancer policy, you should be aware that most such policies require a pathologist's report to certify the diagnosis of cancer. This means that if you are diagnosed as having cancer, you must have this report in order to back up your insurance claim. When you read that in the fine print, it seems reasonable enough, and usually it is. However, it can have peculiar ramifications sometimes, as in the case of a recent patient who was operated on at our hospital for suspected lung cancer. When the chest was opened by an excellent surgeon the cancer was so widespread that he did nothing but close the chest and complete the operation as quickly as possible. He did not take a biopsy and do the pathology because he decided that the diagnosis was quite evident. *Since there was no pathology report, the insurance company that had sold the cancer policy refused payment to the patient for all related claims.* Do you think that was wrong? Well, the family did—they sued the company and found that the position of the company was legal. That is not to say that the company would refuse to pay any and all claims that met their eligibility criteria—which takes us back to the need to be well informed, to read the fine print and to ask questions if you do not understand something.

More than half the total health costs of an individual with cancer are spent in the last six months of life, but of course we cannot often know in advance when this will occur. This may pose a painful dilemma, as illustrated by the following example. Suppose you had worked all your life to save $100,000 in property and other equities that you were planning to leave to your children and other family. Then you were unexpectedly faced with an illness from which no one had ever been cured. By spending an additional $100,000 for the full course of aggressive treatment, however, you might live twelve months instead of four, but in the process you would deplete all your savings—what would you want to do? I am not sure I know how to answer that for myself.

Patients usually are not given that alternative because everything happens too quickly and they are engulfed by a maelstrom of events—going through expensive diagnostic tests and hospitalization, learning of the dread diagnosis and facing prompt initiation of very costly therapies, whether medical, surgical, radiotherapeutic or combinations of all three. In the press of these weighty issues finances are usually not considered until much later. And furthermore, often there is no certain prediction as to which will be the last six months of life until all treatment has failed, and that of course makes it harder to plan.

12: On Reducing the Enormous Economic Burden of Cancer

THE BILL As you receive your medical care you will periodically be presented with various versions of THE BILL. We have moved a long way from the simple fee structure of yesteryear, as quaintly illustrated in Table 6. Unless you are a graduate of a business school or have some equivalent practical experience, trying to understand THE BILL may bring you to your knees! Why is it that the average person, a college graduate, even a physician cannot understand a simple little matter like a hospital bill? I am probably not the right person to write this section because I too need help in figuring out our hospital bills. After many years of bewildered observation of this scene, I have to conclude that THE BILL is constructed for the benefit of the hospital, for it is certainly not for your or my convenience. You thought your insurance covered most of the items for which you are being billed, didn't you? So why are you now being asked to pay by the hospital or why, later, is the insurance company denying your claim?

There are so many possible answers to these questions that we cannot give more than a glimpse into them—for they need to be sorted out on an individual basis. But here are some bits of advice. The hospital bills you promptly, whether or not they give you some, all or no credit for your insurance coverage. The hospital's presumption is that since you are the one who received the services, and since the hospital is not 100 percent certain of its ability to recover payment from your insurance carrier, why not send you both a bill? Indeed, there are circumstances in which your insurance company will refuse to pay—again, this depends on what the service is called and on the fine print. If the doctor puts the wrong terms on a discharge form, this can lead to disallowance of your entire claim. Although you need not pay what your insurance will cover, if you do pay, you will eventually be reimbursed. But meanwhile the hospital has the use of your money, interest-free of course, to help with its cash-flow problem. (Hospitals always have a serious cash-flow problem, by the way, because they are slow to be paid for their very real expenses incurred in patient care.) So do not pay until you talk to the person in the business office whose name appears on your bill—and be sure you understand what is being done. Do not pay until your insurance company pays its part, and then pay the balance promptly so as not

Table 6 *Physicians' Rates: Easton, Talbot County, Maryland, 1876*

For a first visit in the Towns or Villages in which we respectively reside	$ 1.50
For any distance in the country not exceeding one mile	1.87½
From one to three miles	3.00
From three to six miles	3.75
From six to nine miles	4.50
From nine to twelve miles	7.50
From twelve to fifteen miles	9.00
For a night visit, double the above rates	
For twelve hours' attendance in the day time	10.00
For a night's attendance	4.00
For riding in a storm or rain, double the above rates	
For a Consultation	5.00
Subsequent consultation fee	5.00
For extracting a tooth	1.00
For bleeding	.50
For reducing a Fracture or Luxation	14.00
For performing any of the capital operations, from 50.00 to	100.00
For Tapping	5.00
For any of the lesser operations with pocket instruments, from 1.00 to	2.00
For dressing Ulcers, from .50 to	1.00
For applying a bandage where no other operation is performed, from 1.00 to	2.00
For introducing a Catheter	5.00
For delivering a woman, in a natural labor	10.00
For a preternatural or instrumental delivery	14.00
For a Recipe	1.00
For a Recipe, with written directions, from 2.00 to	5.00
For compounding prescription in families where they keep their own medicines, from .25 to	1.00
For administering an Enema, from 1.00 to	2.00
Vaccination, exclusive of visit	1.00
Leeching, each leech, from 1.00 to	2.00

Source: Reprinted through the courtesy of Alice B. Nily of Nily Realty Inc. in Easton, MD.

to incur a service charge. Or if you do not understand the situation clearly, pay only a small portion of your bill—that will usually forestall a visit from a collection agency until things are sorted out. This is just my personal advice—this course of action probably would not be recommended to you by the hospital business office, but it is a stalling strategy that often works. Another surprise for you is that the big hospital bill you received does not cover the professional charges, surgical and anesthetist fees, consultants' fees, payment for radiologists who interpret the x-rays, et cetera. Don't worry, you will see that bill soon enough too.

Suppose the insurance company denies some or all of your claim—what do you do then? Do not assume that they are right and you are wrong—I think they often count on that response. Large insurance companies are usually very impersonal and difficult to deal with for various reasons. One reason is that they may employ some clerks who do not know their business—and this can potentially be very costly to you if you stop there. Go to the supervisor for clarification if you are not satisfied and/or go back to the hospital business office for advice. We often find that an individual can be quite frustrated by struggling with the system, whereas our hospital business office can call on your behalf and straighten out the matter in a few minutes. Many people give up and pay bills they should not be responsible for, either out of ignorance or out of frustration. That decision represents a nice profit for the insurance company. You need not feel obliged to contribute—you probably already gave at the office.

If you look closely at the items on THE BILL, you may wonder why an aspirin tablet can cost $2 and a blood count $30 (it costs half that amount at your doctor's office), whereas the room rate is relatively low. Here you can really get confused because it turns out that reasonable rates bear little relationship to the hospital's expenses. That does not make sense, but then the system is bigger than both of us! Let me briefly try to explain this absurd method of bookkeeping. Certain items are regulated according to the reimbursement formulas mentioned earlier whereas others are not. A university hospital is far more costly to operate than a community hospital yet the room rates need to be similar or people will go only to the cheaper hospital. The room rates are usually published in the newspaper and are therefore widely visible to those who are cost conscious. If the university hospital loses money on its daily, or per diem, bed rate, it has to make up the loss in other areas. Those areas are the Pharmacy, Laboratory and Radiology. I can send blood to outside laboratories who do good quality work but charge only half or a third the cost at the university hospital—in part because they have a much lower overhead. That means that their charges reflect their costs plus profit—they obviously do not need to pay for losses (if any) on hospital per diem or for the indigent patients who cannot afford to pay their large emergency room or hospital bills. But if I do send the tests out, then other charges to my patient will have to be raised to offset that substantial loss of income. So some of the funny bookkeeping is to keep up the appearance of being competitive in price, some is because of reimbursement restrictions, and some is due to a Robin Hood effect, whereby the well-to-do pay more than their share to offset major hospital losses on those patients who cannot pay. This is a real social problem because some highly efficient private institutions who refuse to treat unless you can pass the "green test" will offer services for less, but they leave complicated and indigent patients for other hospitals to lose money on. In the final analysis hospitals do have to have a balanced budget or they close—and then the community as a whole may really suffer.

There have been years when Duke Hospital had over $30 million in uncollectible bills—yet as a private hospital without a state subsidy the hospital obviously needs to balance the budget each year. More and more patients have to pay in advance. And is the system understandable to the layman? No. Is it fair? Given the external constraints of insurance and governmental regulation I would say that it is as fair as we know how to make it. But I am very worried about whether poor people can find the care that they need in this country under the present system.

WHAT THE DOCTOR CAN DO TO REDUCE COSTS Understandably the first concern of any patient is with the accuracy of the diagnosis; once that is certain, the patient wants to get well, by means of whatever therapy affords the best possible quality of life. Patients often assume that once the treatments are done, their previous state of health will be restored and they will once again become productive members of society. In some cases this assumption is justified and in some cases it is not; the patient is not always aware in advance of the outcome. Furthermore, many, if not most, physicians will do everything possible to extend a life regardless of whether the patient will be able to resume former activities and be able to handle the bills without being financially drained. This is not intended as a criticism, for such doctors will justify their medical "full-court press" in terms of not putting a pricetag on a human life. Indeed, it may be virtually impossible to avoid financial hemorrhage if the patient wants everything done to preserve life. At the time of this writing I am caring for a young man who is now dying of leukemia after seven good years, during which the expenses were minimal. However, in the past three weeks alone the costs of maintaining his life have exceeded $90,000—he has had emergency surgery, massive amounts of blood products and hospitalization in an intensive care unit. This is not what (I think) I would want for myself, nor is it in the best interest of society, but this is what he and his family want, even though they know there is no chance for recovery. My task, as his physician, is to do the best that I can to meet his wishes. Who pays for this? He is fortunate to have an exceptionally good insurance policy. Clearly, the insurance rates have to account for these experiences on the part of policy holders, but not everyone can afford the privilege of being covered for such contingencies. What would happen if his insurance coverage ran out at $25,000? Then the estate or the family would end up with a huge bill or the hospital might take a big loss; in the latter case, the loss would have to be passed on to other patients through increased room rates or other charges.

If financial matters concern the patient, and usually they do, they should be discussed with the physician and/or with a representative of the business office. It should go without saying that doctors attempt to conserve patient resources, but so many other factors enter into their decisions that sometimes, unless the patient makes it known that cost is a big problem, the doctor may not stop to think about which of two tests (equivalent in value but different in price) should be used, which treatment to choose if finances are a problem, how many x-rays are absolutely necessary to prove the extent of the disease, et cetera. The new federal regulations on Medicare reimbursement and cost-cutting measures and the private insurance sector have both made doctors more conscious of costs than ever before, but the patient must be a part of the decision-making process as well. The issues cut both ways—if my insurance company were willing to pay for only five days of hospitalization for a given problem and the hospital wanted to discharge me at five days but I felt too sick to go home, perhaps I would be willing to pay personally to stay in the hospital beyond the prescribed period of time—certainly I would if I could afford it.

What can the patient do to help reduce costs? Sometimes the specialist who is caring for the patient works in a different city and the visits involve an expensive commute, possibly loss of a day of work to go to the clinic and perhaps higher costs for all services at the referral or tertiary care center. The patient can ask whether the personal physician in the local community can do some of the work so the patient does not have to go back and forth for everything—in other words, the patient uses the specialists on less frequent visits, those that involve major management decisions. Be sure to ask each of your doctors whether they are in contact with the other and whether they have the records of your most recent visit. Patients can facilitate communication by offering to carry records, x-rays and slides in order to get them to another doctor in a timely fashion. I would rather trust the patient than the mail to carry the vital records anytime!

Doctors, of course, can do a great deal to facilitate cost cutting by encouraging patients to receive some of their health care in the home community, preferably on an outpatient or even home basis. My patients usually receive the majority of their chemotherapy in the office of their personal physician; they receive blood transfusions there if they need them; and they may be treated in the community hospital for complications, not only because the services are cheaper and more convenient but because they can be rendered just as effectively and the quality of medical care is not sacrificed. Also, their family and support systems are close by. My job is to confirm the initial diagnosis, suggest the course of further workup, if any, and initiate treatment. For follow-up and continuing care I have periodic visits with the patient at which the major disease parameters are reassessed and decisions made about progress and any changes in treatment. These decisions are then communicated to the personal physician; if any major problems arise, we discuss them by telephone. If a problem arises that the physician is not comfortable in treating at home, the patient can return to the medical center. Unfortunately, some of the flexibility or freedom of choice that patients have been able to exercise is currently being restricted by Medicare reimbursement regulations— that is a serious new problem.

There are other things that physicians can do to help contain costs. In teaching young doctors I point out that the extent to which we should use expensive tests to evaluate a patient depends upon what use we plan to make of the information. If a decision about treatment depends upon knowing whether the disease has spread to other areas such as the brain or liver, then CT scans or other radiologic studies need to be done even though they are very expensive. If, on the other hand, our treatment would be the same regardless of the information, then I wonder whether the expense can be justified. This is particularly illustrated by lung cancer, in which it really is very important to know whether the disease is localized, because if it is localized it is potentially curable. On the other hand, if we see a patient in the office who has cancer of the lung, detected easily and inexpensively by a sputum examination, and that individual has a readily accessible lymph gland in the neck that seems to be involved, all we need to do is biopsy the node to determine if the disease has spread. This is a simple and inexpensive office procedure. It is not necessary to go further since a positive node biopsy means that the patient is not a candidate for surgery. This seems an obvious point, yet too often I see extra days of hospitalization and very expensive x-rays being used to document the last detail on the extent of disease outside the lung, when in fact that information will not make an iota of difference in deciding the treatment that we use. It is true that the extent of disease involvement will potentially be related to how long the patient is expected to live. But is it worth several thousand more dollars to find out whether the patient has more extensive disease and is expected to live an average of four months, or less extensive disease and might be expected to live eight or nine months? It might be, to the patient. But, too, the burden of making such a decision might be more than some patients would want to cope with. In certain types of advanced lung cancer we have no treatments that do more than alleviate pain and suffering—they do not extend life. In any event, the estimates are no more than estimates and are taken from averages of large groups of patients; they do not necessarily apply to any given individual. For the person under my care I will know soon enough.

There are other things that I can do as a physician to help contain costs. After arriving at a clear diagnosis and plan of action, I can decide which tests I will need to measure the progress of the disease on the one hand, and the effects of treatment on the other. I need to find out which tests will enable me to monitor the size or extent of the tumor and which will tell me whether I'm being sufficiently aggressive—or not aggressive enough—in my use of chemotherapy. The tests I will need to measure the extent of disease might simply be tests to measure the size of the lymph glands or the tumor nodules seen on a chest x-ray; but the tests might need to be more complicated—expensive CT scans, for example—if deep abdominal disease is involved. If the latter, I would make some estimate at the beginning of treatment as to how frequently to measure these lesions, depending on whether the information would cause me to change my treatment. The question of whether sufficient or too much chemotherapy is being given can usually be determined by a physical examination, the patient's report of signs of toxicity and simple blood counts since most of the chemotherapeutic drugs we use cause fairly obvious toxicity, particularly to the white cells and platelets. Some drugs must be followed in more complicated ways, necessitating a more expensive monitoring strategy. If there is a substitute for such drugs that is equally good and less expensive to monitor, I can

12: On Reducing the Enormous Economic Burden of Cancer

make the decision about which to use at the beginning. But there is always the possibility of the unexpected complication, and here it is not possible to plan ahead. The only thing I know to do is to keep cost factors in mind all along.

I can also do some simple things like using generic drugs when they are of equal quality and less expensive (often they are not), using less expensive types of drugs if they are equally effective (they often are), looking for pharmacies that sell the drugs more inexpensively than others (there is a surprising variation, which the patient can also determine by comparison shopping), doing some of my follow-up work over the telephone instead of requiring a visit and not scheduling more laboratory tests than I know I will need, while being prepared to add to the list if the circumstances change. As a general rule, the more experienced the physician, the fewer tests needed to achieve a given goal—I do far fewer bone marrow examinations than young colleagues because my examination of the blood or other facts makes it unnecessary to do those tests; the results are predictable. The expert can often plan the work needed at a lower cost than can a more junior physician. But it takes time and experience to get to that point, and there are other pertinent factors, which will be discussed later. Sometimes expensive drugs or other treatments can be economical in the long run. The use of interferon in hairy cell leukemia is a good case in point. Interferon is expensive but it gets the patient better and thereby saves hospitalization for costly treatment of infection or other complication of uncontrolled disease.

Many oncologists are so well trained as general internists that when complications arise it is not necessary to call in another consultant, and thus a patient who has changing problems is not shuttled about from one specialist to another. Still, if the patient has a problem with which I am not making any headway, then it might be very cost-effective for me to bring in someone who is a specialist in that area.

One of the most cost-effective and sensible ways of going about the practice of oncology is to work in multidisciplinary clinics. It has always bothered me that the kind of care a patient gets depends on which door of the institution or clinic he walks into. We can minimize that problem by bringing different specialists together to evaluate a new patient, jointly decide on the initial treatment strategy and then periodically assess progress. A good example of how that works is our Head and Neck Cancer Clinic where head and neck surgeons, plastic surgeons, radiotherapists and medical oncologists as well as other health professionals (nurses, nutritionists, social workers, psychologists, dentists) all have input in making the initial evaluation. This is of course generally possible in the larger cancer centers, such as at some comprehensive cancer centers, but many physicians have worked out functional associations that can accomplish the same goal. Clearly, in such multidisciplinary clinics one physician has to be in charge of the patient and make sure that all the suggestions are properly coordinated and implemented. Such a multidisciplinary clinic will cost more than seeing a single doctor but far less than a series of consultants. The details vary greatly so I cannot be more specific about the various practices.

A much more difficult task for the oncologist is deciding what type of therapy to use when, as mentioned earlier, this decision has important financial consequences. Sometimes there may be trade-offs: one form of treatment is somewhat safer and less uncomfortable but more expensive than another treatment. For example, Adriamycin and cisplatin are both extremely potent anticancer agents and both have peculiar organ toxicity—one to the heart and the other to the kidneys and intestinal tract. There is evidence that these toxicities can be minimized by giving the drug by slow continuous intravenous infusion rather than by rapid intravenous infusion—which may mean the difference between an expensive hospitalization and an outpatient treatment. This is a dilemma, and it can make the physician uncomfortable to have to bring it to the attention of the patient and family, knowing full well that they want perhaps both the best treatment and the most economical one—and both cannot be had! Or, if a prolonged treatment is given in the hospital, the hospital may suffer a financial loss, which poses other obvious difficulties.

Deciding how aggressive to be with therapy is even more difficult. If I have tried full doses of all of the first-line chemotherapeutic drugs and the patient has not responded, I know that unless an exciting experimental drug is available, there is not much more that is likely to work. Yet I cannot know that with certainty *for this particular patient* until I try everything, although to do so would be costly. To give another example, should we pull out all the stops even though the patient is obviously dying, or do we try to encourage a patient to be managed at home in a pleasant environment among loved ones and seek to provide hospice-type care for the patient? Probably it is clear where my preferences would lie, and I do not mind presenting that choice to the patient if and when it becomes necessary. However, ultimately the patient is the one who must make the decision, which also has to be agreeable to key family members. Some patients want to be treated with everything that is available until the very last breath, while other patients would rather not, even if finances are not a consideration. Remember too that the cheapest treatment may be the least effective one, and we are certainly not advocating that!

HOSPICE AND HOME CARE—WHEN? Home hospice groups have spread rapidly throughout the country to meet the need of many terminal patients to spend their remaining days at home and die in pleasant and familiar surroundings near their loved ones. Home care given by family and friends, visiting nurses and lay volunteers also appears to be less expensive. These programs have had enthusiastic start-up support and financial contributions from members of the community. Most of these fund-raising efforts probably cannot be sustained, however, and *I expect many hospice programs will fold unless stable government and insurance reimbursement mechanisms are rapidly put into place.* There is now legislation that permits hospices to get Medicare reimbursement, but to become eligible under the complex regulations may not be feasible for most of these organizations—it appears that the legislation was deliberately written in such a restrictive manner as to give the impression of, rather than the funds for, support. And even hospices that take Medicare patients must still raise money from the community. Hospice of Northern Virginia reports that it loses $1,400 per Medicare patient. As individuals we need to take an interest in this issue, communicate our desires to elected officials and also petition employers and our private health insurance companies (e.g., Blue Cross–Blue Shield) to provide hospice benefits in their policies. *After all, the benefits in private insurance policies are negotiable, and we should support those companies that offer hospice or comparable home care.*

One of the hardest things I have to do as a cancer specialist is decide when to encourage patients to participate in intensive therapy and when to advise them that that treatment is not appropriate and that simpler treatment can be given at much less expense in the home community. Of course, treatment given in the home community depends on the resources and the physicians available in that community, but certainly many forms of cancer can be treated as effectively by an internist or medical oncologist in a community clinic as they can in a major cancer center. On the other hand, other diseases, such as acute leukemia, require specialized resources and expertise, and the cancer centers have access to the latest forms of experimental therapy, which are not yet available (marketed) to practicing physicians.

For example, for some years interferon was available to us and some other investigators to be used in research, but it had not yet been approved for marketing. This meant that a patient with a form of cancer uniquely susceptible to interferon (and there are some) could not have access to the drug unless the patient came to a research center conducting a study, and that might mean considerable travel, separation from family and extensive expenses. If a patient wishes an experimental treatment like interferon but I already know it is very unlikely to be effective and there is a standard treatment that is more likely to succeed, then my job is to present the facts, which likely will discourage the patient from seeking interferon, not only at our institution, but elsewhere. It is sad how often a desperate patient or family will call all over the United States, keeping their suitcases packed and being ready to go anywhere and at any cost if given even the slightest encouragement. That is a characteristic of the human condition and it should not be surprising; unfortunately it is a characteristic easily exploited by those who offer quack remedies and easy promises (a problem that is discussed further in Chapter 13).

SOCIETAL ISSUES In our society we like to think that access to good medical care is a right regardless of the ability to pay. This idealistic concept is at variance with reality. So let us look at the real situation and see what we, as a society, are doing about costs versus ethics.

First, and not at all parenthetically, we must recognize that in a far-from-perfect world it is often the physician who is asked to make the hard decisions of how much to spend, or which high-tech devices should be used (or not) to prolong (or not) the final days of a dying patient. Indeed, hospital chaplains also are often called upon for advice in helping both doctor and patient with difficult problems.

My own view is that doctors should assess each situation on its merits, taking into account medical factors and the best information that we have from patients regarding their wishes, and use all available resources in coming to a decision. If it is clear to me, for instance, that all possible useful treatment means have been exhausted and the patient is inevitably going to die in the coming weeks or months, then my obligation as a physician is to make that process as painless and as comfortable as possible, and usually that can be accomplished. *It is much simpler not to begin using a respirator or other life-support system than it is to start it and then try to turn it off. This is probably more obvious to a lay person than it is to an eager young physician who has been trained to extend life and who considers death a failure of medical care rather than a natural consequence of life, once health is irretrievably lost.*

One very delicate issue is the use of extensive tests and consultations as part of the practice of what in the profession is called "defensive medicine." We have come to a point in this country (more so in certain areas—for example, New York and California—than in others) where malpractice suits are so commonplace that doctors are constantly looking over their shoulders to see if a lawyer is lurking there ready to claim that not everything possible was done because particular tests were not ordered or certain treatments were omitted (even though of dubious value). Their very real fear of being sued causes many physicians to order tests that they know they do not need in order to make treatment decisions and that could therefore be eliminated, providing substantial savings for the patient (or insurance company, or government). Often, days of unnecessary hospitalization are added on in order to perform these tests or treatments, adding further to the costs of totally unproductive work. In fact, performing unnecessary tests is asking for trouble because sometimes unexpected abnormalities return or laboratory errors arise and then these have to be explained with yet another round of tests or consultations, all of which take more time and money.

Huge malpractice awards are increasingly being given by courts, and these in turn are raising the costs of all types of medical care, including that for cancer. It is impossible to measure the economic impact of this on our nation and on cancer care in particular, but if a plastic surgeon has to pay $100,000 a year in malpractice insurance, then (a) fees will be increased in order to pass that cost on to the consumer, and (b) that physician probably will order unnecessary tests and do other procedures to decrease the likelihood of being sued. We need a no-fault system as in the automobile insurance industry and a cap on the size of awards. Malpractice lawyers obviously object to that suggestion. People's expectations have to be realistic—until better treatments are available some cancers will inevitably result in the death of the patient, but this is not grounds per se for seeking malpractice awards. One of our ablest young surgeons in the community recently gave up active practice because of an exhausting malpractice suit against him—which he *won*. It was said that he became so nervous in the operating room thereafter that he decided to go into medical administration—a real loss to the field. But I should add that malpractice does occur in some instances of providing medical care and that physicians are not always forthright in admitting their own errors and may be reluctant to identify an incompetent colleague. Ironically, if they accuse a colleague of being incompetent that also opens the door for a huge lawsuit. These are not easy problems to solve given our current system.

Another problem of national concern is the role of the Food and Drug Administration (FDA), which is charged with deciding on the efficacy and safety of drugs before they are licensed to be used in the practice of medicine. In the early days of cancer chemotherapy in this country, less than two years elapsed from the time a drug was discovered until it was made available to cancer patients by a doctor's prescription. Now the research required to bring a drug from its first testing to approval by the FDA for marketing may take close to ten years, and the cost may be $70–100 million per drug, which of course must be passed on to the consumer. The process has become slow and costly mainly because of the cumbersome administrative requirements for obtaining approval from the FDA. The same strict FDA regulations that are appropriate for a new cold remedy that might be taken by millions of healthy people also apply to a new anticancer drug—even when it offers a new treatment for a rapidly fatal illness for which no alternative treatment exists. The necessity to meet these formidable FDA requirements limits the sponsoring of new drugs to the large pharmaceutical companies, and they will do so only when they believe they have a product that has sufficient marketability and patent protection to enable them to recover their investment costs and make a profit. (The system works much better for biological products, such as interferon, than it does for classical drugs.)

While high standards are essential to protect the public, that process could be greatly streamlined and substantially reduced in cost. We should find a happy medium between the excessive requirements that now exist in our country and the more casual attitude of certain other nations, which permit marketing of drugs that have relatively little solid scientific foundation. It should not be necessary for our citizens to seek treatment in foreign lands because effective drugs, or even promising experimental drugs, are available there but are not available in the United States. This problem was highlighted recently by the disclosure that a prominent entertainer had to go to Paris to get a new drug for AIDS. Neither Rock Hudson nor any ordinary citizen should be denied access to a legitimate drug for an illness that appears to be uniformly fatal. The FDA has been very difficult to deal with in this regard, and the result is expensive and wasteful. Such restrictions make it attractive to those able to afford to do so to visit clinics outside the United States, many of which are not experimenting with legitimate drugs.

The FDA has changed its requirements for approving new anti-cancer drugs in a way that is likely to block further progress very significantly. It used to be that a pharmaceutical company had to show that a new drug caused remissions in patients with cancer, and this was done by demonstrating shrinkage or disappearance of cancer—at least temporarily. Now the FDA requires proof that the new drug prolongs life or improves its quality—a much more time-consuming and costlier process. The logistic and cost implications of the new requirements will probably cause reexamination of the areas where these companies will spend their resources. It is far less costly to demonstrate that an antihypertensive drug lowers blood pressure and that a sedative causes sleep than to show that a drug prolongs life, which after all depends upon what other drugs are used after the experimental drug study has been completed.

These problems are well known by cancer researchers as well as by the pharmaceutical industry; yet despite promises by recent Presidents to simplify governmental paperwork and bureaucracy, the cost of developing new drugs is constantly rising, partly because of these artificial barriers imposed by government. All of this adds to your cost burden when you become ill.

WHAT COST CURE? What is the cost of curing certain types of malignancies? My colleague Dr. Harold Silberman points out that in the long run it is much cheaper to cure a patient than not to cure a patient. He illustrates the point by showing that a child with acute lymphocytic leukemia who is successfully treated is cured for about $15,000; that a patient cured of Hodgkin's disease, even advanced disease, receives the treatment for an estimated cost of $8,000; and that the very rigorous drug treatment required to cure widespread cancer of the testicle may cost around $10,000. Failure to cure, however, means that a patient gets better and worse, experiencing prolonged ups and downs that require repeated hospitalizations and outpatient costs. Treatment of a child with acute lymphocytic leukemia who is not cured will cost about $40,000; of an adult, about $65,000; the patient with Hodgkin's disease who is not cured will be treated at an estimated cost of $80,000, or ten times the price of the cure. These simple cost analyses do not include the other costs of loss of time from work, travel, lodging and the big factor—loss of potential income over a lifetime if the patient is not cured. Actually, the cynic would point out that the cheapest thing is if the patient dies quickly—since the hospital is paid the same amount no matter how long the period of hospitalization. Fortunately this doesn't happen very often!

PAYING FOR RESEARCH ON YOURSELF The shortage of money to support clinical cancer research is forcing investigators to look at new ways of continuing their work. One such development has generated considerable unrest and discussion within the medical community—asking the patient to pay for individual experimental work done in the laboratory. Dr. Robert K. Oldham, founding director of the National Cancer Institute's Biological Response Modifiers Program, has started a for-profit company in Franklin, Tennessee, called Biotherapeutics, which offers to make monoclonal antibodies and other biological substances that are unique to a particular cancer patient. They have expanded to clinics in other areas, also. The company makes it clear that this is "formative-stage technology" and cautions that there are no guarantees that the therapy will work. Patients who contract to receive such services remain under the care of their personal physician while the research to make these substances for them is conducted over a period of two to twelve months. When the research is completed, and if the patient shows a recurrence of tumor or progression of tumor despite standard treatment, then the developed biological substance could be used as another treatment option. The charge for the monoclonal antibodies and for toxins that are attached to them is $35,000. The charge for "cellular component development" research, which involves interleukin-2, gamma interferon and other biological response modifiers, is $19,400. Some services can cost up to $100,000.

Many physicians and scientists find this approach disturbing, even though the leaders in this for-profit experimentation are highly experienced and qualified. This also emphasizes a point made in an earlier chapter—there is a difference between the services the well-to-do can obtain and those available to others. This is an ethical issue for society to consider. There are certainly many things money can buy, but should access to medical research procedures be one of them? There is also the concern that this approach, while conducted by reputable people in this case, opens the door to other entrepreneurs who are not as capable as Dr. Oldham, and may even legitimize quack remedies by unscrupulous people. The other side of the argument is that if an individual seeks to be treated with interleukin-2, for example, and the existing programs will not accept him or her because they are overcrowded, there is no other way the individual can obtain access to such a substance. A private research outfit such as Biotherapeutics, however, requires no formal approval by the Food and Drug Administration because it is considered to be within the realm of the practice of medicine. It is true that the fees that patients pay are not reimbursed by insurance because the treatment is still experimental. In the long run, Dr. Oldham says he hopes to find ways to fund research for patients who cannot afford the costs. "I think it would be in society's best interest and our patients' best interest if there were both societal research done at the National Cancer Institute and the universities supported by philanthropic money and tax funds, as well as private research primarily supported by patients and corporations and private philanthropy. I think this would broaden our approach to cancer treatment and give the patient more leverage in the system. Right now the problem is that the patient has very little leverage."

I certainly have had patients tell me that they have made great efforts to seek access to experimental programs only to be denied for one reason or another, but I am personally not prepared to take a position on this question just yet. It obviously offers an opportunity for some patients—tempered by the possibility of abuse as well as emphasizing the inequality of access to health care. Nor is it a good way to conduct careful clinical research. But it is an innovative response on the part of the private sector to the very serious shortage of funds to support clinical research for all people in our society. I would not use this mechanism of funding, but it is an innovative alternative.

LESSONS The lessons of maintaining good health cannot begin too early and include a great deal more than brushing teeth and washing the hands. People, and especially children, need to be much better informed than they are, and formal education has so far failed in teaching school children where to go when they need medical information, how to think ahead and make long-range plans, how to protect their health while they have it and how to handle insurance and related financial matters. Do you, for instance, have a will? Have you willed your organs (eyes, kidneys, heart) for transplantation? Do you want to express your wishes regarding the use of heroic measures if you have no hope for recovery? These topics are not well taught in our school system, and attempts to introduce educational materials of this sort often fail because our school curricula are not easily accessible and directors of school systems have not been very responsive to health issues other than drug abuse or sex education. This is a problem for us all because health habits need to be learned early and the school system is the logical place for this process to begin. We should be doing a marvelous job of teaching young people how to care for their health and how to assume continuing responsibility for their minds and bodies. They might make things a bit awkward for some doctors by being able to ask the right questions, but on the whole an informed patient is not only preferable for a doctor but is also far more likely, with the doctor's understanding help, to be cured.

As noted earlier in the discussion of the relationship between cigarette smoking and lung cancer, in 1980 U.S. medical expenditures were about $1 billion for cigarette-related lung cancers. The accompanying loss of productivity was valued at $5.9 billion and the losses from prolonged illness at $446 million, for a total of $7.47 billion in 1980 dollars, or about $10 billion in 1984 dollars. These are the costs of a single (admittedly the most common) cancer, which is largely preventable.

In this regard, the public could productively become more involved in saving costs and lives through cancer prevention. The most obvious need is to provide meaningful educational programs for children to inform them about the dangers of smoking and minimize the likelihood of their starting; we also need more quit-smoking clinics and the like. Further, we need to take steps such as higher taxes on tobacco to see that nonsmokers do not subsidize the health costs of smokers and that government does not subsidize the growing of tobacco or the tax-free sale of tobacco products in federal installations, and we need to protect nonsmokers from passive smoking inhalation in public places. I believe it is time to ban tobacco advertising altogether, or at least the advertising directed to young people, as a public health hazard.

None of the economic costs, high as they are, take into account how much we value human life, nor do they try to put a value on pain and suffering both to the patient and to the family. As a society we do not like to think in terms of the monetary value of human life, yet there clearly are precedents for this. Think about the cost of preserving the life of brain-dead individuals, yet this is done, or of transplanting hearts at a cost in excess of $100,000 per patient when the medical indications are that the recipient can seldom be restored to normal function or to the working ranks. Yet this too is done and publicly, at least, there is nothing but applause for the effort. Many cancer patients can be successfully treated and cured now; many more will be successfully treated in the future through medical advances that are now being developed or through the work of laboratory scientists who are just starting on their research programs. But given its staggering costs, *are we doing enough as a society to support these efforts to prevent and to cure cancer? I think not!*

The funding for cancer research has come primarily from the National Cancer Institute, a part of the National Institutes of Health, and to a smaller but very important extent from the American Cancer Society, followed by other charitable organizations such as the Leukemia Society, the Damon Runyon Society and others.

The National Cancer Institute has recently set a goal of reducing deaths from cancer by 50 percent by the year 2000. The budget of the Institute is in the neighborhood of $1 billion, against the $10 billion lost to lung cancer alone each year. And the purchasing power of this budget has not increased for many years. Yet the polls show that since the 1930s cancer has always been ranked as the disease people are most concerned about, with more than 50 percent of the public considering this the worst health problem that could happen to them. One wonders whether that public concern is being adequately reflected in appropriations directed toward preventing and curing cancer.

With the cutbacks in funding, young scientists who have been training for years are now finding it extraordinarily difficult to go out on their own and become productive. So here we have the contradiction of having spent the money to train young cancer researchers who are capable of making major discoveries, but of now having no way to support the work they could do. By the same token, well-established investigators who have been productive for years are facing crises year after year as they attempt to keep their laboratories going, under at times desperately adverse conditions. The odds of getting a grant application funded to support new studies are only about one in ten or a little better. Not many businesses would want to face the future against such odds every three years or so, regardless of how successful they had been in the past. For significant parts of the year these scientists have to devote full time to attempting to secure research grants to fund their activities—instead of continuing to do their research. This is driving many potentially productive medical scientists into other occupations such as the private practice of medicine or industrial research or even into other fields.

Some scientists are attempting to solve the funding problem by turning to industry or venture capital organizations to fund research, but that approach provides only very limited solutions. Such funding opportunities are limited to those ideas that are most ready to be exploited for commercial gain; the funding is not available for the more basic long-range investigations that are ultimately the backbone of the scientific effort. Thus, cancer research, like other areas of biomedical research, is no longer in a privileged position and is falling behind in the United States, while great advances are being made in other countries, like Japan, that are putting higher priorities on research.

The public needs to determine whether elimination of cancer is a national priority or not. Those of us in the field think that it is, but some elected representatives, including the President, have not been acting accordingly. Fortunately the Congress tries to be very responsive and it is encouraging when leaders such as Representatives Henry Waxman and Joseph Early and Senators Orrin Hatch and Lowell Weicker and others fight for the cancer program. It is ironic that an excellent small research program, the National Large Bowel Task Force, lost its modest funding some two years before President Reagan had his bowel surgery; indeed, many of the questions that reporters were asking after his surgery could have been studied and perhaps answered by the research that had to be curtailed. It seems remarkable that this President has had two different cancers removed (colon, skin) during his administration and yet has shown so little concern for the problems of finding a cure and for treating the afflicted. He leaves this to the budget cutters in the Office of Management and Budget. Fortunately the Congress has other ideas.

Before I leave the subject of funding for cancer research, I want the public to become aware of a small group of fund-raising organizations that purport to be major contributors to cancer research but which are largely self-serving for their organizers— a hoax using a name or location designed to sound like a legitimate foundation, often by taking on a name and a logo that resembles that of known and respected charitable groups. These are run by resourceful fund raisers and the public is not adequately aware that they may give only a small fraction of the money they raise to cancer research and service. It would be inappropriate for me to name them here, but before you assume you are giving to an outstanding charity, ask questions, try to know someone in the organization you give to or check references with a nationally known organization. Lookalikes are common in designer jeans, fancy shoes and now also in charitable institutions.

IS THERE A BETTER WAY? We have identified many of the economic problems that loom large for patients, families and society. The issues are complex and it would be inappropriate to say that we have definitive answers for many of them. But clearly we

12: On Reducing the Enormous Economic Burden of Cancer

as a society believe in a personal care health system, and are struggling with the question of how to pay for the care we ourselves insist upon.

Some general suggestions are in order. Plan ahead—for your individual insurance needs and instructions in case of incapacitation; talk with other members of your family to learn their wishes and needs as well, and by all means have a will drawn up. This is not in the least morbid—on the contrary, it can actually be a pleasure to sort out what you will give to whom. We often hear this from our patients who are nearing the end. For doctors—keep the financial problems of your patient in mind as you order blood tests and expensive x-rays, and as you plan to use potentially costly treatments. If you need it, go for it—but be sure that your patient understands! Do the necessary and avoid repetitious use of tests. For hospitals—simplify the bookkeeping system so the average person can follow it, consolidate all the charges into a single bill and indicate which portions are expected to be paid by the insurance carrier and then do not bill the patient for these costs unless the claim is denied! For society—let us make a conscious decision about whether cancer research and health care are truly priority issues, and do that in competition with other national needs and priorities. I think some percentage, 5 to 8 percent for example, of the costs of health care should go to research. That's how it is done in every successful business that depends on scientific innovation. Our budgeting and health care decisions are now a hit-or-miss affair, and are certainly not always in accord with the public's perception of its priorities. And let us go to some type of no-fault malpractice insurance that eliminates the horrendous multimillion-dollar awards for pain and suffering.

I want to develop some specific suggestions for you to take to your congressional representatives, if you agree, and ask them to help work out the details of our concerns. The main question that has to be addressed is who should be at risk for the financial costs of catastrophic illness? After discussing this with our business manager, Mr. Ralph Hawkins, it seems clear to me that we must move in the direction of sharing these risks in order to meet the high costs of treatment. There are three legs of the chair that need to provide the financial support:

1   The federal and state governments must address the matter of providing even more assistance for the treatment of cancer (and other catastrophic illness).

2   Employers must also provide more of their profits for programs of prevention and treatment of employees. This is done by purchasing health coverage, as described below.

3   The individual participates in a plan of third-party insurance coverage that becomes the primary vehicle to be used in future solution of these problems.

It is important to recognize that whereas the federal and state governments can be asked to provide coverage for the dreaded illnesses that potentially face all Americans, our present tax structure is clearly not able to support a total national health care system. Nevertheless, the essential thing is to provide the peace of mind that comes from knowing that catastrophic illness will not deplete the life savings of the average citizen. Federal and state governments are already spending enormous amounts of money through Medicare, Medicaid and veteran's benefits. These programs could be restructured into a single health care system that provides for catastrophic illness. The insurance plan of the future or, as we will refer to it, the third-party risk, will be in the form of health maintenance organizations (HMO's), individual participation associations (IPA's) and similar mechanisms. This will essentially allow the younger and healthier members of society to pay for those who are less fortunate and who have illnesses such as cancer, in return for similar coverage for themselves should they need it later. The key element of the entire formula is capitation, which simply means that all who participate in the program—i.e., the employer, the patient and, very importantly, the health care providers (hospitals, doctors)—share in the risk. (Dr. Richard Rosen, who practices oncology in Greensboro, North Carolina, strongly disagrees with the idea of capitation and urges people to stay away from a system that encourages underutilization of doctors and reduces the quality of care. All of this is controversial and there are no easy answers.)

Employers must not only pay their part of this insurance coverage but also provide more training for their employees in how to prevent illness and for early detection of curable illness; in turn, employee motivation must be tied to a healthier body and mind. I suggest that incentives be given for healthier employees—along the lines of additional free time, vacations, et cetera.

How much money should the individual pay as the deductible part of the insurance before the other mechanisms contribute? I suggest that an individual with assets of a million dollars should pay more than an individual who has assets of $10,000, much as our tax system is structured. Using a simple formula, each individual could decide how much he or she could afford to pay for health care before it would cause a serious financial drain, and only costs in excess of that amount would be insured. That's really the basis of a catastrophic illness program. After all, illness makes us all equal and the financial burden should not be placed disproportionately on the poor.

Mr. Hawkins predicts that in the future, employees will place a greater value on the type of health insurance offered by the employer, and insurance policies will increasingly become an important tool for companies in recruiting and keeping the best people. And when new health services come along, such as hospice care or other special advances that are not currently covered by insurance, employers will have an opportunity to study these options and try to purchase the best for their employees. For agreeing to participate in such a program, the insured employee gives up certain freedoms, unless he or she is willing to pay for them privately—such as obtaining services above and beyond those provided by the insurance plan. That's a trade-off that probably has to occur in order to obtain a new vitality in the health insurance and care system.

At the present time, and in the foreseeable future, very few families can withstand the financial hemorrhage of a costly bout with cancer. Perhaps we can find more innovative ways to help each other by way of people-to-people programs. Hospice is a great step in that direction, as are Road to Recovery (operated by the American Cancer Society) and other transportation programs to help patients get to medical appointments; pharmaceutical companies that manufacture chemotherapeutic drugs and costly antibiotics need to help the indigent with costly drugs (some do), and food programs such as Meals on Wheels are needed even more widely. Services should be coordinated on a neighborhood basis so that we can try to recapture the idea of neighbors helping each other in an emergency that not only threatens our health but also threatens to make paupers of us in the process. Religious groups are often in a position to help through their social concerns committees, and these need to be expanded to lend a helping hand to our nuclear families. But these are only goals—it is up to individuals to draw up the blueprints for effective action.

Americans are very generous people. We open our hearts and our pocketbooks to nameless victims of hunger, floods, earthquakes and those who need expensive care such as heart or liver transplants. Can all that good "people power" be harnessed to help the victims of cancer and other dread diseases? To give is better than to receive, and these problems do affect us all!

EXPERIMENTAL THERAPY OR QUACKERY: WHAT'S THE DIFFERENCE?

13

TESTING OF NEW DRUGS IN HUMANS As discussed in Chapter 4, cancer chemotherapy is a relatively new field. During the past thirty-five years a tremendous amount of research has led to some notable successes and to promising leads in other areas that have not yet been conquered. This chapter reviews the manner in which new drugs are developed, but it also shows how claims can be made on the basis of improper testing in order to confuse you, and we will explore the unfortunate story of phony claims and quackery.

The discovery of an effective agent is very difficult. Such an agent obviously does not just appear out of thin air. First there must be isolation, usually in pure form, of a chemical that has demonstrated anticancer effects on several cancer cell systems, including transplantable mouse tumors as well as human tumors grown in test tubes and in mice.* There needs to be a reason, or rationale, for using this new drug and usually some idea, even if not exact, as to how the drug acts to kill cancer cells and to be less toxic against normal cells than other drugs. Then it is necessary to do very careful toxicologic and pharmacologic studies of the drug in different animal species, usually including mice and dogs, to estimate the amount of the drug that can be safely given to humans, the route by which it can be given (intravenous, oral, under the skin, into the muscle) and its toxic effects on various normal organs. The maximum tolerated dose (MTD) is first established for animals. This is the amount that when given to an animal is likely to cause serious toxicity, yet from which most animals will fully recover. When amounts in excess of that amount are given, the animal is likely to die; autopsy studies are then done on the animals to determine the causes of death and the effect of the drug on various organs and tissues.

Unique and unusual toxicities are looked for as well as the common ones that occur with most chemotherapeutic drugs, such as inhibition of blood-forming cells in the bone marrow, loss of hair and damage to the intestinal cells or nervous system. Some of these studies are done in dogs because this species handles drugs in a way that is quite similar to humans. This tells us what to look for in patients and how to prevent unpleasant surprises. An interesting by-product of this phase of the research is that some of the information gained from studying side effects can be useful in suggesting other clinical trials for different kinds of cancer. For example, if a drug is particularly toxic to normal lymph tissues, bone marrow or skin, then it may turn out to be effective against cancers that arise from those tissues, such as lymphoma, leukemia or carcinomas, respectively.

*Human tumors cannot be transplanted to mice or to other species except under special conditions in which there is no immunologic resistance. Athymic nude mice are such a unique colony of mice; they have to be kept under germ-free conditions, which is expensive, but they lack the capacity to recognize cells from other species as being "foreign" and thus will not reject them. Human cancer cells can be injected into these mice, they will grow to form a measurable tumor, and the mice can then be treated with drugs to see if the tumor shrinks or even disappears.

13: Experimental Therapy or Quackery: What's the Difference?

Before a new drug is tested with patients, a very careful protocol is developed, taking into account everything that has been learned from the animal and tissue culture studies, in order to determine the maximum tolerated dose in humans. Since there is no way to know for certain whether humans will handle this new drug in the same way animals do, it is important to allow a wide margin of safety, so only a small fraction of the maximum tolerated dose for animals is used as the starting dose in humans. If that dose results in no toxicity to the first series of patients, then the dose is progressively increased until toxic manifestations appear. In this type of study, technically called a Phase I clinical trial, the aims are to learn how to use the new drug, how much of it can be used safely and what the side effects will be when toxic doses are reached.

To justify giving a new drug to patients, there has to be strong evidence that it is potentially useful in humans—evidence, for example, that it has a potent effect against some types of cancer cells, in animals, that are not usually killed by standard drugs. To illustrate, if a new drug is very active in killing lung cancer cells in culture or in animals, where existing agents are not very active, that would justify considering this compound for a clinical experiment. Patients are then chosen for such studies only if they volunteer to participate after they have heard the full details of the proposed program; the formal procedures for this are called obtaining the volunteers' "informed consent." Every potentially dangerous procedure and every complication that can reasonably be anticipated are explained to the patients, and then they are asked to reflect on all this, ask questions and sign their willingness to undergo such a procedure. Understandably, this process often involves long discussions; sometimes we are able to supplement the oral and written explanations with a video made for this purpose. (These very elaborate precautions are generally taken only with experimental research protocols and not with accepted means of medical care. I have sometimes seen patients about to undergo risky heart surgery who, although they have signed an operative permit, have little idea of the risks and problems that lie ahead, and I think that full informed consent should also be extended for "standard procedures" as well.)

Experimental consent forms are often three to six pages long and detail step by step what the procedures will be, itemizing all of the possible risks; they tend to exaggerate the possible risks so that even if they are unlikely to occur, the patient may be forewarned. Of course, we must always be alert to the possibility of a surprise reaction because there may be a type of toxicity that occurs in humans that has never been seen in the animal studies. For instance, I remember many years ago when we were testing a new antimetabolite called azauracil; it proved to put patients to sleep temporarily and to change normal brain waves from waking to sleeping patterns, a reaction that had not been suspected from the animal experiments. Brain waves changed even when the patients were not asleep. This was an entirely unanticipated side reaction of a drug that was very effective in killing tumors in mice and in test tubes, but it caused this drug to be shelved. Fortunately the side effects wore off completely in short order. Another antimetabolite, called 6-propylmercaptopurine, caused our patients to complain of tasting garlic on their breath after taking the drug; this was due to a peculiar chemical reaction that occurred in humans but not in mice (mice probably would not have complained, anyway). The explanation for the reaction was carefully worked out by Dr. Gertrude Elion, who found that humans, unlike lower species, break down the drug in such a way as to produce a normal purine substance that does not inhibit cells plus another that is the essence of garlic, a useless, if smelly, compound! In any event, there was no harm done but we had to chase down this lead, which for a time had looked very promising, and of course the drug had to be abandoned. As it turned out, we learned something important about human metabolism, even though the drug was a failure. Typically something important is learned from a carefully set up clinical study.

Generally speaking, patients who have cancer for which there is no effective means of treatment are the ones who are asked to participate in an experimental study. For example, if a patient has a form of lung cancer for which there is no available effective therapy and this patient is aware that there is not much time remaining, he might be very eager to be among the first to receive a promising new drug. This is the way all drug studies begin; indeed, patients who are now cured of their leukemia owe a debt of gratitude to earlier patients who volunteered to participate in experimental studies before the drugs were known to be effective. This type of clinical research therefore has potential benefit not only for the patient who participates but also for humankind, and fortunately many people perceive this as a great opportunity to make a meaningful contribution!

Patients are not asked to participate in a Phase I experimental study if there is an effective alternative means of treatment available for them, for under most circumstances this would not be considered ethical. For further protection, each research institution has an institutional review board (IRB) that reviews every experimental study to be sure it protects the welfare of the patient. The IRB's are made up not only of health professionals but also of clergy and other concerned lay persons who work together to ensure that all procedures are ethical, as defined by the Helsinki Declaration on Human Rights. Our own experience has been that patients who know they have an incurable form of cancer are generally very interested in trying something new if the consequences have been carefully explained to them and openly discussed with their family members, although occasionally some vocal member of the family will express the wish that you not use his relative as a "guinea pig." To that one prominent researcher replies that guinea pigs will be the first ones cured.

Researchers have sometimes been accused, but they have on only very rare occasions been guilty, of not taking patient safety adequately into account. Several years ago the *Washington Post* ran an "exposé" along these lines, accusing specific cancer researchers of unethical practices with children and adults who participated in clinical studies. This caused consternation and grief for many people, but since the claims were unfounded, they were formally retracted. Still, a great deal of damage was done by those accusations, which were leveled by irresponsible reporters. The controversy paralyzed quite a few doctors who should have been busy with other matters. Then, too, I have known of some researchers who, in their enthusiasm for a new treatment, put considerable pressure on a patient to participate in a hazardous study, knowing that the disease itself is the ultimate hazard. At times I have vigorously urged a young person to stay with a treatment program that had the opportunity for curing him—firm in the knowledge that failure to try meant certain death. Nonetheless, my counsel and belief is that the adult patient should be given the available information, it should be explained with great care and patience, and then the individual must decide what he (not the doctor or family) wants.

If a drug comes through a Phase I evaluation satisfactorily, which means that a safe dose and schedule has been found, the next step is to begin trials to see whether it has significant effects against particular types of cancer. A study will be designed in which perhaps fifteen or twenty patients who meet certain rigid entry criteria and who have a particular kind of cancer, say bowel or melanoma, will be studied with the treatment schedule developed in the earlier trials. The hope is that this (Phase II) evaluation will give some idea as to whether this new drug possesses any effective anticancer activity in humans. Some drugs may be effective in only one or two types of cancer out of more than one hundred, so although the drug may be found inactive in several types of cancer, it still might have important anticancer activity if only the right tumor is chosen. Tremendous professional judgment is required in planning for these studies, which are done only by oncologists who are also established scientific investigators.

If a Phase II study shows that a drug has some effectiveness against a given type of tumor(s), the next question is *how* effective it is, and whether it is more effective than other anticancer drugs that are already available. To answer those questions a Phase III study is designed—patients who have a particular type of tumor and no significant contraindications to the use of either drug are asked to participate in a so-called randomized controlled study. This means that each patient has a 50–50 chance of receiving either the best available established drug for that cancer or the new, experimental one. Neither the patient nor the doctor knows ahead of time which drug is to be used in an individual case, so both drugs have to be acceptable. All patients are treated for a predetermined period of time, such as three or six months, to see what effects the different drugs have. The number of patients per group depends upon the extent of the differences that are anticipated, but sixty to eighty patients per group is not a large number for a study of this nature. If small improvements are being sought, then larger numbers of patients are necessary to achieve statistically meaningful differences, and a definitive study may require as many as 150 or more per group.

It is hard to explain to patients that there is no legal way an investigator or other physician can give an experimental drug to a patient who is not participating in a research study, except in certain extraordinary circumstances that are beyond the scope of this discussion. A doctor who is not participating in an experimental program of this sort cannot gain access to experimental drugs; he can only refer the patient to the investigator responsible for the study. These study designs make every effort to minimize side effects and protect the safety of the individual patient who chooses to participate, but the risks of treatment may be significant, as in the case of bone marrow transplantation. The National Cancer Institute now has a computerized system that can quickly provide information as to which investigator(s) is studying a particular experimental drug. This "PDQ" system is being used to disseminate such information and facilitate patient referral, if that is appropriate. This system looks good on paper but it is expensive and, in my view, still of very limited value. Many times I have been called by a patient who has learned about one of our research protocols and has bags packed and is ready to travel a thousand miles. It may take me a half hour on the telephone to figure out that the patient not only is not a candidate for my study but also is ignoring good advice by home doctors that could be curative. Doctors cannot practice medicine on the telephone nor by remote computer terminals. Still and all, if we can give more information to people, that is a desirable end, for they can make more informed decisions.

Investigators who participate in experimental studies are regulated not only by their hospital review committees but also by the National Cancer Institute and/or by the pharmaceutical company that is developing the drug, and each company in turn is closely monitored by the Food and Drug Administration. All results have to be reported to the sponsoring group, serious reactions must be reported immediately, and all records are open to inspection, with due protection for the anonymity of the individual patients. Thus, if there is a question about the validity of the results, the data can be reexamined at any time by independent reviewers. (In fact, occasional abuses of taking shortcuts and falsifying data have been detected by independent audit, and usually have resulted in severe punishment of the perpetrators. There are rascals in every profession—unfortunately medicine is no exception.) Most of the major cancer centers in the United States are engaged in clinical trials, and it is generally felt that participation in a study of this type is in the best interests of the patient because of the careful thought that has gone into the study. This is not to say that good medical oncology cannot be practiced without experimental protocols; however, experimental studies are not only consistent with outstanding clinical care, they are also essential to further treatment developments—no new treatments will emerge without such efforts! And when discoveries are made they are written up for publication, reviewed critically by other scientists with an opportunity for rebuttal, and published if deemed worthy.

TESTING OF COMPOUND "X"—THE STORY OF KREBIOZEN You can now appreciate the care that goes into the design of clinical studies so that we can best serve the public and minimize the risks of doing so. What a contrast this format for the conduct of legitimate clinical research presents to the circumstances that surround quack remedies! The history of these is so characteristic and repetitive that a new one can be easily identified by an informed public (you), provided you are willing to pay attention to the warning signs I will describe. Unfortunately, desperation and the promise of a cure—the pot of gold at the end of the rainbow—often make sensible people do irrational things, even when the real gold goes into the pockets of scoundrels. The history of krebiozen is instructive in this regard, and the story, though fading from memory, is so typical that it can serve as a prototype of what happens with these quack remedies.

Some years ago Dr. James Holland, reporting on the krebiozen saga in the *Journal of the American Medical Association,* wrote: "My definition of cancer quackery is the *deliberate* misapplication of a diagnostic or treatment procedure in a patient with cancer. Those who misapply diagnostic or treatment methods *unknowingly* may be honestly mistaken, inept, or fools. But the culprit who victimizes his fellowman suffering from cancer, impeding the patient's access to available therapies or constructive investigation, all the while greedily enriching himself, is a quack, a criminal, a jackal among men who deserves the scorn and ostracism of society. Because human life is at stake, he must be controlled."

Listen to the story of krebiozen because it is periodically reincarnated in different forms. In 1949 Dr. Steven Durovic arrived in the United States from Argentina with his industrialist brother, bringing with him a substance allegedly isolated from beef blood that was supposed to be useful in treating high blood pressure. There are no reports documenting that claim, however. He was later introduced to Andrew C. Ivy, M.D., Ph.D., formerly at Northwestern and then Vice President of the University of Illinois; at their first meeting Dr. Durovic told Dr. Ivy that he also had another substance, krebiozen, for treating cancer, but he had only 1 milligram that had been produced from two thousand horses. Dr. Durovic told Dr. Ivy that this was a growth-controlling substance, and this apparently fit with Dr. Ivy's view that growth-controlling substances must be present in the body. Dr. Ivy was a well-known intestinal physiologist, but he had no experience or particular knowledge of cancer as far as is known. Dr. Durovic did not divulge to Dr. Ivy how he made the extract, since it was "a commercial secret," but Dr. Ivy later testified at his own trial that without repeating any of the experiments and without knowing Dr. Durovic as a scientist or looking at his records, he proceeded with the development of this substance, volunteered to take it himself and then injected the first cancer patient with it in August of 1949.

Two years later Dr. Ivy announced at a press conference at the Drake Hotel in Chicago—at which science writers, the mayor, two

U.S. Senators and potential financial supporters were present—the results from treating twenty-two cancer patients. Of the twenty-two, eight were already dead, but in not a single case was cancer listed as a cause of death. Later, however, at Dr. Ivy's trial, it was brought out that those patients had in fact died of cancer. Furthermore, two others of the twenty-two patients had also died of cancer, one seven days and one two days before the press conference. "Dramatic clinical improvement" was listed as the outcome of the treatment for the patient who had died two days before. The patient who had died seven days before the press conference was the wife of a colleague of Dr. Ivy's; this colleague attended the press conference and did not contradict the claims of improvement in his wife; her death was not even mentioned.

Over a period of years the Krebiozen Research Foundation that Dr. Durovic and his businessman brother established claimed to have treated over four thousand patients and claimed improvement in 61 percent of patients with tumors of the brain and spinal cord, 70 percent with metastasis to the brain and 49 percent of patients with breast cancers. When Dr. Durovic and Dr. Ivy were indicted there were interesting disclosures about those claims. For example, Dr. Ivy had kept a research record on a Mr. Taietti, a patient whom he never saw. Dr. Durovic kept Dr. Ivy informed about Taietti through verbal reports, which were then entered into the record. In 1959 Dr. Ivy entered the note that "the patient is remaining well and a recent cystoscopy revealed a normal bladder," and in 1961 he wrote that "the patient is well and active." Yet subsequent investigation showed that those records of 1959 and 1961 were false: Mr. Taietti had actually died on July 12, 1955, of bladder cancer.

Eventually, some physicians became suspicious of the remarkable claims of krebiozen cures, and in March 1963 one physician wrote deliberately to request the drug for a patient who had had "bilateral total pneumonectomy" (the removal of both lungs), which is of course not compatible with life. However, the Krebiozen Research Foundation sent eight ampules of krebiozen and a bill for $76! The National Cancer Institute repeatedly asked the Krebiozen Research Foundation to cooperate in carrying out proper clinical trials, but the Foundation insisted on complete control of the conduct of these trials—which is entirely inappropriate for a scientific investigation.

We had a wealthy young businessman whom we were treating for cancer of the esophagus, usually a poorly responsive cancer, with a new chemotherapeutic drug—and he was doing very well. The cancer shrank, the patient gained weight and felt fine —though we expected that benefit to be temporary. He suddenly decided to go for a cure and get the krebiozen treatment. My colleague Dr. Rundles actually arranged for this patient to go to Chicago and be met by a reputable physician who took him to the program and introduced him to their staff. The patient purchased krebiozen, took his first doses in Chicago and brought the rest back for us to inject him with according to their instructions. When the cancer grew back rapidly the patient was satisfied that he had at least tried krebiozen, and we resumed our former treatment program. Fortunately we were able to help him again for a time, but mainly we had "kept in touch" with him during his krebiozen experience and never made him feel like an outcast because he exercised his notion to give this quack remedy a try. This proved to be a very effective way of working with this intelligent man, who had his own agenda. We didn't like it but we helped him exercise his choice.

When finally a formal investigation was launched by the FDA and the National Cancer Institute, the Krebiozen Research Foundation initially turned over the records of 504 patients who were supposed to be among the best in the Foundation's file. A scientific committee consisting of expert oncologists was appointed to review these cases. They found that only 283 of 504 case records were adequate for interpretation. Of these 283, only two patients had had a shrinkage of tumor; in thirteen instances there were doubtful effects, which were incompletely substantiated and might have been associated with other treatments being given at the same time; and in all the other patients the disease had progressed.

Later, a full-scale investigation was sponsored by the FDA, and a blue-ribbon group of sixty-eight experts reviewed *4,307* patients treated with krebiozen. They found *2,781* (!) records unacceptable for evaluation because of overlapping treatments, lack of proof of diagnosis, inadequate documentation and other flaws. Nevertheless, there were *1,526* patients whose records were considered interpretable; among these there were only *three* in whom it was possible, but not certain, that partial shrinkage of tumor might have occurred! One of these improvements lasted for two weeks, one was in a patient who had had a single breast cancer from which large biopsies were removed, and in the third only a small lymph node was present to begin with. The Krebiozen Research Foundation claimed that their data were misinterpreted by the committee.

Samples of krebiozen were requested by the National Cancer Institute and were analyzed and found to be creatine, a normal constituent of muscle and a common laboratory compound that could be purchased at thirty cents a gram. But when the National Cancer Institute indicated that they needed a large supply of the material for a study, Dr. Durovic said krebiozen could be provided at a cost of $170,000 per gram—a 500,000-fold markup, truly a steal! Other samples that were sent to the FDA for analysis were found to be fraudulently labeled, and some had nothing in them but mineral oil. Drs. Ivy, Durovic, and Mr. Marko Durovic were brought to trial for violation of FDA regulations and for fraud. Despite all the evidence, a jury acquitted them. The whole matter quietly petered out, but there is no telling how many patients who might have been cured with standard treatment were treated with krebiozen until it was too late, like the well-documented case of a woman who had operable breast cancer but was treated for a lengthy period with krebiozen while her disease kept progressing; she died soon after of metastatic cancer.

Even after the phony nature of krebiozen was exposed, patients continued to seek it for some years—until it was replaced by the next substance of this type, laetrile, a well-known chemical derived from the pits of apricots, about which a similarly great mystique developed, complete with international intrigue and unrealistic expectations. There were in fact many honest supporters, including a few reputable scientists, who supported the claims.

Laetrile was finally tested by a qualified group of clinical investigators who found that it did not provide the prolongation of life for cancer patients that its proponents had claimed. The laetrile story was similar in many respects to that of krebiozen except it could be very toxic and cause cyanide poisoning (see below).

OTHER MIRACLE DRUGS—LITMUS TESTS FOR INTELLI-GENT CONSUMERS If you learn the following points you should be readily prepared to identify the characteristics of a quack treatment, whether for cancer or for some other chronic disease. These hoaxes tend to be similar in that people with no background in cancer treatment research suddenly emerge with claims of miraculous cures, using unproven remedies that have not been studied by rigorous scientific methods. The originators often cloak their material in secrecy and refuse to divulge its contents; they claim that others would not be able to do as well because of the manner in which they mix their materials and remedies, and therefore they cannot afford to share the information. They have multiple unusual degrees such as N.D. (Doctor of Naturopathy), Ph.N. (Philosophy of Naturopathy) or Ms.D. (Doctor of Metaphysics)—these may have come from correspondence "schools." Their protocols are not registered through reputable channels and thus are not available for inspection. They discount the need for biopsy verification of the cancer and they discourage or refuse consultation with respectable physicians. Moreover, they do not publish their results in reputable journals and their data are not available to others. Rather, their supporters are often prominent public figures who are totally naive about scientific methods in clinical research. The originators of these remedies generally manage to mix in just a modicum of science, which may even attract outstanding scientists in their own right (like Dr. Ivy), but ones who do not know how to evaluate clinical cancer research. These legitimate scientists then serve to add respectability to the claims.

Since these substances are not licensed, they cannot be sold in the continental United States except under very unusual circumstances, and therefore clinics that can supply them tend to be located in Mexico, the Bahamas, Canada or any other nearby sanctuary that is willing to permit their operation. In fairness, the Canadian government is not at all receptive to such schemes, but sometimes a haven may be found there temporarily. The treatments are expensive, and when patients arrive they are told that no cures can be promised—but of course the publicity suggests that many others with similar problems have been cured, so why not you?

Sometimes the quack remedy is given by itself and sometimes it is combined with more standard drugs, but the claims for improvement are always attributed to the special remedy rather than to the standard drug, which may not even be mentioned. The treatments themselves may be innocuous, as in the case of krebiozen, or potentially quite toxic. Megavitamins, macrobiotic diets, laetrile and serum therapy are among the current favorites.

Victor Herbert, M.D., J.D., of New York estimates that about half of all cancer patients participate in quackery schemes. (That would be much higher than in my experience.) He urges that the touting of such consumer fraud be reported to the district attorney and the state consumer fraud division. Dr. Herbert feels that we are up against an army of some twenty-five thousand people with fraudulent credentials, about half from the so-called American Association of Nutrition and Dietary Consultants. To illustrate the point, for the price of an application and $50, they awarded a beautiful diploma with a gold seal—the types often found in health food stores labeled for "professional members"—to the family dog, Sassafras Herbert (Figure 14). This diploma certifies (sic, or woof!) that Sassafras has been found competent as a professional nutrition consultant. This kind of chicanery is endless—but it sells products or they wouldn't persist.

LAETRILE, SERUM THERAPY, VITAMIN C Even the knowledge that people have suffered cyanide poisoning from taking too much laetrile, while others have gotten severe hepatitis and AIDS virus from contaminated serum from the Burton Clinic in the Bahamas, will not stop the flow of believers. An investigation of the Burton operation seven years earlier recommended that it be closed because its claims were not legitimate, but the government took no steps to close it until the *Miami Herald* broke the story about the contaminated serum, which threatened the tourist trade. At that point the authorities acted to close the clinic. The most remarkable thing to me about these quack practitioners is that they appeal not only to medically unsophisticated people, but also to those who are well educated and very knowledgeable, including physicians and people who can afford the best medical care in the world. Steve McQueen, the well-known film actor, claimed he was getting better day by day from his quack remedy right up to the day he died—he actually believed that and urged other cancer victims to take the same remedy. That people are gullible is hardly news— P. T. Barnum preached that regularly; but it is sad that desperately ill people are especially vulnerable to exploitation. The tragedy is compounded when patients seek out a quack remedy instead of

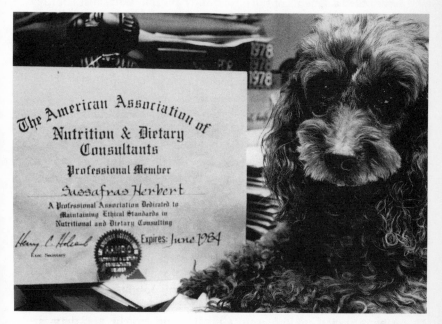

Figure 14 The family dog, Sassafras Herbert, posing with her professional credential from the American Association of Nutrition and Dietary Consultants—an example of how easy it is for charlatans to make themselves look legitimate to the unsuspecting public by purchasing phony credentials. (Photograph © 1983 Marilynne Herbert, photographer)

going to treatment programs that might offer them an opportunity for cure if given in a timely fashion; often by the time they turn back to standard treatments it is too late. In my view there is no meaner crime than to victimize someone who is already a victim of a dread disease, to offer false hope and fleece the person in the process.

Why do intelligent people find quack remedies so appealing? Probably no single answer will suffice. Why do intelligent people act according to what their horoscopes dictate? Why do they pay attention to financial predictions from psychics? Why do people seek medical attention for known serious medical illness like cancer from naturopaths or homeopaths, rather than from well-qualified medical experts? Clearly some of us in the medical profession have failed segments of the public and have not dealt satisfactorily with their problems, so they turn to someone who offers a ready solution. The medical doctor who tells a patient "There is nothing more I can do for you" is probably right about what he can do, but wrong about his approach and wrong about what a really thoughtful doctor could do, even for a patient who is "terminally" ill. *There is always something we can do to improve the situation for our patients; too often they are abandoned by physicians when they are no longer curable or are dissatisfied with a poor state of health that is unlikely to get better. It is just at these times that people are particularly vulnerable to the promises of quackery.* So at least part of the answer to the question at the head of this paragraph lies with the medical profession. And in fairness, part lies in the perfectly natural human reaction to life-threatening circumstances of willingness—indeed, urgent compulsion—to try anything.

The attractions of "help" (vulnerable patients read "cure") are even more seductive. The controversy over the effects of vitamin C is very instructive: this is an example of well-intentioned efforts that are not quackery but represent overly optimistic claims. The discovery of vitamin C won a Nobel Prize many years ago for Dr. Albert Szent-Györgyi; ironically, its more recent notoriety in health matters has come from the claims of two-time Nobel Laureate Dr. Linus Pauling, who has made pioneering contributions to chemistry and to our understanding of sickle cell disease and other genetic disorders. Though not a physician, Pauling earlier champi-

13: Experimental Therapy or Quackery: What's the Difference?

oned the claim that taking large regular doses of vitamin C would prevent the common cold—a most controversial idea in itself that has never been proven. Then he and his colleagues put forth the proposition that taking huge quantities of vitamin C could lengthen the life of patients with terminal cancer. In the opinion of many scientists their claim was supported only by a poorly designed clinical trial that was published in the *Proceedings* of the National Academy of Sciences. Unable to obtain research grants that are evaluated by experts in the field for his proposed studies, Pauling began fund-raising nationwide by his own foundation. Why wouldn't someone give money to support the research of this eminent scientist, who claimed that a relatively harmless vitamin could extend the life of terminally ill cancer victims? The fact that experienced clinical investigators thought the claims were baseless was dismissed by proponents as coming from the conservative and negative views of the "cancer research establishment," who were reluctant to accept any new ideas—particularly from one whose background was so far removed from clinical cancer research.

In time, so much political pressure was brought to bear on the National Cancer Institute that it had to support a well-controlled study of the subject in patients who were terminally ill from cancer. Dr. Edward Creagan of the Mayo Clinic was the senior investigator, and the study was carefully designed so that neither doctor nor patient knew whether the study drug (vitamin C) or an inert substance (placebo) was being given. It turned out that there was almost exactly the same survival rate in both groups of cancer patients—showing a total lack of effect not only on length of survival but also on the other measurable aspects of the illness. A second study (Figure 15) was performed in which vitamin C was compared with placebo in patients who had not previously received chemotherapy, in response to a complaint of Dr. Pauling. This time the patients were studied until the point where their disease progressed—again there was no advantage for those who received vitamin C. In a separate series of controlled studies, laetrile was also tested by this group and found to be of no value. That should be sufficient, but often it isn't.

The American Cancer Society has a committee on unproven methods of cancer treatment that carefully tracks the status of many claims of new treatments. Some may later be proven to be useful. The ACS is a source of such information to the public and can be reached by writing to 90 Park Avenue, New York, NY 10016. However, no one can afford to come right out and call a quack a quack for fear of having to defend a lawsuit. Many of these clinics operate just inside the law and it can be legally dangerous to speak out against them. And their lawyers love for you to accuse their clients of being quacks; they find it useful in a lawsuit. It still behooves the individual consumer to seek out the facts and heed the old admonition of letting the buyer beware. It shouldn't be that way—but it is.

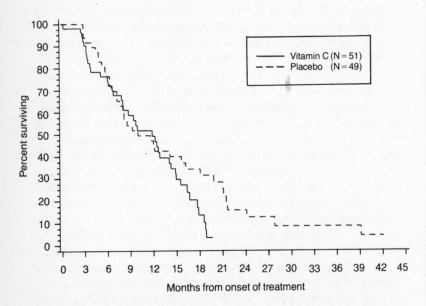

Figure 15 High-dose vitamin C versus placebo—time from beginning of treatment assignment to disease progression in one hundred patients with advanced cancer. The solid line shows data for fifty-one patients given vitamin C. The broken line shows comparable data for forty-nine patients given the lactose placebo. There is no significant difference in the curves. (Data published by Dr. C. G. Moertel, et al.; reprinted by permission of the *New England Journal of Medicine* 312 [1985]: 137)

ATTITUDE: THE ISSUE OF
MIND-BODY UNITY

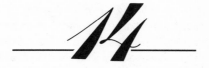

A great deal has been written about the importance of positive thinking in determining the outcome of cancer. The basic claims are that active mental participation in treatment may determine a longer than expected length of survival and an improved quality of life. The ideas are intuitively appealing. There are beginning to be some well-designed investigations of these claims, but the data are still limited. Nevertheless, a great deal has been written about this subject. The public has been quick to take an interest in this field but so far has been exposed to large amounts of fallacious thinking. One could devote an entire book to the subject of the influence of emotions on the body and vice versa. All of us have had the experience of having a cold/flu and the "down feeling" that accompanies such illness, or the contrary, when an accomplishment of some sort left us with a feeling that all was right with the world and with a renewed source of physical and psychic energy. So to treat the mind and the body as separate entities is to do an injustice to the person.

Instead of devoting an entire book (maybe I will when more data are obtained) to this interesting and important subject, let me summarize my view of the status of the field, then critically analyze one prominent example of a controversial program, that of the Simontons formerly from Texas, and conclude with some other illustrative material. First, let's try to separate the wheat from the chaff:

☐ *Does my attitude affect the likelihood of my developing cancer?* There is no convincing evidence that whether a person is happy, optimistic or whatever has any role in determining whether cancer will develop later in life. Psychologist Dr. Lawrence Le-Shan has written books about typical components in the life histories of cancer patients, but experimental evidence for this is obviously hard to come by unless one gathers huge data banks of psychological data on youngsters and then keeps track of them over a lifetime. If there are cancer-prone psychological profiles, this has not yet been demonstrated, but we will discuss this in greater detail. Depression cannot be used as a characteristic to describe patients with cancer after they are symptomatic or know they have the disease. To do so is an error that is commonly made by poorly trained investigators.

☐ *Does attitude affect the length of survival in patients with cancer?* Several partially controlled studies suggest that a positive attitude, expecting improvement—yes, even demanding it at times— may be associated with a longer than expected survival duration. The patient who quietly accepts fate appears not to do as well. This has most frequently been reported in series of patients with breast cancer where the will to live or a "fighting spirit" can be a self-fulfilling prophecy. By the same token, the lack of a will to live is also predictive for a shorter survival. Although the final answers are not all in, attitude does not appear to change length of life.

☐ *Does attitude affect the quality of remaining life?* An unqualified "yes" would probably come from almost every physician and nurse who is involved in the care of patients with cancer. My own experience is rich with stories of patients with cancer and other diseases who lived and experienced life to the fullest after they decided to get on with it and did. To sit around and grieve about our fate is also a kind of death. I often wish the well could learn from our patients who better appreciate the beauty of life *after* learning that it is in serious danger. Of course, their friends and relatives do learn about the power of courage and determination from these amazing success stories.

☐ *Can you "will away" your cancer?* This is a serious claim made by some clinics that specialize in "holistic" approaches. They teach that it is possible to mobilize your immune cells to attack and destroy the cancer. Not only is this a totally unfounded claim, it is also potentially very dangerous in that patients who engage in these programs may be sacrificing a real opportunity for benefit from more standard forms of treatment. We recognize that some of these clinics claim they also use all standard or traditional forms of treatment and merely add on their unique approaches to modify attitude and behavior, and therefore they sacrifice nothing in the process. Such claims are also made by groups practicing with quack remedies—the basic problem is that outstanding physicians generally will not associate themselves with these fringe groups, and it is advisable to have such a physician if the problem is difficult. There probably are exceptions, but I don't know of them.

☐ *Can biofeedback and visual imagery relieve the pain and discomfort often associated with cancer?* Here the expert consensus would be overwhelmingly favorable. We are quite convinced, from extensive experience and familiarity with some excellent published studies, that symptoms such as pain, nausea and vomiting, anxiety and panic can be greatly alleviated by appropriate relaxation and other biofeedback programs.

☐ *Should I believe the claims that holistic approaches cure cancer?* This falls into the same category as willing away your cancer. If you want to believe in magic remedies, there are many out there for sale, just as there are "miracle" diets for weight reduction that ignore basic laws of physics and thermodynamics ("Calories don't count"—indeed!). If the claims are legitimate, they will be reported at major scientific meetings and published in reputable journals—good news travels fast! But the warning signs I hope you will heed are very similar to those described for quack remedies in Chapter 13. I know that some lay people get upset with me for faulting the claims of miraculous cures attributed to one or another of these groups or approaches. Believe me, I would support whatever works even if I don't understand how it works—I believed in the tooth fairy when I was a child and was happy to have my children do likewise. But cancer is a deadly serious adult issue, and we have to keep our wits about us in evaluating the claims.

Getting Well Again is a book often referred to by those who wish to emphasize important nontraditional modes of treatment. The authors' backgrounds are as follows: Dr. Simonton was trained as a radiation oncologist, Mrs. Matthews-Simonton is a psychotherapist and Mr. J. L. Creighton listed himself as a collaborator with the Simontons who had also worked in patient counseling. They operated the Cancer Counseling and Research Center in Fort Worth, Texas, and they claimed to combine traditional medical management with psychological treatment to create the best environment for recovery. They also claimed that their results were "remarkable, with survival rates twice the national norm and, in many cases, [patients] have experienced dramatic remissions or total cures."

Again, they speak not only to the quantity but also to the quality of life. With regard to the latter, the Simontons are to be commended for calling attention to the mind-body connection, pointing out that how persons perceive their situations can be critical to their happiness, and that professionals can help patients by specific techniques that will likely help them feel better. They make the case effectively and, as indicated above, the notions are now quite widely accepted—although they weren't always, by any means. That part is fine, and I support it enthusiastically.

Perhaps my rigorous scientific training can be perceived as a drawback, making it difficult for me to grasp this type of subject matter. However, I do object to their other important claim, which I find totally unsubstantiated, that the length of survival can be significantly increased by the techniques they describe. First, it seems remarkable to me that in a 246-page book they devote less than one page to the data that supposedly provide the scientific underpinning for their important conclusions. Let me take you through the argument by relating this entire section of their book and then critiquing it as a scientist would have to do with any claim of a new advance, regardless of its type. If you are interested in examining the claims, please read the following points from their "Results of This Approach" and my critique that follows them.

The Simontons spent three years teaching patients to use their minds and emotions to combat the course of their diseases. After this three-year period they decided to conduct a study designed to distinguish the effects of emotional and medical treatments on illness in order to prove scientifically that emotional treatment has an effect.

They began studying a group of patients whose illnesses had been proclaimed medically incurable with expected average survival times of 12 months.

During a four-year period the Simontons treated 159 patients who had been diagnosed with a medically incurable illness, and at the end of that time 63 of their patients were still alive. The surviving patients had an average survival time of 24.4 months from the time their illnesses were diagnosed. The Simontons stated that the national norm of life expectancy for this group is 12 months. At the time their book was published a matched control population was being developed. The initial results of the control group indicated that the survival rate of that group was comparable with national norms and that the control group's survival rate was less than half the survival rate for patients in the Simontons' group. Finally, the average survival time for patients in the Simontons' study who died was 20.3 months. The Simontons therefore concluded that the patients in their study who survived up to the time of their writing had lived, on the average, two times longer than patients who received only medical treatment. They also pointed out that even the patients in their study who died still lived one and a half times longer than the patients in the control group.

At the time of the publication of their book, the Simontons reported on the status of the surviving patients in their study as follows: 22.2 percent (fourteen patients) had no evidence of the disease; 19.1 percent (twelve patients) fell under the category of "tumor regressing"; 27.1 percent (seventeen patients) were "disease stable"; and 31.8 percent (twenty patients) experienced new tumor growth.

Critique: On the face of it all of those claims sound favorable. But let's look at them through the eyes of a physician-scientist and examine the problems.

1   It is laudable to conduct a study to distinguish the effects of emotional and medical treatments in order to demonstrate "scientifically" that the emotional treatment was having an effect on survival, over and above that of the medical treatment. That is *the* issue, but it can be studied only by designing a protocol that has the following *minimal* elements.

a   It is necessary to decide in advance what type of patients are eligible to participate in the study, that is, what types of cancer, how advanced (in terms of spread and other medical factors), how sick the patients are when they enter the study, what ages of patients are included, how often they will be seen and followed up—these are all critical issues in such a study. "Medically incurable" cancers come in different varieties, I presume, and each variety carries with it a different life expectancy. Could it be that the "national norm" comprises all varieties, yet the study group consists of patients with longer life expectancies to begin with? Thus, their statement that they have only patients who are deemed "medically incurable" and that such patients would have an expected mean survival time of twelve months is not enlightening in regard to these factors. Indeed, it is a *totally meaningless* statement for a scientific study. That certain types of people select themselves to go to this clinic creates a group that is "biased" and in no way reflects an average population of people with cancer. Quite possibly their characterization of an active and positive participation presupposes an ambulatory patient, or at least a person in reasonably good condition. By contrast, bedridden patients who couldn't travel to Texas would be included in the national norm but may not be represented proportionately in their study group.

b   A properly done study defines the criteria for response in advance. Not every patient who has cancer has tumors that can be measured quantitatively—how the measurements are to be taken and how often they are to be repeated has to be carefully specified. How long the study will last and how long the response must last in order to be called a response are also critical issues. If a small tumor shrinks and disappears but then reappears a month later, that is not a very important result—but it could be rated as an excellent response or as no evidence of disease remaining—if one chooses not to be fussy about such issues. The category "disease stable" also generally offers no benefit to the patient, as we usually evaluate a new cancer treatment. "Tumor regressing" can mean almost anything—this study did not define how much and for how long. Thus the percentage of patients who fall into different categories of response is useless information.

c   Their statement "A matched control population is being developed and preliminary results indicate survival comparable with national norms and less than half the survival time of our patients" is misleading and self-serving. If a study is being developed, we are naturally talking about the potential for obtaining results in the future, *if* the study is done satisfactorily in *all* respects (and that is a big if). One cannot have preliminary results from a study that is being developed—it's like being a little bit pregnant, and there is no such thing. *A properly controlled study would require that all of the patients would be given medical treatment and half of the patients would receive emotional treatment. Which half would get the emotional treatment and which would not would be determined by chance alone and not by the patients or the doctors. The results would have to be coded so that an independent investigator analyzing the data would not know which group is which until after all the data are in and the study fully analyzed.* Admittedly this is very hard to do but clearly it is not the way in which this study was conducted. Critical clinical research is very hard to do, but to ignore basic scientific principles is to create a bias and make it ethically impossible ever to do a proper study. We have seen that mistake made time and again in other areas of medicine.

2   *To count survival from the time of diagnosis to death is irrelevant if we are trying to evaluate treatments that often begin long after the diagnosis is made.* An example might be a potential patient who had a diagnosis of cancer in May 1980, had surgery at that time and developed a recurrence in April 1982. If that person entered into a study then and died in May 1982, he or she lived for one month after the study commenced but two years after the diagnosis. Clearly we are interested in attributing to the new treatment *only* the events for the period during which the patient was receiving it, and not all events from the time the diagnosis of cancer was made. I cannot evaluate the Simonton study in that way based on the information they give us in their book.

3   The authors tell us that over the past four years they have treated 159 patients. We do not know how many were studied in each year. If their studies were the same each year then they would have entered forty new patients annually. (Almost certainly they entered more patients in the last year than in the first since it takes time for a practice to grow.) Assuming an even distribution would mean that only seventy-nine or eighty patients had been followed for longer than two years, and therefore an average survival time of 24.4 months "from diagnosis" makes no sense since half the patients have not even been under treatment that long. By the same token we cannot evaluate the importance of sixty-

three patients' being alive, since they might all have been entered in the last two years while all the other patients are dead. There are other serious problems with the survival data.

a   As we have said, a "national norm" for medically incurable cancer does not exist, and so the notion that this historical control, as it is called, serves as a yardstick for their results is inappropriate. A straw man is being created because they are comparing old data from other groups with data on a different group treated with newer methods.

b   The authors stated that those patients in their study still living had lived two times *longer than* the "control group." What they meant by this, I presume, is that their patients' life expectancy was extended by twelve months beyond that nonexistent "national norm." The status and structure of the "control group" are not at all clear.

c   Without knowing the rates at which patients were entered into a study, there is no possibility of assessing the significance of the statement that sixty-three of 159 patients were living at the end of the fourth study year, as mentioned above.*

*To compute this, our statistician, C. Y. Tso, Ph.D., has made the following assumptions:

☐   The number of patients entering the study per year is uniform over the four-year period.

☐   Survival of any one patient is independent of the survival of all other patients.

☐   Death rate is constant over time for all patients, that is, the survival does not depend on which of the four years the patient entered the study.

From the Simonton data, we estimate the average survival time to be 21 months (median survival to be 14.6 months). Median survival is far superior to average survival because a few long survivals could affect the average dramatically. (For example, suppose we have five patients and four live for one month and one lives forty-eight months—it is not informative to give the average figure [52/5 = 10.4 months].) The authors seemed impressed with the observation that the average survival of the *living* patients at the end of the fourth study year was 24.4 months. It turns

On balance, there is no way in which this study could be classified as "scientific" nor can the results, as described, be said to hold
any measurable significance.

If there were one hundred holistic centers operating on principles similar to the Simontons', and only the most "successful" one
wrote a story, would similar success bless the next such center?

I don't mean for this analysis to be an "overkill" of data summarized in a book. Without the opportunity for the authors to rebut,
that isn't quite fair. Nor do I object to the urging for active participation of patients in their care. But the point that must be understood if you are to make intelligent choices in such matters is that
scientific advances can be made only when studies are carefully
designed and fully analyzed by impartial means. It is easy to make
lofty claims, but when lives and costs are at stake it is imperative
that investigations be careful and follow the "rules." *If anything,
studies that are inadequately set up or are misinterpreted to make a point (no
matter how well intentioned) ultimately serve only to undermine confidence rather
than contribute to supportive strength.*

What about the case reports given in the book, which seem to
suggest the miraculous success of the Simontons' treatment approach? I could critique them individually, and to their credit the
authors themselves provide some disclaimers regarding possibilities that factors other than their treatment were responsible. Some
patients do very well and are cured with traditional treatments, as
we have described elsewhere, and to claim that the emotional
therapy should be credited with *determining* a favorable outcome I
would call assuming the conclusion. If you know the answer, why

---

out that under conditions of the study *the result is inevitable, and it signifies no
benefit from the treatment itself.* In more detail: if we had 159 patients from the
"control group," accrued uniformly over four years, and if at the end of
the fourth year we compute the average survival time of the *living* patients, the result would still be close to twenty-four months. Of course
the *number* of patients living would be smaller, assuming the "control
group" had lower life expectancy. Additional calculations not listed here
tell us that with an approximate confidence of 95 percent, we can say that
the average survival of the thirty-eight or thirty-nine living patients
would be between 19.6 and 28.4 months.

do the study—but we don't! Thus, for me the case reports do not help in substantiating the story—any experienced oncologist could come up with a long series of favorable case reports based on currently available treatments. And sometimes there are surprising cases of temporary improvement that occur spontaneously, sometimes after an infection, sometimes without any other unusual association.

What about the claim by the Simontons (and that of others) that stress has an unfavorable effect on the immune system and on the resistance of the patient to the cancer? From my research I believe it is likely that stress can be quantitated with newer techniques, and that reduction of stress may favorably influence immunity and resistance to cancer. While I believe that this is likely, this is very different from saying it is true, or that reducing stress will prolong survival. *The difference may seem subtle, but it is critical to understand the distinction.* And some of the writings about producing superimmunity are naïve and misleading.

So where do we go from here? Much important information needs to be garnered about the role of emotions in patients with cancer—no one would dispute that point. Nor would anyone dispute the importance of the emotions, that a positive, hopeful and participatory approach is vital to virtually all aspects of prevention and care—that of course is largely the message of my book. The important point is that doctors should employ whatever emotional and supportive treatments are helpful for their patients, using them as part of a total mind-body approach to health care. Nor is any one emotional approach suitable for all patients, any more than is any particular medical treatment—*each and every patient is different and requires unique and thoughtful care.*

It has been claimed that stress causes cancer in humans, but the evidence supporting this claim is quite flimsy. We know that acute or short-term stress usually does not cause much change in the immune system—so individuals who have been on a fast, those who have completed a marathon or space travelers experience very little change in their immunity, and will return to normal in just a few days. So this probably has little or no biological significance. On the other hand, the most severe of the "ordinary" stresses with which people are afflicted is generally the death of a family member such as a spouse—when that occurs there is often a temporary depression (also) of the immune response. After a time it tends to return to normal, but that is not invariably the case.

In mental disorders such as chronic depression, a normal immune response is often lacking. Statistics indicate that bereaved and depressed patients are more likely to become ill and to die than are normal people—but whether changes in immunity are responsible for that susceptibility is not known, nor is whether these conditions influence the growth of cancer. A recent study by Jamison et al. found no relationship between psychogenic factors and length of life in patients with breast cancer.

In animals the situation of frustration and stress can increase the rate of tumor growth, whereas stress without concomitant frustration does not have the same effect. In a recent book entitled *Behavior and Cancer,* Sandra M. Levy, Ph.D., reviews the literature on this subject and on the overall effects of the brain on the processes of immunity. She and others have concluded that there is no question that psychological factors (such as stress) can profoundly change the secretion of hormones due to changes in the brain. We also know that some human and animal tumors are controlled by hormones, and such tumors may either grow or shrink depending upon whether these hormones are lacking or present in excess. The relationship, therefore, between emotions and the brain, since the latter affects immunity and hormone secretion, seems highly relevant to the subject of tumor growth, but precisely how this will work in individual instances is unknown. We doctors have all had patients under our care who appear to be dying within a matter of days, but who simply "decided" to hang on until a particularly important event, such as the marriage of a child, a longed-for trip, a graduation or an anniversary, had taken place. We had one well-known musician on our ward who at times was barely conscious in the terminal phase of cancer, but who miraculously managed to rally prior to the time of a scheduled final fund-raising concert for charity and go on with the show. This was the culmination of her hopes and she was able to perform beautifully; like a delicate butterfly, she died shortly thereafter. There are many well-documented cases of this type, and there are lessons to be learned that are still beyond our understanding.

A number of studies now link coping styles with prognosis. Several studies in both breast cancer and malignant melanoma have shown negative correlations between feelings of apathy, fatigue or helplessness and various factors related to prognosis such as the number of lymph nodes involved with breast cancer, tumor thickness in melanoma and indeed, more recently, even length of survival. Some authors have attempted to characterize these different emotional states into one unifying personality—the "Type C" person: "An individual who is cooperative, unassertive, patient, who suppresses negative emotions (particularly anger) and who accepts/complies with external authorities." The number of patients in such studies is small and indeed the number of studies themselves is low. Nevertheless, the characteristic behavior pattern documented is remarkably consistent. These studies are difficult to perform because of the great number of other factors involved at the same time. Still, it does appear that those who openly express their fears, frustrations and anger are likely to have a better outlook than accepting, uncomplaining patients.

None of the associations mentioned above prove conclusively that emotions control either the likelihood of getting cancer or how fast it will grow. Nonetheless, there is ample evidence to indicate that feelings (anger, frustration, stress, anxiety, helplessness) may affect at least the quality of life and possibly even the quantity of life in patients with cancer. Some of the people who write books about their system of care confuse quantity with quality of life. Definitive answers are hard to attain through studies of such patient populations and there is therefore probably a greater tendency to speculate in this field than in most others.

Clearly we need more information about the specific effects of stress on the immune system and about bringing about stress reduction for patients. Then we need to objectively evaluate how effectively these treatments improve the quality and quantity of life for different classes of patients. My own feeling is that such studies are extraordinarily difficult to organize and conduct in an impartial manner, and they need to be done by capable, experienced clinical researchers, who will design careful studies, impartially analyze the data and move forward the frontier of knowledge. Only then will we get away from the unproductive rhetoric of claims and counterclaims. Fortunately we do have drugs, such as benzodiazepines, that can reduce anxiety, and this at least gives us a tool with which to study the effects of altering this psychological factor. And then behavioral intervention techniques—training in relaxation, hypnosis, et cetera—are also useful tools to study.

A number of books are beginning to appear on the general subject of coping with the emotional aspects of cancer. But remarkably little about cancer has been written for lay people by oncology specialists who take care of afflicted patients all day, every day. Helping to fill that gap was the impetus for this book, in fact. We can read moving personal experiences written by patients who tell stories of their own coping with cancer—experiences that while interesting and provocative are not suitable to be generalized from or considered as authoritative. An interesting book of a somewhat different nature, by psychotherapist Neil A. Fiore, Ph.D., is *The Road Back to Health.* Fiore used his personal bout with cancer as a point of departure for later work with cancer patients, and his discussion of how to become an active and hopeful patient by building emotional support systems with physicians, family and friends is quite informative as well as readable. I would like to quote the opening paragraphs of his 1984 book.

I was a cancer patient. But that alone does not give me the qualifications to write a book, nor does it necessarily mean that I have anything of value to say to you, the reader. There are many valuable books which tell of patients' experiences with cancer, but I want to do more than share my experiences. As a psychotherapist I want to do more than share my experiences. As a psychotherapist I want to help other patients cope with this trauma and return even stronger to the tasks of healthy life.

On June 13, 1974, my doctors diagnosed my condition—I had cancer. Neither my doctors nor my hospital were prepared to treat the emotional or psychological aspects of cancer. Nor could I find a book that dealt with these human aspects of serious illness. Once I began speaking and writing about cancer, patients and their relatives began asking me what they could read. There were books by cancer patients that told their stories. There were books that were studies of how patients seemed to cope with their illnesses. And there were books that speculated about a link between emotional-psychological states and cancer. But there wasn't a single book that I could comfortably recommend to a patient. I couldn't believe that there weren't any books on how to cope with the emotional aspects of cancer.

Neil Fiore's book is a good one on this subject.

Bernie S. Siegel, M.D., has written a very different kind of book, one that is bound to become controversial, on the role of the patient in healing. In *Love, Medicine & Miracles,* Dr. Siegel—Bernie, as he prefers to be called—describes his own transformation from a "mechanical" surgeon to a "privileged listener" who helps patients take charge of their lives and gives them hope to become the "exceptional patients" who are healed of their disease. He gives us many insights into the various attitudes that doctors unconsciously convey to patients and into the importance of doctors' being able to instill hope into their patients. Bernie must be a good doctor and a fine human being. I agree that physicians must learn to project hope at all times, even at what may seem a terminal stage of disease. Dr. Siegel talks about the exceptional patients who made miraculous recoveries and characterizes these survivors as people who invariably made a drastic change toward a more loving and self-reliant attitude. "Exceptional patients refuse to be victims. They educate themselves and become specialists in their own care. They question the doctor because they want to understand their treatment and participate in it. They demand dignity, personhood, and control, no matter what the course of the disease. It takes courage to be exceptional." All of this makes the utmost sense to me in terms of attitude.

Unfortunately, in my view, the book goes completely off the deep end because of a kind of religious fervor or conviction of the author concerning techniques of self-healing that were actually inspired by the Simontons. He accepts these ideas and presents some unsubstantiated observations of his own as dogma, without the slightest recognition that he is assuming, rather than proving, the conclusion. Poor science offends good scientists—just as bad writing or music offends artists. But when that science deals with the lives of patients, the stakes are high, and it is far more than a matter of aesthetics. Once again, the point is that making far-fetched claims is not a contribution, for it is good studies that are needed to lend credence to the notion that genuine progress can be made in this important field. For example, there is no justification for stating that there are no incurable diseases, only unloving patients who cannot cure themselves. That is blaming the victim, just as happens in rape. Dr. Barrie Cassileth, a psychologist who has studied this subject, has helped to care for many determined and motivated patients who fought hard to live—but could not overcome their terminal cancer. Let us not oversimplify a complex problem and thereby do an injustice to patients by blaming them for making anything less than a complete recovery.

The emotional needs of our patients with cancer require expert and sensitive professionals who will help the patient to cope with each successive medical setback, rehospitalization, broken bone, loss of income and inability to take full part in the normal activities of daily living. In an article on this subject for physicians, social worker Joan F. Herman points out that by the time patients reach the advanced stages of cancer they have already lost many parts of themselves, and it is the physician, in addition to the patient, who must face the results of those losses. In offering advice to help physicians to be useful in turn to patients and families, she points out that "most of us are not naturally gifted in the practice of our professions. . . . There are times when the losses are too painful, and we retreat for a while to replenish ourselves. There are other times when we rejoice in the courage of our patients and their families and are renewed. At all times, we struggle with remaining open to the life around us so that we might be permitted to help with the way it is lived." I dare say that each of us who works in this field would agree with those observations.

A word about the long-term survivors of cancer—they are often neglected in our thoughts. They also may have special needs so that they can function normally in society. Dr. Jimmie Holland of

Memorial Hospital in New York states that "successful" survivors need a number of things to ensure their quality of life. These include:

- [ ] *Job*—Stability and normal ability to pursue career goals
- [ ] *Family*—Maintaining the family unit and key relationships
- [ ] *Sex*—Normal libido and performance, satisfaction and fertility (including sperm banking before chemotherapy)
- [ ] *Psychological comfort*—Maintaining a sense of security and freedom from destructive levels of anxiety, depression or preoccupation with illness
- [ ] *Social and leisure activities*—Ability to enjoy hobbies and the absence of social isolation

These are all good points to look for, and I would add only the category of successful integration into the school in the case of children. This is a special problem for them, particularly if they have suffered any brain damage from the treatment of their disease.

A section on mind-body unity in cancer should not end without my observation on the importance of humor in maintaining perspective during an illness. The world is full of examples of suffering, as the book of Job teaches, but a bit of humor always soothes and comforts us and those around us.

CANCER RESEARCH: THE CUTTING EDGE

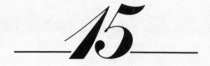

It is hard to believe, but it is true: we have learned more about the control of cells and how they multiply and mature in the last fifty years than in the whole previous history of the world! The breaking of the genetic code in the 1950s led to modern molecular biology, and to the rich discoveries that made it possible to isolate chromosomes and parts of chromosomes, and to move them from one cell to another, to purify certain sequences of DNA and determine their exact composition, to put certain sequences to work as chemical factories to produce rare molecules for use in treatment of human diseases or to make monoclonal antibodies to probe unique properties of cells, and to isolate and identify growth factors that turn cells on and off and regulate their function and ability to divide. Advances in the biological sciences have been at least as impressive as the discoveries in the physical sciences that are illustrated by the accomplishments in computer technology and space exploration.

The cancer researcher has to understand how normal cells are regulated and how the regulation of tumor cells differs, in order to either manipulate the controls and regulate the growth of tumor cells or make them differentiate and behave more like normal cells. Alternatively, another approach is to try to kill tumor cells selectively, without destroying vital normal cells. These are enormous challenges, and there are almost as many different approaches being tried as there are investigators engaged in this type of research.

UNDERSTANDING HOW CANCER AND NORMAL CELLS DIFFER Some researchers concentrate on the outer cell surface, the membrane that separates the cytoplasmic contents of the cell from its external environment. This membrane comes into contact with other cells and provides signals to the inside of the cell that it should stop dividing or that it should continue to divide (normal cells characteristically stop while tumor cells continue to divide when they come into contact with adjacent cells). When normal cells grown in tissue culture touch each other, they communicate their proximity by a process known as contact inhibition, which turns off further cell division. This also operates *in vivo* as with a cut in the skin that stimulates the cells on one side of the wound to grow until contact is made with those from the other side and the process shuts down when healing is complete—the cells don't keep on growing to form a tumor. The outer cell surface is also the point at which growth regulators attach themselves and are selectively bound, thence to be transported to the nucleus of the cell either intact or as altered "second messengers" that provide further signals to regulate the functions of the cell. This outer membrane of the cell permits certain molecules to pass freely, others to pass not at all and still others to be transported on a very limited basis. The gatekeeping decision of what shall pass and what shall be withheld determines whether a chemotherapeutic drug has a chance of entering the cell to cause its effects or whether it will be excluded altogether. These are but a few of the functions and events that take place at the outer cell surface.

There are many ways of studying the cell surface, ranging from new techniques of visualizing the structure of the membrane, to isolating the chemicals that make up its structure, to studying the functional interactions between the chemicals at the cell surface and the receptors that are there to recognize them specifically, to examining the immunologic characteristics of the cell that distinguish it from others, and so on.

The study of growth factors has been a most promising research area in cancer research. Dr. Stanley Cohen of Vanderbilt School of Medicine, an ACS Research Professor, and Dr. Rita Levi-Montalcini were awarded the Nobel Prize and the Albert Lasker Research Award for their work on finding and characterizing Epidermal Growth Factor (EGF) and Nerve Growth Factor (NGF), both soluble proteins that are produced by growing cells and stimulate growth of other cells. These growth factors must bind to receptors on the cell surface and this activates an enzyme, tyrosine kinase, which in turn stimulates cell growth. The specific biochemical steps are also common to the effects of a number of oncogenes, by mechanisms that are being unraveled at a very rapid rate. Tyrosine kinase, for example, is coded for by a known oncogene.

Some researchers start at the inside of the cell and investigate the switches that activate certain genetic information within the nucleus of cancer cells, which makes growth factors for example, that may not usually be turned on or expressed in normal cells, even though that information may be potentially available. Other researchers are trying to isolate specific genes that perform vital functions, such as the synthesis of immune globulin proteins, in order to discover how these go awry in a malignant disease of the plasma cells called multiple myeloma.

Imagine a situation in which a particular normal cell (plasma cell) type goes astray and becomes malignant. In health we rely upon normal plasma cells to produce immune antibodies and protect us when we come in contact with foreign antigens or specific chemicals on the cell surface, such as blood group factors or those on the cell wall of disease-causing bacteria. In cancer, it may be that only one of millions of plasma cells undergoes malignant transformation; then it begins to produce identical daughter cells and gradually to replace the other normal plasma cells, as well as other normal blood-forming cells in the bone marrow. These abnormal plasma cells produce peculiar immune globulin proteins that are characteristic of multiple myeloma; these proteins have no useful effects in terms of immunity, but rather can cause harm to the patient when they are produced in very large numbers. For example, the proteins can clog up the kidney tubules and cause kidney failure. Malignant plasma cells multiply and can spread beyond the confines of the bone marrow and may infiltrate any of the organs of the body. In the process they are likely to cause destruction of bones and so much loss of mineral substance that so-called pathological fractures occur with little or no traumatic provocation. In perhaps half of the patients treated for multiple myeloma we are able to kill sufficient numbers of plasma cells with chemotherapy to at least partially restore these patients to health and improve their chance for longer survival, but only very rarely are we successful in curing such patients. In fact, I am now following a great character who certainly lived well since he was cured of myeloma many years ago by the use of chemotherapy by one of my colleagues. There are less than a handful of such examples, and although the available treatments are improving, they are still not as effective as they need to be. Researchers have come to recognize some of the properties of the transformed plasma cell, and we know how its chromosomes become rearranged, but we do not yet have any insight into how those changes can be reversed, if that in fact turns out to be the best thing to do.

NEW TECHNOLOGIES AND NEW INSIGHTS In the past few years we have learned about the presence of oncogenes—genetic materials that are invariably present in certain forms of cancer and are also found in viruses that may be responsible for inducing those cancers. And Dr. Robert Weinberg of MIT has described his recent discovery of "antioncogenes": the *loss* of this genetic material predicts that a child will get retinoblastoma, a rare tumor of the eye. This is the first demonstration that certain portions of DNA protect against getting cancer. We have a complex biological system in which oncogenes are genes that promote cancer when they are inappropriately activated or armed by carcinogens. By contrast, antioncogenes are genes that promote cancer when they are inappropriately lost or inactivated. As we learn more about the molecular details of cancer cell formation it is likely that some totally new approaches to cancer prevention will emerge. For example, we may soon be using molecular methods to predict the likelihood of getting colon cancer, and that would be a great help for early diagnosis.

The technology involving DNA chemistry is exploding. There is even a debate about attempting to determine the sequence of some three billion nucleotide building blocks in human DNA; possibly this could be accomplished by automatic chemical sequencing. This would be a powerful tool to determine how normal and cancer cells differ—but developing it is going to take time and money. As noted in Chapter 7, cancers that have been linked to exposure to a virus include the African Burkitt's lymphoma, which is linked to the EB virus; nasopharyngeal cancer in the Orient, which is linked to this same virus; and liver cancer, also in the Orient, which is linked to the hepatitis B virus. But now the evidence is not only by association (epidemiology) but is also strengthened by direct evidence of viral nucleic acid's being present in such cancer cells but not in normal cells.

The first large attempt at a practical application of the latest information about viruses in the etiology of cancer will be a clinical trial conducted in Asia with a vaccine against hepatitis B virus. In that region of the world, hepatitis B infection is very common, and liver cancer arises years later in the same population. Indeed, the liver cancer (but not the adjacent areas of normal liver) contains the DNA base sequences derived from the hepatitis B virus. Therefore, the hope is that by preventing this type of virus infection in the first place, we will also be able to prevent the later occurrence of cancer. This is a very attractive approach because vaccination is so effective and inexpensive in preventing infection, but it will take years to determine whether this approach is effective in preventing cancer. If it is, then further tests of EB virus and other suspected cancer-causing viruses can be performed.

In the case of animal tumors caused by specific viruses, we already know that immunization against the virus can prevent the cancer from occurring; this is quite clear in the case of the very common leukemia that occurs in cats and for which there now is a vaccine. This is quite an advance for cat lovers. And there are some interesting relationships between the virus that causes leukemia in cats and the family of HTLV viruses that can cause a kind of leukemia and also AIDS in humans, though the cat virus is not infectious to people. The cat virus impairs immunity in infected animals much as do the human viruses, showing the central role of particular lymphocytes in immunity and certain leukemias, as shown by Drs. Myron Essex of Harvard and Robert Gallo of NCI. If we can bring our knowledge of viruses in humans up to the point of our knowledge of viruses in animals, we will have made great progress; this is clearly happening from one day to the next. Every single week when I pick up a scientific journal I read of important new discoveries with oncogenes and new insights into the processes by which cells become cancerous.

I recently heard Dr. Philip Leder (Harvard) deliver a Lasker Award lecture in which he showed how cells with rearrangement of the L-myc oncogene could be transplanted into other mice all of whose female offspring would develop breast cancer. There may be profound relevance of this finding to the genetic susceptibility of some women to breast cancer.

The manner by which chemicals cause cells to change into malignant cell types is beginning to be understood for the first time. Specific receptors for tumor-promoting agents have been identified on the cell surface; these are activated when that agent is physically bound to the receptor and that bonding in turn generates a chemical signal that activates cellular processes that might lie quiet indefinitely if not stimulated. We are also beginning to realize that more than one factor may interact with the cell, explaining why it generally takes more than one transformation event to change a normal cell into a cell that is capable of producing a tumor. It used to be thought that chemicals could cause cancer under certain conditions and possibly viruses could as well, but there was no recognition of a possible link by which some combination of chemicals and viruses could interact ultimately to trigger malignant cellular transformation. The possibilities for interaction between viruses and oncogenes on the one hand and chemical carcinogens on the other is now beginning to be elucidated and a pattern has begun to emerge. New information also raises the possibility that chemicals, including certain nutrients, can be found that prevent the development of cancer even after normal cells have been altered by carcinogens. This new and exciting field is called chemoprevention, and scientists are developing potent drugs that seem to work in experimental (animal) systems.

Each piece of the story represents an independent piece of research done by an investigator working in a laboratory using his creative skills, but also benefiting from the work that others have done. Scientific meetings, both small and large, afford investigators opportunities to exchange information that is at the very cutting edge of science, long before the information can be published in a medical journal. All this is still at the earliest stage of exploration—as are many other lines of investigation in cancer research. We must, and should, and do, always have hope. But it is terrible when such lines of investigation are given a great deal of oversimplified publicity at this earliest time, resulting in misplaced hope and battered confidence for thousands. There have been too many examples of premature press conferences, and it all can happen so innocently. But not all of the investigators' findings will hold up; the experiments must be reproduced, not only by the laboratory that made the original discovery but also by other workers, who may turn up flaws in the methods or come up with quite different findings. That's the way it goes in science. Up to a point duplication is important, even necessary, but once the evidence is conclusive it is important to disseminate that knowledge quickly lest there be wasteful replication. Research tends to move along at a slow but orderly pace until some major new insight is added; then a great flurry of discoveries is likely to follow, bringing us to a new level of understanding.

MONOCLONAL ANTIBODIES FOR DIAGNOSIS AND TREATMENT As new features of the cell are recognized, new tools become available to sharpen our understanding further. For example, the recognition that cancer cells possess certain antigenic patterns makes it possible, using a new technology called hybridoma research, to produce very specific monoclonal antibodies that recognize one particular antigen and no other. Several practical applications may come from such research. For instance, it is possible to attach radioactive labels onto these monoclonal antibodies and inject them into an animal that harbors tiny nests of tumor cells; the antibodies will "home" specifically to these cells and because the antibody molecules are carrying radioactive tracer labels, they can be scanned by image-detecting devices, which can pinpoint the microscopic metastases. *Such metastases are too small to be identified by any other technique.* These discoveries raise many exciting new opportunities for both diagnosis and treatment.

Instead of attaching radioisotopes, it is also possible to attach very toxic chemicals to the antibody molecules, using the latter like a modern-day Trojan horse to carry lethal chemicals directly to the specific cancer cells that the antibody molecule will recognize. The front end of the antibody molecule contains the specific recognition site for latching onto the tumor cell, and the back end carries the lethal substance, much as a nuclear warhead is carried along by its rocket engine and programmed steering. Among the lethal substances being tested is a portion of the ricin molecule, ricin being one of the most potent toxins known—but it will not kill cells that lack the recognition site to which its carrier antibody is bound. (The complete ricin molecule is the poison that is thought to be used by the KGB in its political assassinations—in that case injected without benefit of antibody!)

Numerous obstacles must be overcome before this treatment approach can be effectively used with cancer patients, but it is a wide open new avenue for researchers. The obstacles include the fact that tumor cells have variable characteristics (heterogeneity) and not all of them necessarily have the antigen recognition sites on the cell surface at all times. Thus, a treatment using a charged or toxic monoclonal antibody would kill only those cells that are bearing sufficient numbers of antigen sites to permit a critical interaction to occur; the treatment would leave behind those cells that do not meet that requirement. Another problem comes from the propensity of cancer cells to change their antigenic makeup and thereby protect or camouflage themselves to resist this type of immune destruction. A third problem lies in the possibility that at least some types of normal cells may share antigens with tumor cells and thus be susceptible to being destroyed by the chemicals aimed at the tumor cells; this could possibly cause serious damage to normal tissue. There is also the possibility that the toxic chemical substance will not bind with sufficient tightness to its antibody carrier, and tiny amounts might leach off.

There is another problem, which Drs. Amos, Peacock, Buckley and I discovered long ago, and that is the effect of excessive amounts of tumor antigen, more than can be "destroyed" by antibody molecules. Years before monoclonal antibodies were discovered, we treated patients with human isoantibody that happened also to react and destroy leukemic cells of certain patients. Dr. Amos had found that women who had been through multiple pregnancies produced antibody against a large array of antigens on normal white blood cells and we could type them to find which had powerful plasma antibodies that also reacted and killed leukemic cells from my patients with chronic lymphocytic leukemia. We then purified this globulin antibody and infused it into the patients, watching excitedly when most of the leukemic cells disappeared and lymph glands shrank, but then we observed that the disease gradually returned. The problem, we found, was that there were far too many leukemic cells to kill with the antibodies than we could harvest from the women donors, and the matter was dropped until others found out how to make almost limitless amounts of antibody by the hybridoma technology. The other problems mentioned earlier also need to be solved before we can hope to cure patients of this chronic lymphocytic leukemia. And these are just a few of the barriers that must be overcome before useful applications can be expected in the clinic. But the monoclonal antibody work is progressing nicely in colon and some other cancers, and the next few years should be most enlightening.

One of the newest approaches to the use of antibodies directed against specific substances present in tumors was reported by Dr. Stanley Order of Johns Hopkins and by radiotherapists at several institutions. An antiferritin antibody was prepared by immunizing various types of animals with an iron-containing protein called ferritin, a substance that is present in high concentration in and around tumors. The researchers then attached radioactive iodine to the antibody and gave that to 105 patients who had liver cancer (hepatoma). By so doing they were able to show that the antibody was concentrated in areas of tumor in the liver and it carried with it the radioactivity, which then served to destroy the surrounding tumor tissue. About half of their patients had a partial remission, defined as 50 percent or greater shrinkage of tumor size, for at least a period of time before the disease recurred in most patients. There are other ways of combining this treatment with radiation therapy or with chemotherapy, and there are also other types of radioactivity that could be attached to the antiferritin, which would give it the possibility of improving its efficiency in killing cells. Although it is premature to suggest this as a routine treatment, it certainly is of interest as a first step in treating difficult cancers of this sort, since we have little else that is effective against liver cancer.

KILLING BY LYMPHOCYTES—THE INTERLEUKIN-2 STORY

There is great current interest in immune therapy using the patient's own lymphocytes to kill the tumor cells. Dr. Steven Rosenberg and his colleagues at the National Cancer Institute have reported on their first series of patients so treated and they are optimistic, although it is far too early to put this into perspective. The fascinating technique works something like this. Tumor cells from the patient are placed into many tiny sterile dishes to which are added normal lymphocytes from the blood of the patient. Lymphocytes are white blood cells composed of many different subgroups; some of them, present perhaps only in a tiny amount, can have the capacity to kill tumor cells. When such cells are found they can be stimulated to multiply by adding a normal growth factor for lymphocytes called interleukin-2 (IL-2), and large batches of cells can be grown that have this same property of killing tumor cells. These test-tube-grown lymphocytes are then returned to the patient, and they are continually stimulated to grow by treating the patient (not just the test tube) with interleukin-2.

The idea to identify killer cells and cause them to multiply is very clever, and there are some even newer ways of isolating potent lymphocytes that gather around cancer cells. The technology is complex and terribly costly at this point, and side effects are quite severe, but it is a new lead that perhaps can be exploited much further. The first public announcement of the new treatment was properly published in a good journal and was immediately followed by a deluge of calls from hopeful people—most of whom could not be accommodated by the study. At that time only eight patients per month could be so treated, but many hundreds applied each day. The programs were expanded at other centers as rapidly as resources would allow. Remember that this is not yet proven as an effective treatment, it has not yet cured a single patient, and it is still very toxic. Why, then, is such a treatment even announced? The answer is simple—we live in a free society where, we hope, the free exchange of well-documented scientific information may lead to improvements in all areas. Premature press conferences and headline-seeking reporters unfortunately exaggerate these early findings, and do a great deal of damage to vulnerable people. In such circumstances there is no way to stop the unhappy avalanche of people seeking help where none yet—and it is a very important yet—exists. *We plead for restraint and responsibility in reporting such news;* all of us in science feel that this is in the public interest. The issues are delicate because the public also has a right to know and to be informed.

In an update of the interleukin-2 story, I heard Dr. Edward Bradley from Cetus Corporation and his clinical collaborators discuss results on over eight hundred patients treated with IL-2 at various cancer centers. They and others are not finished with the laborious work of finding the best way to give this substance to optimize its anticancer effects and hold down its considerable toxicity and there are many things to be tried before large-scale anticancer studies are appropriate. Low doses of IL-2 are well tolerated, however, even on an outpatient basis, as also reported by scientists like Dr. West in Memphis. High doses, by contrast, cause extreme toxicity and virtually all patients receiving them need to be treated in an intensive care unit—and then there have been some who died from treatment. On the positive side, there have also been very impressive results in patients who failed to respond to other types of treatment and/or have forms of cancer that rarely respond to established drugs. Bradley, West and other workers are hopeful that this substance can become important in time, once some of these questions are answered. And for the fortunate patients who have responded, the future is a good deal brighter than it was.

Tumor Necrosis Factor (TNF) is a soluble protein that kills cancer cells grown in tissue culture tubes to a greater extent than it kills normal cells. Furthermore, although some kinds of cancer cells may be resistant in tissue culture, they can be made sensitive by adding chemotherapeutic drugs; unfortunately, that also renders normal cells susceptible to killing by TNF. More to the point, when the cancer is in a mouse instead of a test tube, it can often be dramatically destroyed by TNF—with or without added chemotherapy. Beneficial effects of TNF are also increased by adding interferon. TNF acts differently in the animal than in the test tubes, destroying blood vessels that feed the cancer. It is still too early to know for sure, but preliminary studies in patients have taught us how much can be given and what its toxicity is, and it does cause a lot of toxicity. Scientists are working hard to find better ways to use this interesting drug before we are ready to talk about its use outside of a research setting.

At a recent meeting of the Society for Biological Therapy, I was delighted to see close cooperation between many excellent scientists working in a large number of biotechnology and pharmaceutical firms with researchers who are more traditionally based in universities and research centers. In the past it seemed that the biotechnology groups were only interested in investing in short-term projects; now at least some recognize the need for longer lasting commitments. All of this is new and the final chapters have yet to be written until we see the follow-up in this area of research.

TURNING CANCER CELLS BACK TOWARD NORMAL It seems that at an early time in its life cycle a cell has to "decide" whether to divide and produce two daughter cells or to mature and never divide again, a process called terminal differentiation. Normal tissues need to have a balance of both processes in order to replenish dying cells. As mentioned earlier, cancer cells appear to be arrested in their maturation process but they retain the capacity to divide. Cancer researchers are beginning to find that at least some types of chemical substances can induce cancer cells to undergo the maturation (differentiation) process, that is, to revert from being cancer cells to being normal cells and doing whatever they should have done in the first place, at least in test tube situations. There is now considerable hope that safe chemicals having this property of making cells revert can be found and used to treat cancer. A tremendous amount of excellent research is being done in this area.

Just as promising is the possibility that such substances might be effective in preventing the malignant transformation from occurring in the first place. This could be particularly important for individuals who are at high risk for cancer, such as smokers; they might be willing to take a chemoprevention pill daily, even though they may be unable to give up smoking.

This research area is called chemoprevention, the idea being to find substances to take that will prevent, or at least delay, the onset of cancer. The process to be blocked goes something like this. We are exposed to a carcinogen, a cancer-causing chemical, that has to be metabolically activated or "armed" by normal cells to a reactive product that rapidly binds to DNA and leads to a stable change—a process called initiation. The conversion of an initiated cell to a premalignant or fully malignant cancer cell may take decades in humans, and it may occur spontaneously or by action of other substances called tumor promoters. It is difficult to block the process of initiation, largely because it happens so quickly, but it is possible to interfere with the second step, or promotion. There are now many chemicals that can prevent or delay cancer from forming in animals exposed to carcinogens, but many are too toxic to give to healthy people over a period of years. However, some chemicals, such as vitamin A derivatives and vitamin E, are emerging as candidates for clinical trial, and the NCI is planning large-scale testing of some of these in the near future.

Ideally, this is what we want to do—identify people who are at a high risk for cancer and have them take a non-toxic compound that prevents it from occurring. We are still a long way from being able to achieve that goal, but at least the principles are established.

EXPERIMENTAL CHEMOTHERAPY As we learned earlier, chemotherapeutic drugs are designed to interfere with the ability of the cancer cell to divide, grow and perform its functions. There are many drugs that do this to a greater or lesser extent, depending also on the cancer type. Unfortunately, one of the most striking characteristics of cancer cells is their ability to adapt to toxic chemotherapeutic drugs, so that if the cells are not killed in the initial course of treatment, they become resistant to a drug's effects and eventually the drug becomes totally inactive against the cancer cells, although it continues to be toxic to normal cells. *Curiously, normal cells never seem to become resistant to chemotherapy, and this fundamental biological difference has not been fully explained.* However, the ability of cancer cells to acquire resistance is beginning to be explained in molecular terms, and as we progressively define the mechanisms by which this happens, we find new avenues for designing chemotherapy that will destroy these resistant cells and be harmless to normal cells. The idea is actually to exploit the adaptability of cancer cells and have them commit suicide by the very property that has protected them thus far. A number of chemicals have been designed for this purpose, and some ingenious approaches are in various stages of testing.

I think it is entirely feasible to take advantage of the adaptability of cancer cells that enables them to become resistant to chemotherapy. Our own laboratory group (and others) are doing research along these lines, with the aim of actually causing types of cancer resistance to standard drugs that will, in turn, make the cancer cells susceptible to new drugs. The beauty of this is that normal cells are spared because they are not capable of developing the same metabolic adaptations. This is called collateral sensitivity, and it is the opposite of the process of collateral resistance—which sometimes occurs when cancer cells resistant to one drug simultaneously become resistant to other drugs.

Let us put the subject of drug resistance into another perspective. When we use chemotherapy to treat a patient with cancer, we expect one of three possible outcomes: we hope to cure the cancer, but if not, we may shrink the tumor temporarily, or have no effect on it at all. In the first instance there is no problem, of course, but in the other two circumstances the cancer cells are resistant to chemotherapy. Resistance can either develop spontaneously or as a result of adaptation to the drugs. In the case of a tumor that shrinks temporarily and then recurs and is resistant thereafter, it is likely that the initial exposure to the drug killed off the cells that were sensitive and allowed the resistant ones to grow back and take over permanently. Alternatively, it is possible that the resistant cells were not there from the start but developed as a result of a permanent mutation that protected that cell (and all of its offspring) against further damage from chemotherapy. In the case of a cancer that fails to shrink in the first place, we assume that the original cancer cells were spontaneously resistant to the drugs.

Numerous laboratories are studying ways in which cancer cells can become resistant to drugs that need to accumulate inside cells to kill them. To prevent being killed, a resistant cancer cell can have a mechanism by which it selectively fails to pump the drug into the cell, and if the cell acquires this property of keeping the drug on the outside, there is no way in which the cell will be damaged or killed. Another means by which a cell can become resistant to a drug is to increase the number of critical enzyme molecules that have to be blocked in order to destroy the cell. A very important process called *gene amplification* was described by Robert Schimke, Ph.D., and his collaborators at Stanford, who showed that some fraction of the cells that are exposed to low doses of a drug (methotrexate) will eventually become resistant to that drug. This is because they activate the genes that produce the enzyme dihydrofolate reductase—the enzyme target that must be blocked for the drug to kill the cell. Thus, even if methotrexate can enter the cell in a normal fashion, there is simply too much of the enzyme within the resistant cell for the drug to knock out all of the enzyme molecules. We know from the work of Dr. David

Goldman at the Medical College of Virginia that almost 100 percent of the enzyme has to be inhibited in order to kill a cell, but this becomes impossible when there is far more enzyme to be inhibited, as in the case of gene-amplified cells. By the way, the fundamental discovery of gene amplification has very broad biological applications outside of the field of cancer too, in areas as remote as cell resistance to other types of drugs and evolutionary selection.

These are some of the ways in which a cancer cell can become resistant to a given drug such as methotrexate—and there are other ways too. As mentioned, many researchers are working on means of circumventing these types of resistance by the use of different inhibitors that will kill cancer cells that are resistant to methotrexate by various means. Indeed, some promising drugs are being tried, and it is reasonable to predict that some will be successful.

Another form of resistance to drugs is not specific to a given drug, but rather causes a cancer cell that is resistant to drug A also to become resistant to drugs B, C and D—which may be different classes of chemicals altogether. This type of resistance is called *pleiotropic drug* resistance. Dr. Victor Ling of Toronto began a line of research showing that the development of this type of resistance is associated with the production of certain cell-wall chemicals called glycoproteins. The chemical substances appear to be responsible for preventing the accumulation of drugs in the cell. Various approaches are being used in order to interfere with the ability of cancer cells to produce these glycoproteins, or to block their effects, in an effort to prevent the emergence of this type of resistance. One approach that is showing some promise involves the use of "calcium channel blockers," which are drugs commonly used to treat heart disease. In the laboratory such substances have been found to reverse the resistance of cancer cells to chemotherapy drugs, and clinical trials with some of these drugs are under way.

An interesting new line of research indicates that resistance of cancer cells to chemotherapy may be related to the ways normal cells protect themselves from the effects of chemicals that can cause cancer or even cell death. Dr. Charles Myers and colleagues at NCI have demonstrated that elevated levels of certain enzymes (protein kinase C, glutathione transferase) are present in drug-resistant cancer cells—possibly these are switches that determine resistance. In my opinion there is no more important research priority than to learn to overcome the problem of drug resistance.

Scientists are working at a feverish pace to learn more about the initial biochemical events that stimulate cells to become cancerous. The oncogene story gives us exciting new insights into how viruses can cause some cancers, and may also show us how chemical carcinogens activate specific regions of DNA to initiate the process of transformation of normal cells into cancer. This research is at such a fundamental level that it is difficult to predict how the information can be exploited, but it is safe to say that it will be used for the prevention of cancer.

The ultimate therapeutic test of course is in the treatment of patients. Clinical studies testing new approaches with patients require just as much scientific expertise as do the basic investigations, and they pose an additional problem—people cannot be standardized the way mice can be inbred genetically, nor the way cancer cells can be grown in cell cultures. It is the individual variations in patients that ultimately determine how much of a chemical can be given before the point of tolerance is reached. Thus, clinical trials using new drugs or other approaches require a combination of the skills of scientific inquiry, excellent medical practice and an understanding of pharmacology, physiology and human behavior. Research designs that involve several different types of specialists are hard to organize. One promising avenue for treatment of certain cancers (i.e., head, neck and rectal cancers) involves medical, surgical and radiation oncologists, all of whom need to plan and work out treatment programs. By working together we are finally beginning to cure some patients who were previously deemed incurable.

Research in better means for cancer prevention is moving forward slowly but surely. There are now good scientific reasons for thinking that drugs that block estrogen function (e.g., Tamoxifen) may be able to prevent breast cancer from occurring in women who are at high risk. We think the means are at hand but safety and effectiveness still need to be proven.

Some types of experimental treatments are unique to clinical medicine while others involve attempts to extend what has been learned from more basic scientific models to see if the lessons are applicable to humans. Certain experiments are successful in animals but cannot be reproduced in humans, because of different enzyme systems or control mechanisms, or differences in the way in which the drugs are handled by human tissues. One such approach that is right at the interface between test tube research and clinical application is the stem cell assay technique. By this method cancer cells are removed from patients, cultured in flasks and different drugs tested to see which are effective. A drug that is not able to kill cells in culture will not usually kill them in the patient—that part of the prediction is good. However, an effective drug in culture is not necessarily effective when given to the patient. So we have part of the solution to the problem of prediction but not all of it by any means. The complexities of clinical research are very great—one cannot just try out new drugs by testing them in patients and seeing what happens. Anything but a rigorous approach is potentially life threatening to patients and also likely to miss vital information. The ethics of clinical investigation are constantly under scrutiny. Fortunately, new epidemiological and biostatistical techniques are maximizing the amount of information that can be learned from patient groups and pointing the way to new leads that have not been previously suspected. Computers and sophisticated data analyses show a great deal of promise in helping us to distinguish patients who are likely to respond to a given treatment from those who will not, so that we can give the treatment only to the former and spare the latter the toxicity of an ineffective treatment. This has to be done for each disease since there are some types of cancer about which we already have the capability to predict, but many others for which the data are still incomplete.

We urgently need innovative work on the psychosocial and behavioral aspects of cancer. How can we better motivate people, particularly the underprivileged, to learn about cancer and take the necessary steps to look after their own health from the standpoints of prevention, early detection and treatment? Not only will lives be saved but, for many, the quality of life can be improved. I predict that such research on behavior modification will be a rewarding new frontier not only for cancer but for health care generally.

Americans currently spend $440 billion on health care services for the sick and only $8 billion to find cures or how to stay healthy. We need to do more to build on our enormous research potential.

HOPE FOR TOMORROW

In 1971 the administration of President Richard M. Nixon inaugurated a national plan for what was called the War Against Cancer. This plan called attention to the emergency facing our nation, and it provided new resources and stimulated bright young people to go into cancer research. There was great excitement surrounding that plan, which was perceived as a real national commitment to get on with the job of finding causes, alleviating suffering and discovering cures. We have made tremendous progress since then in waging that war, but much more remains to be done. We are encouraged when we note that some spectacular clinical progress, especially in the treatment of childhood cancers, is a product of the research of the past—and that the fruits of the tremendous research advances of the past five to eight years have yet to be harvested. At the same time we are mindful of the continuing crisis in funding for cancer research, one of whose results is that many researchers who are trained and ready will be halted before they proceed with their work.

There are other important crosscurrents of public policy as it impinges on the cancer story. The most obvious threat to progress is the retrenchment of federal research programs, which are likely to bear a major burden in the drive to balance the budget. Since health research programs are not exempted from budget cutting, while many other programs are relatively protected (e.g., defense, social security), there will be great pressure to cut back on the remaining programs. Cutbacks will inevitably delay progress in cancer research and will affect the near-term goals of prevention and cure. The unanswered question of who will pay for research with patients under new federal and insurance restrictions is already slowing this important arm of the cancer effort. Then, as other health funds become squeezed even further, the impact on clinical research is likely to be enormous.

Clearly there needs to be a renaissance in public policy on health research. Assuming there is no slowing in our activity, what can we predict for the near future? Scientists in general, and cancer researchers in particular, deplore the word "breakthrough" because they recognize that major advances usually follow many small steps that eventually culminate in an important discovery. Even a brilliant insight such as the recognition by Watson and Crick of the double-helical structure of DNA was based on laborious interpretation of careful biochemical and physical-chemical studies of DNA made by other scientists. We are also well aware that while certain applied technologies can be carefully planned in advance and deadlines set, such as for space exploration, the development of fundamental information is far less predictable. Nonetheless, we can be sure that good scientists who are adequately funded and equipped and who work in a scholarly and exciting environment will ultimately advance the frontiers of science by one means or another.

"Prophesy is difficult, especially of the future"—Chinese proverb With these caveats about uncertainty, what can we predict will happen in the field of cancer research by the year 2000? The National Cancer Institute has set a goal of reducing deaths from cancer by 50 percent—a tremendously ambitious goal given that all the efforts that have gone before have only just begun to result in a drop in mortality from cancer in certain age groups. Whether this can be achieved is not known, but it is an essential goal. Certainly, greater attention to the principles of cancer prevention, discussed earlier, is expected to have a major impact on cancer-related mortality. If Americans can simply decrease their cigarette consumption, as has been done in Great Britain, that alone could be responsible for meeting half the goal. However, we need to find more effective means of public education and behavior modification in order to realize that objective. Continued efforts at control of urban pollution and reduction of carcinogenic substances in the workplace will also be important in cancer prevention, but probably less so than one might imagine.

The National Cancer Institute's goal of reducing cancer mortality by 50 percent by the year 2000 is based partly on better means for prevention, for screening, for monitoring the results of treatment and for improving accessibility to the latest treatments for the average American. Committees are now at work in each of these major areas. The key preventive measures in these calculations require a 50 percent reduction in smoking from 1980 levels and the adoption of a prudent low-fat, high-fiber diet by all Americans. Looking at treatment alone, it is believed that *by fully applying state-of-the-art treatment, we can save 50,000 more lives per year than are now being saved by treatment, and that does not even take into consideration advances or new treatments that are sure to be available by the year 2000.* By that we mean extending the reach of current knowledge and technology to those who are either uninformed, uninspired to try or unable to afford the current costs. Some of the kinds of advances that are being counted on in making estimates based on current knowledge, and the projections as to the number of lives that could be saved, are presented in Table 7 and summarized in the text below.

☐   *Breast cancer:* It is predicted that improved techniques for evaluating the extent of the disease will be used for 100 percent of patients with breast cancer, instead of just 50 percent, as at present. There will also be an increase in the percent of patients diagnosed in the early stages, from 40 percent to 70 percent. A decrease in the side effects of extensive surgery

Table 7 Estimates of Lives Saved in the Year 2000 by Provision of State-of-the-Art Therapy for Selected Cancer Sites*

Site/Type	No. of Deaths in Year 2000 under 1985 Survival	No. of Deaths under State-of-the-Art Treatment	No. of Lives Saved	Reduction (%)
Prostate	36,685	21,266	15,419	42.0
Breast	53,023	45,465	7,558	14.3
Colon	51,826	41,450	10,376	20.0
Rectum	22,466	13,641	8,825	39.3
Lung, small cell	40,376	37,407	2,969	7.4
Bladder	13,618	11,625	1,993	14.6
Melanoma	19,778	14,891	4,887	24.7
Cervix	2,872	2,089	783	27.3
Corpus uteri	2,604	1,907	697	26.8
Lymphoma (DHL)	3,093	1,377	1,716	55.5
Ovary	12,030	11,114	916	7.6
Testis, nonseminoma	477	320	157	32.9
Childhood				
Acute lymphocytic leukemia (ALL)	852	565	287	33.7
Acute myelogenous leukemia (AML)	195	149	46	23.6
Medulloblastoma	601	301	300	49.9
Adult ALL	6,223	4,745	1,478	23.8
Subtotal	266,719	208,312	58,407	21.9
All other sites	374,906	374,906	0	0.0
Total all sites	641,625	583,218	58,407	9.1

*Prevention and screening activities are held constant at 1980 levels.

Source: *Cancer Control Objectives for the Nation: 1985–2000*, NCI Monograph Number 2, 1986. This is the report of the National Plan Development Committee (chaired by Dr. Paul Engstrom).

296

with improved quality of life is predicted for patients with localized breast cancer, due to more conservative surgical approaches. There will be an increase in the use of combined chemotherapy and surgery in patients who need both because their disease has extended outside the breast and involves the lymph glands (nodes) under the arm. This is expected to be a major benefit to women who are in the postmenopausal age group, and the five-year survival of this group of patients is projected to rise from 66 percent to 72 percent. That sounds like a small improvement, but it translates into many lives saved because this disease is so common. It appears that oncologists have been less aggressive in treating older women with chemotherapy, and that may be why there has been less improvement than in younger women with comparable involvement of lymph glands at the time of surgery. An overall gain of over 11,000 lives is anticipated by bringing all of these more modern techniques to the care of the average patient.

☐ *Colon cancer:* By the year 2000 an increase in five-year survival from 41 percent to 51 percent is expected simply by better definition of the extent of disease and use of more modern surgical and pathologic techniques. For rectal cancer the five-year survival is expected to increase from 38 percent to 59 percent by early detection in more patients and by improved treatment for localized disease.

☐ *Testicular cancer:* By the year 2000 an increase in five-year survival is expected for all stages of cancer of the testis, especially for advanced cancer; and aggressive clinical treatment should increase the overall five-year survival from 78 percent to 94 percent. This is an uncommon type of cancer so the number of additional lives saved is modest; however, all are young men who, if cured, will have an additional fifty years of life expectancy. And every life is important!

☐ *Prostate cancer:* There will be improved control of localized cancer of the prostate, and the proportion of patients diagnosed at an earlier stage will increase. By the year 2000 the five-year survival is expected to increase from 48 to 59 percent.

□ *Cervical cancer:* There will be an increase in the use of new limited-surgical techniques such as cryosurgery, as in the use of radiation pellets in the tumor area for patients with localized disease, as well as improved screening to detect disease at an earlier stage. By the year 2000 there should be an increase in five-year survival from 61 percent to 67 percent. For uterine cancer the survival rate for black patients is currently only 46 percent, and this is expected to increase to 76 percent.

□ *Adult leukemia:* There will be an increase in the complete response rate to 60 percent and an improvement in five-year survival from 5 percent to 25 percent. For patients with the adult form of lymphoma, the five-year survival is expected to increase from 33 percent to 60 percent by means of state-of-the-art chemotherapy.

□ *Childhood leukemia:* It is expected that the common type of childhood leukemia will be cured in 75 percent of cases, up from 65 percent at present.

The combination of these and other expectations for improved treatment is anticipated to save some 50,000 lives annually (Table 7). *There are also plans for decreasing the incidence of the other cancers through effective educational and other programs listed below.*

SUMMARY OF YEAR 2000 (AND SOME 1990) OBJECTIVES FROM NCI

Prevention Objectives for Smoking

□ By 2000, the prevalence of all persons aged twenty-one years and older who smoke will decrease from 33.8 percent in 1983 to 15 percent or less.

□ By 2000, the prevalence of youth who begin to smoke by age twenty will decrease from 36 percent in 1983 to less than 15 percent.

Prevention Objectives for Diet

□ By 2000, the per capita consumption of dietary fat will decrease from the 38 percent of total calories that it was in 1976–80 to 30 percent.

☐ By 2000, the per capita consumption of dietary fiber in whole grains, fruits and vegetables should increase to 20 to 30 grams per day from the 8 to 12 grams per day that it was in 1976–80.

☐ By 2000, the prevalence of obesity will decrease from 20 percent of all persons to 5 percent.

Objectives for Occupational Exposure to Carcinogens Specific objectives for the year 2000 related to occupational exposure were not defined during this effort. Rather, a set of objectives for the year 1990 were outlined in concert with the prevention objectives of the Department of Health and Human Services ("Public Health Reports," 1983).

☐ By 1990, all firms with more than five hundred employees should have a plan of hazard control for processes, equipment and installations associated with established or suspected carcinogens.

☐ By 1990, at least 25 percent of workers should be able, prior to employment, to state the nature of their occupational health and safety risks and the potential consequences; they should be informed of changes in these risks while employed (in 1979, an estimated 5 percent of workers were fully informed).

☐ By 1990, the majority of workers should be routinely informed of lifestyle behaviors and health factors that interact with factors in the work environment to increase risks for occupationally induced cancers.

☐ By 1990, at least 70 percent of primary health care providers should routinely elicit occupational health exposures as part of patient history, and should know how to interpret the information for patients in an understandable manner.

Year 2000 Screening Objectives

☐ By 2000, the proportion of women aged fifty to seventy who receive an annual breast examination plus mammography will increase from 45 percent for examination alone and 15 percent for mammography to 80 percent.

☐ By 2000, the proportion of women aged twenty to thirty-nine who receive a cervical Pap smear every three years will increase from 79 percent to 90 percent and of women aged forty to seventy from 57 percent to 80 percent.

Those are the formal projections from NCI and its advisory committees. On a more fundamental level, one that requires new knowledge, it seems quite likely that means will be found to reduce the transformation of normal cells into malignant cells. This is one of the more exciting areas of research today: the possibility of so modifying cells has already been clearly demonstrated in animal systems and in tissue culture systems but the principles remain to be demonstrated in humans. To do long-term cancer prevention studies with chemicals that may have some side effects of their own is a very difficult task, and it takes many years of research and follow-up. However, by the year 2000 such studies should be well along, and I predict that people who are at high risk for developing cancer will be taking regular doses of cancer-preventing chemicals by that time. It is also quite likely that we will know more about substances in the diet that promote cancer and those that lessen the risk. We seem close to having the necessary knowledge (see also Chapter 7).

A real potential by the year 2000 is the use of the differentiating agents we mentioned earlier to return cancer cells back to normal growth patterns; possibly we may also be using these in patients who already have established cancer. There are already some models for accomplishing this goal in animal tumors and in human cancer cells exposed to these drugs in test tubes. The drugs that are successful are generally still too toxic to use in humans, but the principle has been established and now we are looking for safer chemical derivatives. After all, in theory the ideal differentiating agent might have no toxicity at all to normal cells, a very exciting notion and one that will be extensively pursued if research money is available.

A number of interesting biological substances are now being developed, and these will be modified for ultimate use in cancer treatment. We have spoken about the interferons, some of which have already demonstrated their beneficial effects. There is reason to believe that their use in conjunction with other types of anti-cancer agents will add to their effectiveness. There are a variety of other biological factors (interleukins and bone marrow growth factors, among others) that will soon be tested in humans also. Monoclonal antibodies for most tumors could potentially be developed. Particularly exciting is the possibility that a monoclonal antibody could be developed for the specific cancer of a patient and then be coupled with a toxic drug that would recognize and react only with cancer cells, killing them selectively (see Chapter 16). Much of the technology for this is already available, but there are still major problems: not all of the cells within a cancer have a sufficient number of antigens to react with these antibodies, and furthermore, some normal cells also seem to cross-react with the antibodies and are thereby killed. There will surely be some major clinical trials in the coming years to test this approach. By the year 2000 such testing should be very advanced.

Basic scientists are working at a feverish pace to learn more about the initial biochemical events that stimulate cells to become cancerous. The oncogene story gives us exciting new insights into how viruses can cause some cancers, and may also show us how chemical carcinogens activate specific regions of DNA to initiate the process of transformation of normal cells into cancer. And the discovery of antioncogenes gives us another new target for controlling cancer. This research is at such a fundamental level that it is difficult to predict how the information can be exploited, but it is safe to say that it will be used for the prevention of cancer. We know that it requires more than one event for cancer to develop, and therefore there must be a way to block the process of malignant transformation before it has become irreversible. And chemoprevention (see Chapter 15) is one such way that is being tested.

Among the exciting areas of cancer research is the discovery that some types of cancer cells, for example, those in small cell lung cancer (SCLC), produce chemical substances (peptides) that stimulate their own growth. This auto-stimulation, or autocrine stimulation, first described by Drs. George Todaro and Michael Sporn of NCI, contrast with hormone growth factors that are secreted by normal glandular tissues such as the pancreas (insulin), adrenals (corticosteroids) and pituitary (ACTH, growth hormones, et cetera). These potent substances are distributed by the bloodstream to affect even distant tissues. SCLC cells can be grown in tissue culture systems, and they are quite literally cellular factories that produce a large number of growth-regulating substances. One of these is a polypeptide substance called bombesin, which a decade ago was discovered in the skin of a South American frog, of all places. In any event, monoclonal antibodies prepared against the bombesin molecule will interfere with the growth of these cancer cells. Clinical trials are now being developed to see if it will be possible to develop a unique approach that would be directed at limiting growth by blocking an important regulatory substance.

There are some new, exciting and important insights into the problem of the profound weight loss (cancer cachexia) some patients experience. I have seen patients even with small tumors drop in weight from 170 to 100 pounds over the course of several months, an uncommon amount for such cases. These tumors apparently cause the secretion of a protein-like substance that produces loss of body fat and muscle tissue, which creates a metabolic imbalance that has some resemblance to the condition of poorly controlled diabetes. It turns out that certain types of scavenger cells (macrophages) produce a hormone-like substance that seems to cause the same kind of effects on tissue that one sees in the condition of cachexia. Originally called cachectin, it appears to be the same material as the tumor necrosis factor (TNF) discussed in the previous chapter. These substances are presumably produced because the cancer cells secrete another very potent molecule called endotoxin, which in turn causes normal macrophage cells to produce cachectin (or TNF). This could have great practical significance because it is possible to produce anticachectin (TNF) antibodies to neutralize this substance; when injected into mice, these antibodies protect them from the deadly effects of endotoxin. These substances can all be produced in large quantities by new methodology, so the potential to prevent the common complication of tissue wasting in cancer patients seems quite promising. (Curiously TNF under certain circumstances can cause cancers to shrink, and some animals can be cured. This is another of those biological substances that we have to learn more about.)

One recent accomplishment of cancer researchers has been the discovery that a family of viruses can cause a particular type of human leukemia. Another member of this human lymphotropic leukemia virus (HTLV or HIV) is the agent that causes the disease AIDS, as discussed in Chapter 11. Curiously, the disease itself had not even been discovered when this type of cancer research began, but the background information was available to apply to AIDS research soon thereafter. Now there is a rush to find a vaccine for this virus, to prevent AIDS. Scientists working on cancer chemotherapy have also turned their attention to designing drugs that kill viruses or at least inactivate them, and for the first time in history there is a successful treatment for the herpes virus. A team of scientists from the Burroughs Wellcome Company discovered acyclovir, a potent viral inhibitor. No fully effective inhibitors are yet available for the HTLV virus group, but there are some very promising candidate drugs that are already undergoing clinical testing, including AZT, another drug from the same company. There is now reason to be hopeful that we will be able to successfully treat HTLV infections, whether they cause AIDS or a type of leukemia. And there are encouraging experiments to suggest we might be able to stimulate certain lymphocytes to prevent the progression of AIDS in an infected patient and set up a "carrier state" in which the person can coexist with the virus, as with some kinds of hepatitis. The social problems of isolating infectious patients or testing possible carriers will probably not be resolved in the near future, and may get worse, because of severe conflicts between constitutional rights to privacy and the health of the public. And unless we find effective treatment and prevention we can expect to lose hundreds of thousands of lives during the 1990s in this country—and far more in Africa.

We will continue to find new chemotherapeutic drugs, particularly those that will kill "resistant" cancer cells, and one of these days we will get lucky. If it seems paradoxical to speak of luck in the thicket of the scientific testing that is the normal environment for research, let me assure you that luck does indeed play a part.

Success can come as readily on test number one as it can on test ten thousand and one. The heart of discovery is being willing to go the distance. And because of the discoveries from diligent clinical research, it is now possible to cure some relatively uncommon but widespread cancers with chemotherapy; and it is just as likely that we will find chemicals to cure some of the more common cancers. Indeed, I think it is only because we have been "unlucky" to date that that has not already happened. We might just as well have discovered a cure for a common cancer rather than an uncommon form of cancer. Another practical approach is that we are developing better means of figuring out what biochemical process we want to inhibit within the cell, of monitoring the amount of drug needed to do the job and of planning more effective dosage schedules. The discovery of other new substances that cause destruction of tumor blood vessels (tumor necrosis factor or TNF) or stimulate the body's defense mechanisms such as with interleukin-2 should enhance the effects of our chemotherapeutic drugs.

Hyperthermia, another relatively new tool, destroys cancer cells with heat; when used with chemotherapy, it is a technique that also increases the amount of chemotherapeutic drugs that can reach a tumor. Hyperthermia takes advantage of the observation that cancer cells are slightly less able to withstand high temperatures than are normal cells, and therefore various heating devices have been made literally to cook the cancer. This works quite well for superficial tumors, say of the arms or legs or neck, but the technology does not yet exist to achieve really selective heating deep into the chest or abdomen. The problem is that whereas a piece of meat can be heated very precisely in a microwave oven, a piece of live tissue or a cancer has blood vessels that act as a cooling system or radiator. This whole subject is being attacked very vigorously now, and by the year 2000 I expect the logistics of doing this will be solved and that this will be very helpful for certain types of cancer.

Laser beam therapy also has promising applications for cancer treatment. It is being used for precise removal of tumors in some areas of the body. Moreover, one can give the patient certain types of chemicals (e.g., hematoporphyrins) that, when activated by a particular wavelength of laser beam, become very toxic to the cells they are in; this can be used to kill cancers of the skin and some other areas.

Among the very practical hopes for tomorrow is that you and society as a whole will become better informed and less afraid of the unknown. We also can do a better job of rehabilitating patients who have been cured of cancer, we can clearly develop means of saving limbs that previously had to be amputated, and we can help educate employers that people who have been cured of cancer are every bit as valuable as employees who have never had the disease. We need to eliminate social and occupational discrimination of the cancer patient, including the child who is in remission or has been cured. We are making great progress in finding means of combating the untoward effects of both the cancer and the treatment—we can predict, for example, that within the next five years complications such as nausea and vomiting following cancer chemotherapy will become very uncommon. In fact, with aggressive use of what we already know, the problem is being solved. More effective management of pain is also predictable, partly through lay and professional education and partly by research. Some advances will also be applicable to diseases other than cancer, as witnessed by discovery of the virus that causes AIDS, treatment of gout and successful chemical management of graft rejection, which makes possible organ transplantation.

In all, the future is brightening up really for the first time in history: instead of the problem of cancer getting worse and worse, we seem to have turned the corner! Let us hope we may again come to a time when professors of medicine have to make special efforts to bring their medical students to see patients with cancer because it has become a rare disease. Let us hope and pray that this happens for our children and grandchildren, yours and mine. Amen.

EPILOGUE: VIEW FROM THE OTHER SIDE—A PERSONAL EXPERIENCE

I hope you can also learn from my experience as a patient in two discrete instances, then and now—five years ago and today! All of the chapters of this book were written and until yesterday I had almost forgotten the "then" part of the story. It's funny how often we forget unpleasant events in our lives. Six years ago, while attending an out-of-town meeting with other hematologists (blood specialists), I went to the restroom after a coffee break and urinated what looked like almost pure blood. Standing nearby was a colleague—when I told him what had just happened he said that sometimes a blood vessel ruptures in the urinary passage (urethra) and brisk bleeding starts, stops and no one ever figures out why. That sounded comforting, but nonetheless I resolved to have it checked upon returning home a few days later. But since the bleeding had stopped spontaneously by then and I felt fine, I "forgot" to check it out then and there. (Denial is a very powerful psychological means of coping.) Three months later a second episode of bleeding forcefully brought me to my senses—and to face reality. Within a couple of days Dr. David Paulson, an excellent specialist in urinary surgery (urology) and a close professional colleague of mine, had me in the hospital to remove a large tumor from the bladder. The operation was very successful, although the postoperative course was unpleasant for a time because of the need to wear a catheter to collect urine for about ten days. Since then I have been healthy.

It had been a frightening experience—having general anesthesia and surgery for the first time, fear that the disease might have spread and threatened my life, or that the treatment might call for more radical surgery on my bladder, which would cause other profound physical and psychological changes. I had been afraid and did not share that with my family. It was a big relief when it was over and everything turned out well. I knew it might recur.

Thereafter, I followed the advice of having regular examination of my bladder through an instrument called a cystoscope, which permits the doctor to visualize the lining of the bladder. The examination is uncomfortable, more for men than for women, but it takes just a few minutes (and it takes me a bit of courage to go). At first the examinations were every three months, then four and then six. Talk about happiness!

Yesterday, *January 21*, I had a regular six-month checkup and Dr. Paulson found another tumor in the bladder—this time a very small one, however. I was crushed to have to face surgery again, because of the uncertainty that is always present and the postoperative discomfort of wearing a catheter (hollow tube) pushed through the urethra to drain the bladder until healing takes place—and then resuming the routine of three-month checkups, if everything is OK. And what if it isn't? Seeing my worry immediately after hearing the news, Nick, Dr. Paulson's able assistant, told me that they take these tumors out all the time and everything works out fine. "Trouble with you, Doc, is that you know too much." I think he's right!

This is going to be only minor surgery—intellectually I know that very well. Still, I didn't sleep well last night, got up early and worked furiously at home on a lecture for later this week. The surgery is next week, and two trips needed to be cancelled. First things first. But this is really such an inconvenient time for this to happen—my schedule is full and the day of moving to a new job and to another city is fast approaching. So then I went out and ran five miles and felt better. How could I be sick and do that much exercise in a normal fashion? I have to reason with myself that there can be something tiny that is wrong that can be potentially life threatening if not tended to promptly. Fortunately I will not ever repeat the mistake of waiting. Since I am nearing completion of this book at this moment, perhaps the next few weeks will be worth recording to share the follow-up with you.

January 22. Woke up early again and worked on my lecture. Went into the hospital late, which I almost never do, and on an impulse I stopped at the shopping mall and bought a case of tennis balls—tennis being my favorite sport. On the way back to the car I passed a new men's clothing store and stopped by to look. Ordinarily I would never just browse in a store, but this time I was not in a hurry. Ended up buying a new suit and a sport jacket—something I might buy once every twelve to eighteen months on a weekend or in the evening—certainly not on a working day. Felt fine and went on to work at the hospital. Later in the day I went to see Dr. Paulson and asked for more details about the proposed surgery, since I did think of some other questions. He explained that this time the recovery should be much easier since less surgery needs to be done, and I should be in and out of the hospital in a couple of days. That's good, because the weather is unusually mild and I'd like to use the tennis balls soon after I recover. My family now knows about the surgery and that it should be very minor—but they're not used to seeing me out of order and they are concerned about possible serious consequences.

January 23. Went to an important meeting of antifolate drugs to learn what others are doing and to present the research work of our research team with an interesting new compound made by Burroughs Wellcome Company. The conference was excellent, my own presentation went well, the location near Tampa, Florida, was delightful, but I came back early (January 25) to get everything ready to go to the hospital. Would have liked to participate in a free afternoon in which they were having a tennis tournament—something I always enjoy. Not this time—too much else to arrange at home.

January 27. Went to work in the a.m.—one of those mornings where many nuisance things arose. Fortunately, I had a delightful note from one of my former patients who is doing remarkably well, and that brightened my day. Visits, gifts and cards from relatives and close friends were cheering me up.

At 2:30 p.m. I was admitted to the Duke Hospital as a patient and in short order had a cardiogram (EKG), blood tests, urine sampling, talks with my surgeons and workup by the intern. The nurses were all very nice and helpful and assumed that I knew nothing about what would be done—I'm glad they did. In this circumstance I am a patient, not a doctor. They gave me some material to read about the surgical routine (I thought it a bit too technical for lay people to follow). Dr. Paulson came by and assured me that the odds greatly favored this being a simple problem that would be cured—I felt better after that conversation. The anesthesiologist who will be responsible for getting me to sleep, managing my vital signs during surgery, and waking me after surgery came to talk with me about any other conditions I might have or other medications I might be using—fortunately I am very healthy and take no drugs. I reminded him that I had similar surgery five years before and that whatever they used for anesthesia then worked well and might be useful again. I'm glad I told him about that because the old chart that contained that information had not yet reached my ward and he was unaware of it—thereafter he sought and found the pertinent information. (Doctors should always use the old information and sometimes they need to be reminded that it is available somewhere—if an important x-ray was taken a year earlier at another hospital, it could be very important to have it brought in for comparison.)

January 28. I was awakened at 4:30 a.m. by a loud noise in the hallway. I often wonder why they put signs outside of hospitals that say "HOSPITAL—QUIET" when it's often much noisier in the halls.

I showered, shaved and got prepared. I was given a relaxant shot at 6 a.m. and was taken off to surgery on a stretcher at 7 a.m. I was calm and confident by that time. The preparatory surgical area was crowded but businesslike. Nurses and anesthetists started my intravenous fluids and antibiotic drugs, gave me a drug to put me to sleep and had me breathe through a mask. At the beginning of this process I concentrated on a pleasant topic—a hoped-for vacation trip—and went peacefully off to sleep. I woke up in the recovery room about one and a half hours later feeling quite well. Had discomfort because I couldn't urinate and had brief but very painful bladder spasms. They gave me some antispasmodic drug, which provided relief, and sent me back up to the ward. Once they helped me to my feet I passed some pure blood, but then the urine began to clear and later that morning it was back to normal pale yellow. Ah, the beauty of clear yellow! I dozed off after having a pain shot and by early afternoon was hungry and ate a good lunch. My doctor came by about 3 p.m. and said that the operation had gone very well and that a small tumor had been removed. We would have to wait a few days for the pathology. He asked if I would like to go home—I was half-dressed before we finished the conversation. Tubes were disconnected, pulling a bit of hair from here and there, and I was discharged. The orderly who was to wheel me to the exit was slow in coming so I got my friend to help me with my suitcase, briefcase and some nice flowers and fruit—I walked to my car in the parking lot and drove home.

This is the morning after surgery and I am working in my apartment but I feel very well. A few aches here and there but no need to take anything other than the antibiotics that were prescribed. Now I have to await the pathology report, be checked over tomorrow and probably return to my work schedule. It does create anxiety not to know what the pathologist will find—since those findings hold the key to my follow-up risks and treatment.

January 30. Woke up feeling fine. Just a tinge of blood in the urine—this is to be expected off and on for a while, I was told. Drove into my office, then was checked by Dr. Paulson. The pathology report was very favorable. The tumor was a small Grade I (low-malignancy) intraepithelial carcinoma, which means it involved only the outermost layer of tissue and should be no threat to my life at all. These tumors can come back periodically so the plan is for me to be checked with cystoscopy every four months—I just wrote it down on my calendar as a reminder, so I won't be late. What a relief that it's over! I went home, jogged my five-mile route slowly, showered and fell asleep exhausted. Watched my son play a high school basketball game at night. It feels good to have this behind me and look to the future.

February 2. Doing fine. Still a few uncomfortable feelings after urination but nothing serious. Working full-time and concentrating quite well. Ran my five-mile route in my normal time. That tells me that my body is healed—and that feels good.

APPENDIX 1: HELP IS FOR THE ASKING

There are a great many people and organizations whose business it is to provide you with needed services and information for and about cancer. In this appendix we describe some of the national organizations and their local chapters, the cancer centers, how to reach them and what they can do for you. The directors of these organizations change from time to time and the type of services they offer also is subject to change. However, these are good places to start if you need help, and as you begin making inquiries you will find additional ways of answering your questions and solving your problems. If you have no questions now, you may prefer to skip this section but keep it available for future reference for yourself or your friends.

AMERICAN CANCER SOCIETY The largest organization that is specifically geared for providing services and information is the

American Cancer Society (ACS). ACS is a health agency that has over two million volunteers dedicated to the fight against cancer, which they wage by providing monetary support for research and education (professional and lay), patient services and rehabilitation programs, and by dealing with important issues of cancer causation such as tobacco. The national office of the American Cancer Society is at 90 Park Avenue, New York, NY 10016. It in turn has some fifty-eight chartered divisions and almost three thousand local units; the local units are prepared to provide assistance to their constituencies.

As you might expect, the national office administers the overall research program, distributes its medical grants and fellowship programs according to the advice of leading authorities in this country and provides leadership with programs for public (adult, youth) and professional education. There are divisions in all of the states plus certain additional metropolitan areas; units are organized to cover counties in the United States. When you need information you can reach the local units in most areas of the country by looking up the American Cancer Society in the telephone directory and asking for the person in charge of providing patient services or whatever you need. They try to answer many of your questions by telephone and have printed materials available on many subjects. These are available free of charge at the unit offices. They cannot give you direct information about a specific patient—that has to be done by a doctor—but they can help you find medical resources. The local units of the ACS conduct the service activities that provide information and counseling for the patient and family members. They have special programs for rehabilitation of patients who have had mastectomy, laryngectomy (removal of the vocal cords) and ostomy (removal of portions of the bowel), and they have a loan closet that often can provide much-needed supplies and equipment for patients being cared for at home, such as walkers, food blenders, bedpans, wheel chairs, et cetera. A new program (Road to Recovery) provides transportation services for patients who have difficulty in going from home to the doctor's office or hospital to receive treatments.

I worked as a volunteer for the Durham, North Carolina, local

Appendix 1: Help Is for the Asking

unit for over twenty years; this is one important way for lay and professional people who wish to render a service to others to become involved. If you do not need the ACS, or other volunteer health agencies, to do something for you, perhaps you can do something for them by giving of yourself. Then, too, if you wish to have an educational program presented to a civic or church group, you can ask the ACS to schedule this for you through their Public Education Program. I have spoken to numerous civic groups at their luncheon meetings, many experts are available throughout the nation, and all types of free programs can be prepared for your group, given some advance planning. Informational pamphlets are available about most aspects of cancer—contact your local chapter or divisional office. The addresses for the divisions are listed on the following pages.

ALABAMA
402 Office Park Drive, Suite 300
Birmingham, AL 35223
205-879-2242

ALASKA
1343 "G" Street
Anchorage, AK 99501
907-277-8696

ARIZONA
634 West Indian School Road
Phoenix, AZ 85013
602-234-3266

ARKANSAS
5520 West Markham Street
Little Rock, AR 72203
501-664-3480-1-2

CALIFORNIA
1710 Webster Street
Oakland, CA 94612
415-893-7900

COLORADO
2255 South Oneida
Denver, CO 80224
303-758-2030

CONNECTICUT
Barnes Park South
14 Village Lane
Wallingford, CT 06492
203-265-7161

DELAWARE
1708 Lovering Ave., Suite 202
Wilmington, DE 19806
302-654-6267

DISTRICT OF COLUMBIA
University Building, South
1825 Connecticut Ave., N.W.
Washington, DC 20009
202-483-2600

FLORIDA
1001 South MacDill Avenue
Tampa, FL 33609
813-253-0541

GEORGIA
1422 West Peachtree Street,
N.W.
Atlanta, GA 30309
404-892-0026

HAWAII PACIFIC
Community Services Center Bldg.
200 North Vineyard Blvd.
Honolulu, HI 96817
808-531-1662-3-4-5

IDAHO
1609 Abbs Street
Boise, ID 83705
208-343-4609

ILLINOIS
37 South Wabash Ave.
Chicago, IL 60603
312-372-0472

INDIANA
9575 North Valparaiso
Indianapolis, IN 46268
317-872-4432

IOWA
Highway #18 West
Mason City, IA 50401
515-423-0712

KANSAS
3003 Van Buren
Topeka, KS 66611
913-267-0131

KENTUCKY
Medical Arts Bldg.
1169 Eastern Parkway
Louisville, KY 40217
502-459-1867

LOUISIANA
Masonic Temple Bldg.
 7th Floor
333 St. Charles Ave.
New Orleans, LA 70130
504-523-2029

MAINE
Federal and Green Streets
Brunswick, ME 04011
207-729-3339

MARYLAND
1840 York Road
Timonium, MD 21093
301-561-4790

MASSACHUSETTS
247 Commonwealth Ave.
Boston, MA 02116
617-267-2650

MICHIGAN
1205 East Saginaw Street
Lansing, MI 48906
517-371-2920

MINNESOTA
3316 West 66th Street
Minneapolis, MN 55435
612-925-2772

MISSISSIPPI
345 North Mart Plaza
Jackson, MS 39206
601-362-8874

MISSOURI
3322 American Ave.
Jefferson City, MO 65102
314-893-4800

MONTANA
2820 First Ave. South
Billings, MT 59101
406-252-7111

NEBRASKA
8502 West Center Road
Omaha, NE 68124
402-393-5800

NEVADA
1325 East Harmon
Las Vegas, NV 89109
702-798-6877

NEW HAMPSHIRE
686 Mast Road
Manchester, NH 03102
603-669-3270

NEW JERSEY
2600 Route 1
North Brunswick, NJ
 08902
201-297-8000

NEW MEXICO
5800 Lomas Blvd., N.E.
Albuquerque, NM 87110
505-262-2336

NEW YORK
Long Island
535 Broad Hollow Road
(Route 10)
Melville, NY 11747
516-420-1111

Manhattan
19 West 56th Street
New York, NY 10019
212-586-8700

Queens
112-25 Queens Blvd.
Forest Hills, NY 11375
718-263-2224

Upstate
6725 Lyons Street
East Syracuse, NY 13057
315-437-7025

Westchester
901 North Broadway
White Plains, NY 10603
914-949-4800

NORTH CAROLINA
222 North Person Street
Raleigh, NC 27611
919-834-8463

NORTH DAKOTA
Hotel Graver, Annex Bldg.
115 Roberts Street
Fargo, ND 58102
701-232-1385

OHIO
1375 Euclid Ave.
Cleveland, OH 44115
216-771-6700

OKLAHOMA
3800 North Cromwell
Oklahoma City, OK 73112
405-946-5000

OREGON
0330 S.W. Curry
Portland, OR 97201
503-295-6422

PENNSYLVANIA
Rt. 422 & Sipe Ave.
Hershey, PA 17033
717-533-6144

Philadelphia
1422 Chestnut Street, 2nd Floor
Philadelphia, PA 19102
215-665-2900

PUERTO RICO
Avenue Domenench 273
Hato Rey, PR 00918
809-764-2295

RHODE ISLAND
400 Main Street
Pawtucket, RI 02860
401-831-6970

SOUTH CAROLINA
2214 Devine Street
Columbia, SC 29205
803-256-0245

SOUTH DAKOTA
1025 North Minnesota Ave.
Sioux Falls, SD 57104
605-336-0897

TENNESSEE
713 Melpark Drive
Nashville, TN 37204
615-383-1710

TEXAS
3834 Spicewood Springs Road
Austin, TX 78759
512-345-4560

UTAH
610 East South Temple
Salt Lake City, UT 84102
801-322-0431

VERMONT
13 Loomis Street
Montpelier, VT 05602
802-223-2348

VIRGINIA
4240 Park Place Court
P.O. Box 1547
Glen Allen, VA 23060
804-270-0142/
800-552-7996

WASHINGTON
2120 First Ave. N.
Seattle, WA 98109
206-283-1152

WEST VIRGINIA
240 Capitol Street, Suite 100
Charleston, WV 25301
304-344-3611

WISCONSIN
615 N. Sherman Ave.
Madison, WI 53704
608-249-0487

Milwaukee
11401 West Watertown Plank
 Road
Wauwatosa, WI 53226
414-453-4500

WYOMING
Indian Hills Center
506 Shoshoni
Cheyenne, WY 82009
307-638-3331

NATIONAL CANCER INSTITUTE The National Cancer Institute (NCI) supported a very extensive information network operated by the comprehensive cancer centers, called the Cancer Information Services (CIS). This was an effective means of providing answers to general questions in layman's language, prepared by a trained staff of health professionals. They were available to provide information on the causes of cancer, methods of detection, availability of various types of treatment and rehabilitation programs, counseling services, financial aid and resources available at the local level. Unfortunately, the National Cancer Institute is phasing these programs out because of federal budgetary restrictions. In some instances the comprehensive cancer centers still provide free information of this type, but because this is a diminishing program in many areas, we will not list the names and numbers of all of the services. Most of them are advertised in local telephone directories under Cancer Information Services; if you don't find such a listing, perhaps your local ACS can give you a toll-free number at which you can reach one of the existing Cancer Information Services. The NCI does operate a trained volunteer- or staff-operated toll-free cancer-information system, which you can reach by dialing 1-800-4-CANCER. They answer callers' questions, provide the latest facts about or risks for different types of cancers and treatments, and so on. When I called to ask for materials for use in writing this chapter, they were quite helpful to me.

The National Cancer Institute is one branch of the National Institutes of Health (NIH), which in turn is run by the Department of Health and Human Services (HHS). By the way, the NIH probably represents the greatest success story among all federal programs in this country because of its many accomplishments in health research, in which the United States has become preeminent in the world; the present director of NIH is my friend and former colleague Dr. James Wyngarden. The director of the NCI is Dr. Vincent DeVita and the address is NCI, National Institutes of Health, Bethesda, MD 20014. NCI deals largely with cancer research, and also with initiating experimental service programs aimed at providing the latest in information no matter where you live. One of the programs developed by the Cancer Control Branch of NCI is the so-called Physician Data Query (PDQ) system, which physicians can use to find out who is doing research with the latest treatment, or with particular drugs or on particular illnesses. Your physician can contact the National Cancer Institute to get further information about this system. Since 85 percent of patients with cancer are treated by community physicians, a delay of even a few months in transmitting information could cost lives; the PDQ system is designed to minimize such losses. Also, each institution engaged in research programs can register these with the NCI, and all of the information is then made available by means of this computerized network. Thus your doctor in California can contact a physician-researcher at Memorial Sloan-Kettering in New York (or wherever) to find out more about a particular research program, and also whether your type of problem would be suitable for this new approach. The system also lists the accepted treatments for that condition. PDQ, still a relatively new program, seems to be gaining in popularity, although I personally have some serious reservations about the wisdom of advertising or announcing some of these highly experimental programs on a nationwide basis before the projects have been evaluated in a critical fashion. And the notion of using computers to select treatments for individuals with cancer will have to be proven useful, in my opinion. But my experience in using the system is limited, so I should reserve judgment, especially since many others are quite enthusiastic.

The Public Information Office of the National Cancer Institute is also available to provide all types of information and educational materials on research and patient services. They are extremely helpful and you can write them at the Office of Cancer Communications, National Cancer Institute, Building 31, Room 10A30, Bethesda, MD 20014 (301-496-6631).

The NCI also has a clinical treatment program at its Clinical Center in Bethesda, Maryland, and its oncologists are engaged in an ever-changing series of studies. The Center generally will take only patients who are referred from other physicians, and you must be eligible for a particular type of ongoing study. This is *not* a general hospital. One of its unique aspects is that patients who are accepted for these studies are treated free of charge. The telephone number of the Patient Referral Service is 301-496-4891; your doctor can call to get additional information regarding whether there is a program that would be of interest to you.

In addition to ACS and NCI, a number of other organizations are prepared to give help to cancer patients and their families. The list and a brief description of each follows.

CANDLELIGHTERS, 2025 EYE STREET, N.W., SUITE 1011, WASHINGTON, DC 20006, 202-659-5136 Candlelighters is an international network of groups of parents of children with cancer. Some children are newly diagnosed, some are in remission, some are in relapse, some are in treatment, some are long-term survivors, some have died.

Believing "It is better to light one candle than to curse the darkness," Candlelighters have these goals:

☐   To link parent to parent, family to family, group to group

☐   To ease frustrations and fears through sharing of feelings and experiences

☐   To exchange information on research, treatment, medical institutions, community resources

☐   To break down the social isolation of families

☐   To provide guidance in coping with childhood cancer's effect on a child, on parents, on siblings, on a family

☐   To identify patient and family needs so that medical and social systems respond adequately

☐   To seek consistent and sufficient research funding

☐   To be an emotional support system of "second families" for each other

Locally, Candlelighters serve as an informal forum where parents share feelings, experiences and information on family life with a child with cancer.

Some groups have youth auxiliaries for teenage cancer patients and teenage siblings of children with cancer.

Groups sponsor crisis phone lines, buddy systems, parent-to-parent contacts, professional counseling, self-help groups and social functions where families meet and relax in supportive settings. Groups also offer babysitting or transportation; serve as clinic waiting-room aides; or sponsor blood banks, in-hospital visits, or the establishment of residences for families of children on extended care away from home.

The Candlelighters Childhood Cancer Foundation is a nonprofit organization whose free services and publications are supported by tax-exempt donations and a grant from the American Cancer Society, Inc.

NATIONAL HOSPICE ORGANIZATION, 1901 N. FORT MYER DRIVE, SUITE 902, ARLINGTON, VA 22209, 703-243-5900 The idea of hospice is to provide support and care to patients who are terminally ill, say with weeks or months of life expectancy, and assistance not only for the patient but also for family and friends.

Hospice has grown rapidly throughout the United States, now numbering well over 1,200 programs, and quite possibly your county has a hospice organization that you can find in the telephone directory or through the American Cancer Society. Most of these programs provide services in the home; they will first send in trained nurses to evaluate the needs of the individual situation, as well as volunteers who have varied and suitable talents and who will provide help almost any time of the day or night. Some of the hospice programs utilize beds in the hospital or nursing home and provide care in that setting, either solely there or in addition to the home-care part of the program. Wherever their services are provided, they emphasize the quality of survival rather than its length, and they are very concerned that the patient be as free of pain and other discomfort as possible. Hospice staff can be extremely helpful in providing counseling on how to help the patient with cancer (or other illness) deal with emotional problems, nutritional problems, legal problems (wills), preparation for a funeral, organ donation, or in providing companionship for a patient and respite for a tired family member. They help with whatever the patient and family need. Prerequisites to participation in the program are referral from a physician who believes that the patient is in a terminal phase of the illness, and a clear understanding by the patient that the *goal of care in hospice is comfort rather than cure.* This does not mean that a patient who is in a hospice program cannot also receive full medical treatment at the same time. In cases of mental incompetence, certain steps need to be followed before the patient can be deemed eligible.

By writing to the national office you can obtain a list of inexpensive publications about hospice.

LEUKEMIA SOCIETY OF AMERICA, INC., 733 THIRD AVE., NEW YORK, NY 10017, 212-573-8484 This is a fine national voluntary organization particularly concerned with providing services for patients with leukemia and lymphoma. The Society can provide guidance about referral services in the community, and can sometimes help with payment for drugs that are used in treatment, blood transfusion, transportation to and from a doctor's office and other costs. The Society also supports research and training. There are chapters in Alabama, Arizona, California, Colorado, Connecticut, Delaware, the District of Columbia, Florida, Georgia, Illinois, Kansas, Louisiana, Maryland, Massachusetts, Missouri, New Jersey, New York, Ohio, Pennsylvania, Rhode Island, Texas, Virginia and Wisconsin. If you cannot find a chapter in your local telephone directory, contact the national office.

Financial assistance up to $750 a year per person is given by the Society to outpatients being treated for leukemia, the lymphomas, multiple myeloma and preleukemia. Outpatients are those not confined to a hospital, although they may be treated at various times at a hospital.

Aid is limited in all cases to expenditures not covered by other sources. However, patients receiving federal, state, county and local aid, Social Security, Blue Cross, Blue Shield or Medicare may still be eligible for aid from the Leukemia Society. The services covered within the $750 limit include:

☐ Drugs used in treatment and/or control of leukemia and allied diseases as determined by the national Patient-Aid Committee, and dispensed by approved drug sources

☐ Processing, typing, screening and cross-matching of blood components for transfusions; fees for transfusions of red cells, leukocytes and platelets

☐ Transportation to and from a doctor's office, hospital or treatment center to the extent specifically approved by the national Patient-Aid Committee

☐ Initial induction x-ray therapy designed to cure the patient in amounts up to $300 for patients with Hodgkin's disease

☐ Initial induction x-ray therapy in amounts up to $300 for cranial (not spinal) radiation for children with the acute form of leukemia, and adults with acute lymphoblastic leukemia.

An application form may be obtained from local chapters.

REACH TO RECOVERY, AMERICAN CANCER SOCIETY, 90 PARK AVE., NEW YORK, NY 10016 This program offers assistance to patients who have breast cancer. Trained volunteers who themselves have had breast cancer are available to lend emotional support and furnish information to patients facing similar problems. I have found it very helpful at times to have one of these skilled volunteers visit a patient who is facing breast surgery. Further information about this program can be obtained from your local ACS office.

COMPREHENSIVE CANCER CENTERS If you need to obtain information about medical services, special types of surgery or radiation programs, or about the availability of specialists in particular types of cancer, it's probably useful to contact the comprehensive cancer center in your area. There are some twenty comprehensive cancer centers in the United States, and they are in a position to provide all of the services that are generally needed and information concerning them. A full complement of specialists usually work at each center, and if you are willing to get on the telephone and possibly make several calls, you can usually obtain the information you want about the availability of services there. The following list gives the names of these comprehensive cancer centers, which are among the leading cancer institutions in the United States, and the addresses and telephone numbers of their directors. Your request will probably need to be forwarded to a specialist in a particular field.

Director, Comprehensive Cancer Center
University of Alabama at Birmingham
University Station
1824 Sixth Ave. S., Room 214
Birmingham, AL 35294
205-934-6612

Director, Jonsson Comprehensive Cancer Center
UCLA Medical Center, Room 10/247
Louis Factor Health Sciences Bldg.
10833 Le Conte Ave.
Los Angeles, CA 90024
213-825-8727

Director, Kenneth Norris, Jr., Cancer Research Institute
University of Southern California
Comprehensive Cancer Center
P.O. Box 33804
1441 Eastlake Ave.
Los Angeles, CA 90033-0804
213-224-7722

Director, Yale University Comprehensive Cancer Center
School of Medicine
333 Cedar St., Room WWW 205
New Haven, CT 06510
203-785-6338

Director, Georgetown University/Howard University Comprehensive Cancer Center
Georgetown University Medical Center
3800 Reservoir Road, N.W.
Washington, DC 20007
202-625-2042

Director, Papanicolaou Comprehensive Cancer Center
University of Miami Medical School
1475 N.W. 12th Ave.
P.O. Box 016960 (D3-4)
Miami, FL 33101
305-547-5757

Director, Illinois Cancer Council
36 S. Wabash Ave., Suite 700
Chicago, IL 60603
312-346-9813

Director, Johns Hopkins Oncology Center
600 N. Wolfe Street, Room 157
Baltimore, MD 21205
301-955-8638

President, Dana-Farber Cancer Institute
44 Binney Street
Boston, MA 02115
617-732-3214

Director, Meyer L. Prentis Comprehensive Cancer Center of Metropolitan Detroit
110 East Warren Street
Detroit, MI 48201
313-833-0710

Director, Mayo Comprehensive Cancer Center
Mayo Clinic
200 First Street, S.W.
Rochester, MN 55905
507-284-3413

Director, Roswell Park Memorial Institute
666 Elm Street
Buffalo, NY 14263
716-845-4400

Director, Columbia University Cancer Center
College of Physicians & Surgeons
701 W. 168th Street, Room 1601
New York, NY 10032
212-305-6730

President, Memorial Sloan-Kettering Cancer Center
1275 York Avenue
New York, NY 10021
212-794-5845

Director, Duke Comprehensive Cancer Center
P.O. Box 3814
Duke University Medical Center
Durham, NC 27710
919-684-2282

Director, Ohio State University Comprehensive Cancer Center
410 W. 12th Ave., Suite 302
Columbus, OH 43210
614-293-8619

President, Fox Chase Cancer Center/University of Pennsylvania Comprehensive Cancer Center
7701 Burholme Ave.
Philadelphia, PA 19111
215-728-2570

President, The University of Texas System Cancer Center
M. D. Anderson Hospital and
Tumor Institute
Houston, TX 77030
713-792-6000

Director, Fred Hutchinson Cancer Research Center
1124 Columbia Street
Seattle, WA 98104
206-467-4675

Director, University of Wisconsin Clinical Cancer Center
600 Highland Ave.
Madison, WI 53792
608-263-8600

OTHER CANCER CENTERS A variety of clinical and nonclinical cancer centers receive financial support from the National Cancer Institute for clinical programs or to investigate new methods of treatment or for nonclinical research programs. Although the clinical centers that have research programs are probably of more interest to you, we will list them all, by state.

Southern Research Institute
Kettering-Meyer Laboratory
Birmingham, AL

University of Arizona Cancer Center
Tuscon, AZ

Cancer Research Center
City of Hope National Medical
Center
Duarte, CA

La Jolla Cancer Research Foundation
La Jolla, CA

Northern California Cancer Program
Palo Alto, CA

Cancer Research Institute
University of California School of
Medicine
San Francisco, CA

AMC Cancer Research Hospital
Lakewood, CO

Cancer Center
Goodwin Institute for Cancer
Research, Inc.
Emory University School of
Medicine
Atlanta, GA

Cancer Center of Hawaii
University of Hawaii at Manoa
Honolulu, HI

Mountain States Tumor Institute
Boise, ID

Northwestern University Cancer Center
Chicago, IL

Rush Cancer Center
Chicago, IL

University of Chicago Cancer Research Center
Chicago, IL

Ephraim McDowell Community Cancer Network, Inc.
Lexington, KY

James Graham Brown Cancer Center
University of Louisville School of Medicine
Louisville, KY

Frederick Cancer Research Center
Frederick, MD

New England Deaconess Hospital Cancer Research Institute and Shields Warren Radiation Laboratory
Boston, MA

Cancer Research Center
Ellis Fischel State Cancer Hospital
Columbia, MO

Eppley Institute for Research in Cancer
University of Nebraska Medical Center
Omaha, NE

Institute for Medical Research
Camden, NJ

Cancer Research and Treatment Center
University of New Mexico
Albuquerque, NM

Cancer Research Center
Albert Einstein College of Medicine
Bronx, NY

American Health Foundation
New York, NY

Mount Sinai Cancer Center
New York, NY

University of Rochester Cancer Center
Rochester, NY

Cancer Research Center
University of North Carolina
School of Medicine
Chapel Hill, NC

Oncology Research Center
Bowman Gray School of Medicine
Winston-Salem, NC

The Cleveland Clinic Cancer Center
Cleveland, OH

The Milton S. Hershey Medical Center
Specialized Cancer Research Center
Pennsylvania State University
Hershey, PA

Cancer Institute
Hahnemann Medical College and Hospital of Philadelphia
Philadelphia, PA

Children's Cancer Research Center
The Children's Hospital of Philadelphia
Philadelphia, PA

Fels Research Institute
Temple University Medical Center
Philadelphia, PA

University of Pennsylvania Cancer Center
Philadelphia, PA

The Wistar Institute
Philadelphia, PA

Clinical Radiation Therapy Research Center
Division of Radiation Oncology
Allegheny General Hospital
Pittsburgh, PA

Memphis Regional Cancer Center
Memphis, TN

St. Jude Children's Research Hospital
Memphis, TN

Oak Ridge National Laboratory
Oak Ridge, TN

Clinical Cancer Center
University of Texas Medical Branch
Galveston, TX

MCV/VCU Cancer Center
Virginia Commonwealth University
Medical College of Virginia
Richmond, VA

CANADIAN CANCER SOCIETY, 130 BLOOR STREET W., SUITE 101, TORONTO, ONTARIO, CANADA M5S 2V7, 416-961-7223 This is also an excellent program that provides the services listed below.

Practical Assistance

□   Dressings, prostheses and wigs

□   Volunteer drivers to and from treatment

□   Long-distance transportation for people in need

□   Ostomy supplies and equipment

□   Medical/hospital equipment loans

□   Drugs for the control of symptoms associated with the disease

□   Information on other available assistance

□   Accommodation for outpatients away from home

□   Educational material on diets, adjustment and other practical areas

Emotional Support

□   Mastectomy Visiting Program. Women who have themselves had breast cancer and have been specially trained visit mastectomy patients to offer temporary prostheses, demonstrate exercises and provide a sympathetic ear.

□   Can Surmount. One-to-one visiting of cancer patients by people whose own lives have been touched by cancer

□   Coping with Cancer. Group discussions for patients, families, friends

☐   Access to books and pamphlets on emotional adjustment to cancer

EUROPEAN GROUPS A number of groups in Europe are studying new treatments and also working in collaboration with U.S. scientists. The principal organization is known as the European Organization for Research on Treatment of Cancer (EORTC); its headquarters is at the Institut Jules Bordet, 1000 Brussels, Belgium. EORTC conducts various types of specialized programs throughout Europe.

CANCER PROGRAMS APPROVED BY THE AMERICAN COLLEGE OF SURGEONS The American College of Surgeons maintains a certification program intended to monitor the quality of care to cancer patients rendered in hospitals in the United States. These programs are regularly monitored by physicians, usually once every three years. I recently served on such an accreditation board, which brought me into contact with a number of cancer programs in community hospitals as well as in university hospitals. The directory of approved programs is available from the Cancer Program, American College of Surgeons, 55 E. Erie Street, Chicago, IL 60611. Because there are well over seven hundred of these, we will not list them individually. Being accredited means that the hospitals are considered to provide quality, up-to-date care with respect to diagnosis and treatment, they hold regular educational conferences to upgrade their physician staff, and they provide necessary paramedical services as well. They must meet certain quality standards, offer a broad range of services and keep careful records of their work.

There are many good hospitals that have quality programs for cancer patients but are not listed with the American College of Surgeons because, for one reason or another, they choose not to participate in this program. However, it is some comfort to know that your hospital is accredited because it means that the hospital has been willing to expose its programs to an outside review and has at least met certain minimum standards.

ADDITIONAL SOURCES OF INFORMATION You can find articles about cancer in your local public library; most of these are listed in the *Reader's Guide to Periodical Literature* or in the *Public Affairs Information Service:* there you can find relevant publications through the subject index. In the medical libraries at most universities and colleges and in some public libraries you can also consult the *Index Medicus,* which lists articles in about 2,500 medical journals. This is somewhat overwhelming, but the National Library of Medicine has a program called MEDLARS, which is a computerized system that can provide lists of articles if you request that particular topics be searched out for you. This is a very thorough information system that draws on an enormous number of possible citations. In practice, however, it is difficult for a lay person to gain access to medical libraries, so you may find your doctor or ACS a better place to go to get additional written information.

If you have questions for the Food and Drug Administration, you can write to its Office of Consumer Inquiries, FDA, 5600 Fishers Lane, Rockville, MD 20857 for information about federal regulations on drugs, food additives and the like. For questions about potential hazards of commercial products, you can write to the Consumer Product Safety Commission, 5401 Westbard Ave., Washington, DC 20207; the toll-free telephone number is 800-638-2666. The Environmental Protection Agency provides information about hazards in the environment other than those of industry; for such information you can contact the Public Information Center at 401 M Street, S.W., Washington, DC 20460. The Industrial Union of Metal Trades, a department of the AFL–CIO, is also interested in industrial exposure; the address is 815 Sixteenth Street, N.W., Washington, DC.

APPENDIX 2: LEGAL ASPECTS (MONEY, WILLS, ESTATES, ORGAN DONATION, FUNERALS)

Cancer, like other chronic or life-threatening illnesses, affects how patients and families cope with their present circumstances and how they plan for the future. The issues are often of agonizing seriousness, and it can be difficult to find answers at times of crisis.

The disease—or the side effects of treatment—may alter a patient's ability to maintain normal routines of daily living or to handle personal or family affairs. For example, the primary breadwinner may be unable to continue working, thereby reducing or eliminating household income; or an aged parent may no longer be able to manage his financial matters. The family may find that the disease now makes practical and legal concerns more urgent.

Practical and Legal Concerns of Cancer Patients and Their Families: A Handbook for Caregivers was developed by our Social Services Group at the Duke Comprehensive Cancer Center and written by Margaret DeLong, J.D., R.N.; Lou Paules, M.S.W., A.C.S.W.; and Carolyn McAllaster, J.D., as legal consultant, in response to the questions raised by our patients regarding life issues affected by their disease or treatment. In this appendix, with appreciation to the authors, I will present the handbook's major recommendations for your consideration, with the hope that this will assist you in taking action on the items that are important to you. It is intended to provide basic referral information about agencies, policies and professionals. It is *not* meant to be a substitute for legal advice from your own experienced lawyer; therefore it would be wise for any patient to consult a lawyer, even in circumstances in which it is not required. An attorney's advice can be useful and not necessarily expensive. Remember that patients from states other than North Carolina should contact a lawyer or agency familiar with the laws of their own state.

The information that follows was originally based on North Carolina law as of March 1982; it has been revised and updated as of May 1984. State or federal laws may change, so up-to-date information will be needed. North Carolina General Statutes (the laws established by the General Assembly of North Carolina) are cited in the text when references to particular laws seem helpful. Copies of the state general statutes can be found at law school libraries and most county courthouses. You would need to refer to comparable sources to learn the law in your own state—do not assume that each state's laws will be the same, although federal law of course is applicable everywhere. It may seem parochial for me to refer to North Carolina laws in writing a book for people outside the state. And yet this state is advanced in regard to these issues—not all states have comparable laws, but I hope calling attention to the need and citing the statutes may stimulate lawmakers in some states to fill the void. Also, there is no central repository that we can refer to in order to give you information pertinent to each of the states.

WHERE TO GET LEGAL SERVICES For people who need a lawyer but do not have one, the North Carolina Bar Association has a statewide *Lawyer Referral Service;* other states also have such a service. You can usually find it listed in the Yellow Pages under Lawyer or Attorney Referral Service. This service does not provide free legal help, but for a $20 fee it does promise a client a half-hour consultation with a lawyer in your community who specializes in your type of problem. Many problems can be resolved and questions answered within thirty minutes, but more time can be arranged if necessary. (To find a participating lawyer in a particular location in North Carolina, call the statewide toll-free telephone number [1-800-662-7660] between 9:30 a.m. and 4:30 p.m. on weekdays.) Lawyers who wish to participate in this program submit their names, and the lawyer recommended to you will be one who specializes in the field of the particular problem involved. The service also can send you a very simple paper about living wills (see below), which will inform your doctor and family what your wishes are regarding the use of extraordinary life-support measures in case there is no hope for recovery.

Federally funded *Legal Aid Offices* provide free legal services to people who cannot afford a private attorney. Legal Aid can represent eligible clients in civil (noncriminal) matters, such as application for welfare assistance, housing or consumer problems. Anyone who thinks he may be eligible for free legal services should ask for his local or state Legal Aid Office. The telephone number can be obtained from the telephone directory or the statewide toll-free CARELINE number (1-800-662-7030). In addition to legal services, Legal Aid can often provide referral to other types of agencies and resources, to help you deal with problems such as how to pay for medicines or deal with Medicare insurance problems. When I called them I was surprised to learn how much help they might give to families who have problems related to serious illness. This service is available for all. Some other states provide comparable services.

WHAT ARE YOUR SOCIAL SECURITY BENEFITS? Social Security provides retirement and disability benefits for workers who have contributed to the Social Security program, and for their survivors or dependents. To receive *full* cash retirement benefits, a person must (1) have paid into the Social Security system, and

(2) be at least sixty-five years of age. He can also receive reduced retirement benefits at age sixty-two. A blind or disabled person can receive full cash disability benefits. To qualify as disabled, he must have a mental or physical condition that will keep him from working for at least twelve months.

Various family members of a retired, disabled or deceased worker may also qualify to receive monthly benefits. The following family members may be eligible:

□   A wife or husband who is sixty-two or older
□   A spouse who cares for a child who is under sixteen or disabled
□   A dependent unmarried child who is either under eighteen, or over eighteen and disabled, or a full-time student under twenty-two
□   A widow or widower who is sixty or older
□   A widow or widower who is fifty or older and becomes disabled less than seven years after the worker's death
□   A divorced parent who is sixty-two or older
□   A dependent grandchild whose parents are dead or disabled

To find out about eligibility requirements, call the local Social Security Administration (listed in the telephone directory), or write to the Division of Social Services, Disability Determination Section, in your state capital.

To apply for Social Security benefits, a person or his representative should go to the local Social Security Administration Office. If he cannot go in person, a telephone interview can be arranged. It may be necessary to provide the following information in applying for Social Security benefits, so be ready:

□   The Social Security number of the worker and of his dependents or survivors
□   The worker's birth certificate
□   The worker's death certificate (if he has died)
□   Proof of relationship to the worker, such as a marriage license or birth certificate
□   Proof of enrollment in school if a child is dependent and over eighteen

If a person's claim to Social Security benefits is denied, he may ask the Social Security Administration to reconsider it, but this must be done within sixty days after the denial. If the claim is again denied, further appeals are possible. An attorney's advice would be very helpful.

MANAGING THE AFFAIRS OF SOMEONE ELSE If a family member has become unable to manage his own affairs, or if it is expected that he soon will become unable to do so, it is necessary for someone else to take over this responsibility. There are several ways that this can be done.

Power of Attorney Power of attorney involves a written declaration, by someone (the principal) who is of sound mind, authorizing another person to act as his agent. This agent does not have to be a lawyer. He can be a capable and trustworthy relative or friend; or the agent can be an institution such as a bank. Because the principal gives up some significant rights when he grants a power of attorney, it is very important for him to have complete confidence in the agent.

The declaration of a power of attorney can grant as much or as little authority as is desired—from handling one particular transaction to handling a range of affairs. One example of this that may be helpful would be an elderly person who grants one of his children the power of attorney to use the parent's bank account to pay the parent's bills.

A power of attorney continues indefinitely unless it is limited by special terms or the principal revokes it, becomes incompetent or dies. (In the legal sense, being incompetent means that the person is not mentally able to manage his own affairs or to exercise certain civil rights, like voting. A court procedure is required before a person can be found to be legally incompetent.) North Carolina law provides a special procedure for establishing a durable power of attorney that continues even after the principal loses competency (#32A-8 et seq.).

When it is possible that a person with a chronic illness may become unable to make important decisions or handle his affairs, it is advisable to set up a power of attorney early. This is important because waiting until the person becomes incompetent requires a much longer and more costly procedure to establish a guardianship of that person.

To arrange a power of attorney it is necessary to consult a lawyer.

Authorizations for Bank Transactions Most banks allow their customers who have checking or savings accounts to authorize another person to make transactions within those accounts. In some cases the bank simply provides a card that the account owner signs along with the person who will now handle the account. The card is valid until the owner revokes it or dies. Because banks do not monitor the use of funds by the authorized person, the owner of the account should give this power only to someone he trusts. This person does not have to be a relative.

Representative Payee for Social Security Checks If a person is incapable of handling his Social Security checks, another person may request authority to manage that transaction. This person becomes the representative payee; his name will appear on the checks, and he has the power to deposit or cash the checks. To ensure that this power is not abused and that the money is used in the interest of the intended person, the Social Security Administration requires that the representative payee keep records of how the money is spent.

Before this arrangement can be made, a physician must sign a Social Security form stating that the Social Security beneficiary is either mentally incompetent or physically cannot handle his affairs. The arrangement may not be used with a physically handicapped person who is fully mentally competent and can sign his name or make an X.

The person who asks to be named as representative payee must file an application with the local Social Security Administration Office. The appointment of a representative to receive Social Security checks takes forty to sixty days, so it is helpful to anticipate this situation and save the time.

Appointment of a Fiduciary for VA Benefits The Veterans Administration may appoint someone to handle the VA checks of a person who is incapable of managing his benefits. The one who is appointed is known as a fiduciary. Before this arrangement can be made, the person entitled to the VA benefits must be declared incompetent by the VA on the basis of an examination by the VA or a private physician's statement that the person is incompetent. The VA selects the fiduciary on the basis of the facts in each case, the amount of income and estate to be administered and the incompetent person's needs. To ensure that this power is not abused and the funds are used in the interest of the person intended, the VA regularly visits with the incompetent and the fiduciary to review accounts. Appointment of a fiduciary can take sixty to ninety days. To learn more, contact your state Regional VA Office.

Incompetency and Guardianship A guardian should be appointed if an adult has become mentally unable to manage his affairs, and no other person has been given legal authority to handle these affairs. A relative or friend of the person petitions the clerk of superior court in the person's home county to have him declared incompetent and to have a guardian appointed (#35-2). During the court process, an attorney, called a "guardian ad litem," represents the allegedly incompetent person in order to protect his rights. The clerk of court holds a hearing before a jury. During the hearing, evidence that the person is unable to make decisions concerning himself, his family or property is presented. A physician must describe the person's illness and give an opinion as to whether or not the person is mentally capable to manage his or her affairs. The doctor may do this in person or provide a notarized affidavit (sworn written statement). If the court agrees with the evidence, it appoints a guardian to be legally responsible for the incompetent's financial and/or personal needs. If either the person who petitioned the court or the person who was declared incompetent disagrees with the decision, he may appeal. The services of an attorney should then be obtained.

Appointing a guardian is a much more expensive and complicated procedure than establishing a power of attorney. Thus, if a person is ill but not yet incompetent, establishing a power of attorney early may help avoid extra costs and time in court at a later date.

WILLS

What Is a Will? The best way for a person to make sure that his money and possessions go to the people he wants to receive them when he dies is to write a will. In North Carolina, to make a will that will hold up in court, the person who makes the will (the testator) must be at least eighteen and of sound mind (#31-1). He must sign it voluntarily and without undue influence by others.

A typical will might:

☐   Name an executor (the person who carries out the directions and requests of the will). Often this is a trusted relative, friend, attorney or the trust department of a bank.

☐   Name a guardian for any minor children

☐   Specify how real property (real estate) and personal property (such as money, jewelry and trust funds for minors) are to be distributed

☐   Specify funeral wishes

Kinds of Wills The preferred form of will is one that is prepared by an attorney. The testator signs the document in the presence of at least two witnesses, whose signatures are certified by a notary public (#31-3.3, #31-11.6). Attorney fees for this service can be reasonable; the testator can ask in advance what the charge will be.

A will that is handwritten by the testator is called a holographic will (#31-3.4). To be valid in North Carolina, this kind of will must be written entirely in the testator's handwriting and must be signed by him. In addition, it must be found in a safe-deposit box or another place where the testator kept valuable papers. A holographic will need not be witnessed when it is written, but after the testator dies, three witnesses must certify that the will is written in his handwriting. One witness must testify that the document was found among the testator's valuable papers. These witnesses may be beneficiaries (persons included in the will).

North Carolina law also recognizes oral wills. An oral will is valid in regard to personal property, like money or jewelry, but not real estate (#31-3.5). It is a statement made by the testator while in his last illness or in imminent peril of death. An oral will must be spoken in the presence of at least two witnesses who are not beneficiaries. It loses its effect if it is not acted on within six months after it was spoken or if the testator recovers from his illness or is rescued.

Guardianship of Minor Children Most doctors and social workers can relate horror stories of instances when the parent died without providing for minor children, and the children went into undesirable situations. The court cannot know what you intended if it is not stated legally. A person who has minor children should name a guardian for his children when making a will—and discuss this with the proposed guardian in case there may be a problem. If he dies without doing so, *the court may appoint anyone who is legally qualified and is willing to serve as a guardian.* Under North Carolina law a surviving spouse, if not somehow disqualified, is preferred over anyone else as guardian. But if there is no surviving spouse, the court will prefer the person named by the will as guardian if he is legally qualified (#33-3, #33-4, #33-5).

Like a parent, a guardian is responsible for a child's well-being. The guardian will be expected to provide guidance in educational and moral matters and, if designated, in financial matters as well. Guardianship ends when the child reaches eighteen.

Changing a Will States have different laws about what constitutes a legally valid will. Therefore, a will written before a person moved to North Carolina should be reviewed by a North Carolina attorney and rewritten, if necessary. In this mobile society this is a pitfall that is easy to overlook.

A person should review his will from time to time to be sure that it states present wishes. Circumstances change, and a will that may have been right for a person and his family several years ago may now need revision. The person you originally selected for guardianship may now be old, infirm or unwilling to serve in that capacity.

There are important rules for changing a will. One should not draw a line through a paragraph or write anything on the will. Such an action may make a will invalid. If changes need to be made, the testator should have his attorney prepare a "codicil," which is a separate document explaining the changes. This document is formally signed and witnessed just as for the original will. If substantial changes are needed, a new will may be advisable.

Where to Keep a Will A will should be kept in a safe place where it cannot be lost or destroyed. The clerk of superior court in each North Carolina county has a place for people to file their wills for safekeeping, free of charge (#31-11). If a testator stores his will in a safe-deposit box, upon his death someone from the clerk of court's office is authorized to remove it, although nothing else in the box may be removed.

It is extremely important for a testator to let his executor and family know where his will is kept. A North Carolina resident who dies without making a will is said to have died *intestate:* or, *if a will cannot be found, the state will assume that there is none and distribute a person's property according to North Carolina law.* Because this results in distributions that are so variable from state to state, we will not describe the North Carolina statutes—but what the law provides in your state may surprise you.

LIVING WILLS I get a lot of questions about a Living Will; what it is, how to obtain it and how it should be prepared. The lawyers of North Carolina have prepared a pamphlet for our citizens, and I will summarize here its major points and give you the example they provide for those who wish to use it in our state. Basically a Living Will states the wish to have a natural death, and having a Living Will permits you to make certain choices now when there is no doubt about your mental competency. It is a way to retain control over what happens at the end of your life, even when you are not able to express yourself. It is a legal document in our state, and it recognizes that an individual has a right to a natural death (#90-321). If an individual uses this means to express a desire that his or her life not be prolonged by extraordinary measures, and if the attending doctor determines that the individual does have a condition that is terminal and incurable, and this is confirmed by another physician, then extraordinary means may legally be withheld or discontinued. Extraordinary means are any medical procedures that the attending doctor judges would merely postpone the moment of death by artificially maintaining or substituting for a vital bodily function.

The form to be used may be obtained from any attorney; citi-

THE LIVING WILL

NORTH CAROLINA COUNTY OF _____
DECLARATION OF A DESIRE FOR A NATURAL DEATH

I, _____, being of sound mind, desire that my life not be prolonged by extraordinary means if my condition is determined to be terminal and incurable. I am aware and understand that this writing authorizes a physician to withhold or discontinue extraordinary means.

This the _____ day of _____, 19____.

Signature: _____

I hereby state that the declarant, _____, being of sound mind signed the above declaration in my presence and that I am not related to the declarant by blood or marriage and that I do not know or have a reasonable expectation that I would be entitled to any portion of the estate of the declarant under any existing will or codicil of the declarant, or as an heir under the Intestate Succession Act if the declarant died on this date without a will. I also state that I am not the declarant's attending physician or an employee of the declarant's attending physician, or an employee of a health facility in which the declarant is a patient or an employee of a nursing home or any group-care home where the declarant resides. I further state that I do not now have any claim against the declarant.

Witness: _____

Witness: _____

CERTIFICATE

I, _____, a Notary Public for _____ County hereby certify that _____, the declarant appeared before me and swore to me and the witnesses in my presence that this instrument is _____ Declaration Of A Desire For A Natural Death, and that _____ had willingly and voluntarily made and executed it as _____ free act and deed for the purposes expressed in it.

I further certify that _____ and _____, witnesses, appeared before me and swore that they witnessed _____, declarant, sign the attached declaration, believing _____ to be of sound mind; and also swore that at the time they witnessed the declaration (i) they were not related within the third degree to the declarant or to the declarant's spouse, and (ii) they did not know or have a reasonable expectation that they would be entitled to any portion of the estate of the declarant upon the declarant's death under any will of the declarant or codicil thereto then existing or under the Intestate Succession Act as it provided at that time, and (iii) they were not a physician attending the declarant or an employee of an attending physician or an employee of a health facility in which the declarant was a patient or an employee of a nursing home or any group-care home in which the declarant resided, and (iv) they did not have a claim against the declarant. I further certify that I am satisfied as to the genuineness and due execution of the declaration.

This the _____ day of _____, 19____.

_____
Notary Public

My commission expires: _____

zens of North Carolina may use the form included here. A Living Will must be witnessed and signed in accordance with state law, and must be certified by a notary public. Witnesses cannot be related to the person making the Living Will or be potential heirs to the estate. The attending physician or employees of the physician or hospital cannot witness such a will, and witnesses can have no claim against the estate of the individual.

People often wonder if they can change their mind once they sign a Living Will, and the answer is yes. You may revoke a Living Will by destruction of the original and all copies of the Living Will, or by communicating your intention to revoke the Will at any time and regardless of your mental or physical condition. This intention should be communicated to all interested persons, including your doctor, either by you or by someone acting on your behalf. It is important to note that a Living Will is not a substitute for a regular will because it makes no provision for your personal belongings or property after your death, and thus it should not be confused with a Testamentary Will.

When no declaration has been made, under some circumstances North Carolina law allows the withholding or removal of extraordinary life-support measures from a person whose condition is terminal, incurable and irreversible. Brain death (that is, the ceasing of all brain functions) is one guide that can help to determine when a person is dead or when artificial life-support measures may be withheld or removed. The decision in this case is in the hands of the physician and close family members or the guardian. This law is subject to change and also it is not applicable in other states, where different but related laws may be in effect.

PLANNING FOR FAMILY SECURITY

Trust Funds A trust is a legal arrangement by which a person called a trustee controls and manages property (assets) for the benefit of other people (who are called beneficiaries). Someone who wishes to set up a trust generally designates as trustee a financial institution, such as a bank, or a reliable person who is knowledgeable about financial affairs and investments. A person may choose to create a trust to begin at his death for the benefit of his dependents. Naming a trusted friend or family member as a trustee for any property left to minor children in a will is often advisable. A person may also create a trust for his own benefit if he does not want to manage his property or cannot do so. If the assets are sizable, it may be wise to name a commercial financial institution as trustee. The institution will charge a fee.

An attorney or a financial institution should be consulted to determine whether establishing a trust fund is wise.

Insurance Policies To protect his family in the event of his death, a person should periodically review any life insurance policies he has. Family circumstances may have changed through births, deaths, marriage or divorce. Changes in the policy's provisions should be made by an insurance agent.

It is also wise to look into any outstanding mortgages or loans that the person has. If these debts are covered by credit insurance, the insurance will pay any balance due if he dies. This tax-free payment may be made either to the family or to the company that made the loan. The original copy of an insurance policy must be presented along with a death certificate before any payment can be made.

Insurance policies should be kept with other important documents in a safe place where they can be reached by those who may need them.

Gifts A person may prefer to make gifts or to transfer property during his lifetime rather than through a will after death. It is important to know that some large gifts may be subject to a federal or state gift tax when they are made. In a few instances, if the gift is made within the three years before the giver dies, the gift may later be subject to estate and inheritance taxes. Parents also may wish to make gifts of cash, securities or insurance to their minor children. These gifts are subject to specific laws (#33-69). Again, an attorney's advice will be helpful.

ANATOMICAL GIFTS North Carolina law permits an adult of sound mind to designate that when he dies, his body or any body part—such as the eyes or kidneys—be given for the purpose of scientific research or organ transplant (#90-220 et seq.). This person is called a donor. Those who may receive such gifts (donees) include hospitals, educational institutions and designated individuals in need of organ transplants.

A wish to make an anatomical gift may be included in a will, but a separate written copy of the wish should also be made, because a will might not make the gift known in time for it to be useful. It is wise to let the executor and next of kin know about these wishes so that the bequest will not be unexpected and perhaps upset the bereaved family.

The simplest way to make the gift is for the donor to carry an anatomical gift card that has been signed in the presence of two witnesses, who also must sign the card. The donor may always revoke such a gift, but should be careful to follow the directions given by the donee for withdrawing the gift. These gift cards are now often provided at the time of obtaining a license to drive a motor vehicle—this seems fitting since motor vehicle accidents provide an important source of organs for transplantation.

A medical center or other donee may reject an anatomical gift, and families should have alternative plans or funeral arrangements in case the donee does refuse the donation. The donee who accepts a gift of the entire body must, subject to the terms of the gift, authorize embalming and use of the body in funeral services if the surviving spouse or next of kin so requests. If the gift is a body part, the donee must remove it without unnecessary mutilation. In some cases, certain costs connected with caring for and transporting the body are borne by the donee.

The law gives the surviving spouse or next of kin the right to offer the deceased's body as a gift at the time of death unless the deceased has made a contrary request. Also, if the surviving spouse or next of kin does not want to carry out the wishes of the deceased in regard to the gift, he or she can revoke the donation.

PLANNING A FUNERAL A person may find it helpful to plan his funeral and to express his wishes in writing. Written plans relieve family members, already under considerable stress, from the added burden of making arrangements and wondering whether their decisions are what the deceased would have wanted. Funeral wishes may be included in a will, but a separate written copy should be kept somewhere else to prevent delays. A family member should know where this document is kept.

Joining a memorial or funeral society is one way to simplify funeral arrangements and make them less costly. A memorial or funeral society is a voluntary nonprofit group that helps its members plan funerals at reasonable cost. Some of these groups meet regularly and have programs that deal with quality of life, how to be involved in making decisions about medical care and control of the use of life-support systems. I was invited to give a talk at a regional meeting about attitudes of doctors who care for patients who are dying. The members were thoughtful, highly intelligent and very serious about looking after their own and their families' needs. They represented many different occupations and religious beliefs. For more information, contact your local society or write to the Continental Association of Funeral and Memorial Societies, 2001 S Street, N.W., Suite 530, Washington, DC 20009. The telephone number is 202-745-0634. This group can provide information about wills, organ donation, funeral practices and the locations of the two hundred associated societies in the United States and Canada. Hospice programs can also be helpful in providing some of this information and information about family-support systems. Hospice programs can also be helpful in making funeral arrangements since they are involved in comforting and helping the whole family to cope.

Ceremony Each family has its own preferences, traditions and religious values that determine which type of ceremony suits it best. Funerals are services held in the presence of the body; the casket may or may not be left open for viewing. They are usually held in a church, chapel, funeral home or at the gravesite. Memorial services do not include the presence of the body and may be held wherever desired. Generally memorial services are less expensive than funerals. Whether the body is to be buried, cremated or donated may affect the choice of ceremony.

Cost Cost varies according to the type of service and where it is held; the choice of vault, casket or urn; whether the body is embalmed; whether it is prepared for viewing and whether some funeral-home services such as limousines or flowers are used. North Carolina law does not usually require that a body be embalmed. It does require funeral directors to disclose the costs at the time the funeral arrangements are made (#90-210.25).

There are usually charges for cremation services. If an earth burial is preferred, a person may wish to buy a cemetery lot in advance. He can thus choose the cemetery and site he wishes, and spare the family this task while they are bereaved. A funeral director can help with buying a burial plot and may even make a cash advance.

WHEN DEATH OCCURS

Whom to Notify After a person dies, family members or friends need to contact:

- A doctor to complete the death certificate; get several copies of the certificate
- A director for a funeral or memorial service
- Insurance companies, including the automobile insurance carrier for possible immediate cancellation
- The executor of the estate or a lawyer
- Income sources. If the deceased had been working, contact the employer and/or business partners. If he was receiving benefits, contact the appropriate agency—such as the local Social Security Office, the VA or the county social services department. Check whether any income for survivors is available.
- Trade union or fraternal organizations
- Credit union and banks. Check whether the credit union has an arrangement that increases the amount on deposit by an assigned percentage or offers a death benefit.
- Companies that receive mortgage or installment payments. Some companies have an insurance clause in the credit document that cancels the debt at death. If a balance remains to be paid, ask the creditor whether payment may be delayed if necessary.
- Post office, utility companies, and the landlord if the deceased lived alone

Disposition of the Body The right to take possession of and dispose of a dead body belongs to the surviving spouse or next of kin. If the deceased has been divorced, the right goes to the next of kin. This right includes authorizing anatomical gifts or autopsies.

Either the doctor or the funeral director files the death certificate and the notification of death. Medical information and cause of death must be certified by the physician and must be included in the certificate. The death certificate must be filed within five days at the register of deeds' office in the county where the decedent died (in some counties it is filed first with the county health department).

If a death occurs naturally at home with no doctor present, the family's attending physician should be called to verify the cause of death. If this can be done it is much easier, but if no physician is available, the local medical examiner will be asked to certify the death. The funeral director, the local rescue squad or the police can contact the examiner. The funeral home will not remove the body unless a physician or the medical examiner has been contacted.

A body may be transported in any vehicle, not just a hearse or an ambulance. If the body of a North Carolina resident is to be carried over the state line, it must be accompanied by a burial transit permit, which is issued by the health department or the medical examiner. To transport a body from one locale to another, the funeral director at the place where the body is to be sent may send a vehicle for the body; if the distance is great, the funeral director in the place where the death occurred may prepare the body and send it in a casket by air to the designated place.

A permit, which the funeral director obtains, is required before a burial or cremation can be performed. Embalming is required only if there is to be a considerable delay before burial.

Autopsy There are many misconceptions about autopsies, and yet they are very important to medical knowledge. If there is a question as to the cause of death or the nature of the illness, the physician or the family may request an autopsy. If a physician asks for an autopsy, the next of kin may grant or refuse permission, except in cases in which a medical examiner is required by law to perform an autopsy. If the person dies at home but the body is transported to a medical center for autopsy, the transportation cost is usually borne by the family. *I do recommend that the autopsy examination be performed whenever possible because it is quite likely that something useful will be learned that can later be of help to someone else.* Studies show that in one-third of autopsies some significant additional finding will be discovered. This is so important for furtherance of knowledge that we can all express our wishes in advance, as with organ donation. Much of what we now know about disease processes was learned by careful study of diseased organs. The autopsy can be done expeditiously and it need not delay the funeral—although occasionally funeral directors find it a bit inconvenient, and I have seen some of them discourage the family from obtaining a funeral on that account. When a person is dead there is of course no pain and the body is treated with respect, just as in an operating room. Most religious leaders encourage the procedure as a means of potentially helping the living.

Bank Accounts Frozen Whether funds can be withdrawn from a bank account that belonged to a deceased person depends on the type of account. If it is a joint account with a survivorship clause, the surviving depositor has access to half of the account but the other half is frozen until the estate is settled (#41-2.1). After any debts of the deceased are paid, the surviving depositor receives the remainder.

If a joint account has no survivorship clause, all funds are frozen. If the account is solely in the name of the deceased, all funds are frozen as well.

Access to Safe-Deposit Box All contents of the deceased's safe-deposit box (except for a will) are held by the bank until the will is probated unless the contents are released by the State Department of Revenue. When a will has been stored in a safe-deposit box, the executor or the family should ask the office of the clerk of superior court in the county where the deceased lived to send someone to remove only the will. This court employee will also inventory the contents that have monetary value, such as jewelry, titles to automobiles or life insurance policies. These items may not be removed before probate without a release from the Department of Revenue. To obtain such a release, the clerk of court must send a copy of the safe deposit box inventory to the Department of Revenue, which then sends authorization for release to the bank or the executor of the estate (#105-24).

Death Benefits Under Social Security regulations, the surviving spouse or the children who are eligible for survivor benefits during the month in which the deceased died may receive a lump sum of $255 for funeral expenses. The survivor must apply for this benefit at the local Social Security Administration Office and must present a certified death certificate and some form of proof of relationship, such as a marriage license.

Under VA regulations, family members are entitled to certain benefits when a veteran dies. The Veterans Administration Office should be contacted for information.

Some trade unions, fraternal organizations and railroad companies award death benefits to family members. Inquiries should be made to any such organization to which the deceased belonged.

SETTLING AN ESTATE

Probate The term "probate" means the court procedure by which a will is proved to be valid, and it is commonly used to refer to all matters and proceedings involved in settling an estate. Under North Carolina law, property cannot be distributed until the will has been probated by the clerk of superior court in the county where the deceased lived (#31-12 et seq.).

Certain kinds of property are transferred automatically at death without regard to the probate process. But this property may be subject to estate taxes and/or the debts of the person who died. Examples of assets that may transfer automatically at death are life insurance proceeds, jointly held real estate, joint bank accounts, trusts and savings bonds owned jointly. Requests can be made for release of some joint bank accounts so that the surviving depositor can immediately draw a portion of the funds from the account. If the spouse needs funds from life and accident insurance policies, the insurance company(ies) should be notified immediately and asked to send the appropriate forms. Reliable companies will usually offer as much help as possible in preparing and processing the forms.

If a person dies without a will and leaves personal property worth no more than $10,000, his heirs may take possession of this property thirty days after the death by obtaining an affidavit from the clerk of superior court in the deceased's home county (#28A-25-1). The office of the clerk of superior court can be helpful in directing this matter.

Personal Representative A personal representative is someone whom the clerk of court makes responsible for settling the decedent's (deceased's) estate (#28A-4-1). If the decedent has named an executor (the person to carry out the requests) in his will, then with court approval this person becomes the personal representative. If the decedent did not name an executor and did not leave a will, the court names a personal representative, called an administrator. Under North Carolina law, a surviving spouse has first priority, if legally qualified, to be the administrator.

The personal representative must prepare an inventory of all the decedent's assets. He also pays all claims and debts against the estate before distributing assets to beneficiaries (#28A-19-6). If there are insufficient funds from which to pay debts, payments are made in the following order:

1 Allowance for the surviving spouse or children for the year following death
2 Costs for administration of the estate
3 Claims that have a specific lien on property
4 Funeral expenses up to $1,000
5 Taxes and preferred debts
6 Judgment liens
7 Hospital and doctor bills for the deceased for a period of up to twelve months; wages due an employee of the decedent
8 All other claims

Legal Rights of a Survivor In North Carolina every surviving spouse is entitled to an allowance of $5,000 for support for one year after the decedent's death (#30-15). This $5,000 may be paid in cash or in personal property, and it is to be paid regardless of how many debts are outstanding against the estate. If there is a will, the allowance is deducted from the property that the surviving spouse inherits. Each surviving child under eighteen is entitled to a year's allowance of $1,000, subject to certain reductions (#30-17). Application for these allowances must be filed with the clerk of superior court within one year of the spouse's death. Survivors are entitled to keep up to $7,500 worth of property used as a residence and $2,000 worth of household items regardless of any claims by creditors (#1C-1601).

An attorney's services will be very helpful in applying for all such benefits.

Dissent from a Will Generally, the person who makes a will has the right to disinherit persons, including children, who would otherwise inherit property if the testator had died without a will. But, at least under North Carolina law, a surviving spouse may not be entirely disinherited (#30-1). A surviving spouse can dissent from (disagree with) the will. An attorney should be consulted about this procedure. *If there is something unusual about the will, say a close relative is to be disinherited, then I think it is very important for the individual to discuss this with the relative so that the reasons are clear and the surviving relative(s) who do inherit are not blamed for influencing the decedent at the last minute, or questions are not raised about the competency of the individual.* It is easy to make a mess for the family by not tending to this matter thoughtfully.

Estate and Inheritance Taxes Estate and inheritance taxation is a complicated area of the law, and the provisions change often. It is enough to say here that both the federal and state governments impose estate taxes when the estate is above a certain size. An attorney, an accountant or the State Department of Revenue should be consulted on these matters.

Income Tax Returns The Internal Revenue Service has the right to audit an income tax return for three years after the return was filed. A decedent's tax records should be kept for at least that long.

A record of all taxable income and deductions for the current tax year (or for the prior years, if such returns have not yet been filed) should be kept. The decedent's personal representative may have to file income tax returns for the decedent's estate covering the year of death.

GLOSSARY

Ablative therapy   A treatment to totally remove part of the body.

Acute   Occurring suddenly or over a short period of time.

Adenocarcinoma   A cancer starting in glandular tissue.

Adjuvant chemotherapy   The use of anticancer drugs in combination with either surgery or radiation as part of the initial treatment of cancer, before detectable spread, in order to prevent or delay a recurrence.

Aflatoxin   A highly potent chemical produced by a fungus that can contaminate grains and nuts stored in warm, damp areas and that is capable of causing liver cancers in humans and animals.

Agent   A substance that causes some changes.

AIDS   Acquired immunodeficiency syndrome.

353

Alimentation The act of giving or receiving nutrients.

Alkylating agents Chemical compounds like nitrogen mustard that have anticancer properties.

Alopecia (al-o-pee'-shah) Hair loss, partial or complete; a common side effect of chemotherapy drugs.

Amenorrhea (a-men-o-ree'-ah) Abnormal absence or stoppage of menstruation; may be a side effect of chemotherapy.

Amino acid Any one of a group of organic acids that are the building blocks of proteins.

Analgesic Medicine given to control pain.

Anemia A condition in which there is a lack of red cells in the blood, causing tiredness, shortness of breath and pallor.

Angiogenesis Development of blood vessels.

Angiosarcoma A malignant tumor formed by the proliferation of endothelial and fibroblastic tissue, the kinds of cells that normally line blood vessels.

Anorexia Loss of appetite.

Antibody A protein substance, specifically a globulin, formed by the body to neutralize specific foreign substances such as bacteria, viruses, alien tissue and other antigens.

Antiemetic A drug used to reduce nausea and vomiting.

Antigen Any substance that causes the body to produce antibodies with which it reacts; these may be soluble toxins or chemicals from the surface of cells such as blood-group substances, or from bacteria.

Antimetabolite A substance bearing a close structural resemblance to a normal chemical required by the body; it is processed like its normal counterpart and exerts its effects by interfering with the utilization of the essential metabolite (any substance produced by metabolism). An antimetabolite can resemble an essential vitamin, amino acid or building block for DNA.

Aspirate To suck off fluid with a syringe.

Astrocytoma The most common cancer that develops in the brain in adults.

ATP Adenosine triphosphate, a chemical found in all cells, which provides the energy that drives other chemical reactions. ATP is essential in order for muscle cells and other cells to perform their normal functions.

B-Cell Subgroup of cells produced in the lymph system, responsible for secreting circulating antibodies.

Benign A term used to describe a tumor or tissue that is not malignant or cancerous and that therefore does not spread.

Biopsy Removal, generally for microscopic examination, of tissue from the body for purposes of diagnosis. An *excisional* biopsy removes the entire suspicious tissue; an *incisional* biopsy removes only a small portion.

Blood-brain barrier A physiological barrier to the free passage of materials back and forth between the bloodstream and the fluids bathing the brain.

Blood count A test measuring the number of red cells, white cells and platelets in a blood sample.

Bone marrow The spongy inner core of the bone that harbors blood-forming cells; the blood-forming property is usually inhibited by chemotherapy.

BSE Breast self-examination.

Cachexia (ka-keck'-see-ah) The wasting away of the body often seen in advanced cancer.

Cancer A general term used for over one hundred different diseases characterized by uncontrolled cell growth of abnormal cells that grow locally or may spread to distant sites.

Carcinogen A cancer-causing agent. Carcinogenesis is the causation of cancer.

Carcinoma Cancer that originates in the epithelial tissue (glands, skin and lining of the internal organs) of the body. Most cancers are carcinomas (80–90 percent).

Carotenoids Fat-soluble, yellow-to-orange/red pigments universally present in plants; believed to be anticarcinogenic either in themselves or through their conversion product, vitamin A.

CAT scan A computerized x-ray system that gives very detailed pictures.

CEA Chorioembryonic antigens.

Cell line A mass of genetically identical cells grown from an originating cell in a culture medium under laboratory conditions.

Cervix Neck of the uterus or womb.

Chemotherapy The treatment of disease, especially cancer, with chemicals or drugs.

Choriocarcinoma A rare but rapidly growing malignancy of so-called trophoblastic cells primarily formed by the abnormal proliferation of cells from the placental epithelium. Almost all cases arise in the uterus, following an abortion, so-called uterine mole or normal pregnancy; now largely curable with chemotherapy.

Chorionic gonadotropin The gonad-stimulating principle from human pregnancy urine.

Chromosome A structure in the nucleus containing a linear thread of DNA (and protein covering) that transmits all genetic information to characterize the function of individual cells. Abnormalities in chromosome number or structure are common in cancer cells.

Chronic Lasting a long time (as opposed to "acute"), said of a condition.

Clinical Pertaining to direct observation and care of patients, as opposed to research.

Cobalt therapy Radiotherapy using radiation from a cobalt machine.

Codon The basic unit of genetic code. Each codon, a sequence of three nucleotide bases in a gene, is translated into one amino acid during protein biosynthesis.

Colonoscope Instrument for examination of the colon (large intestine).

Combination chemotherapy Use of two or more anticancer drugs, together or sequentially, for the purpose of adding together effective cancer-cell killing without adding appreciably to dangerous side effects.

Combined modality treatment   The use of more than one type of anticancer treatment (surgery, radiotherapy, chemotherapy) together.

Complete blood count (CBC)   A laboratory procedure that determines the number of red cells, white cells and platelets in a sample of blood.

Craniopharyngioma   A tumor of the pituitary gland at the base of the brain.

Cruciferous vegetables   Members of the mustard family (Cruciferae), including broccoli, cabbage, cauliflower, brussels sprouts, kohlrabi and turnips; in their raw form believed to protect against colorectal cancer.

CT scan   Computerized tomogram.

Cytology   Scientific study of the appearance of cells to determine their origin, structure and functions.

Cytoplasm   The protoplasm (consisting of nucleic acids, proteins, lipids, carbohydrates and inorganic salts) of the cell that exists outside the nucleus and is the site of most of the chemical activities of the cell.

Cytotoxic drugs   Drugs that inhibit or kill cells in the body, such as anticancer drugs.

Daughter cell   Any cell formed by the division of a mother cell.

DNA   Deoxyribonucleic acid, the type of nucleic acid that carries genetic information for all organisms except for the RNA viruses.

Dysplasia   Abnormal development in size, shape or organization of cells. This property is determined by microscopic examination of biopsy or other tissue, as in a Pap test.

Dysuria   Pain on passing urine.

Edema   An abnormal accumulation of fluid in tissues of the body that causes swelling; can be a side effect of therapy with hormones such as cortisone derivatives.

Endocrine gland   A gland that secretes hormones into the bloodstream.

Endocrine therapy   The use of hormones to treat a disease.

Endoscope   A flexible scope that can be passed into body passages to look for tumors—used for examination of the colon, the esophagus and stomach, the bladder and the bronchial tubes. Can also be used to obtain a biopsy of a tumor or other suspicious lesion.

Epidemiology   The study of factors that influence the frequency and distribution of diseases, such as cancer, in an effort to find the causes and therefore prevent them.

Epithelium   The skin, and the membrane-like tissue lining those internal organs that have external connections (digestive and respiratory tracts, reproductive system, etc.).

Etiology   The study of the cause of a disease.

Fibrocyst   A fibrous tumor that has undergone cystic degeneration or one that has accumulated fluid in the interspaces.

Genome   An organism's entire complement of DNA, which determines its genetic makeup.

Glioblastoma   A highly malignant brain cancer in adults.

Granulocytes   Infection-fighting cells in the blood.

Hematuria   The presence of blood in the urine.

Hepatitis   Inflammation or infection of the liver; can be acute, subacute or chronic in its clinical course.

Hepatocellular   Affecting the liver cells.

Hepatoma   A primary cancer of the liver.

Heterogeneous   Exhibiting variable characteristics; heterogeneity is a common property of cancer cells even within a single tumor mass.

Histology   The study of tissues to diagnose disease.

Homogeneous   Alike or similar in properties—like normal cell characteristics.

Hormonal therapy   Administration of natural or synthetic hormones in order to manipulate hormone levels in the body; this can cause a tumor to stabilize or shrink.

Hormone A substance formed by one organ of the body, which is carried (for example, by the bloodstream) to another organ and stimulates the second organ to function.

Hybridoma An immortal cell line formed by a process of cell fusion, usually prepared for the purpose of synthesizing specific antibodies in large quantities.

Hyperalimentation The infusion (drip) of highly nutritious fluids containing protein and lots of calories into a vein or into the stomach.

Hypernephroma A cancer of the kidney in adults.

Immunoglobulins Proteins that function as specific antibodies.

Immunology Branch of science dealing with the body's resistance mechanisms against disease or limiting the damage caused by the invasion of a foreign substance.

Immunosuppression Prevention of formation of a normal immune response; a consequence of certain forms of cancer, AIDS or intensive chemotherapy. Can be temporary or permanent.

Immunotherapy An experimental type of therapy used to stimulate the body's own defense mechanisms to control cancer or to kill cancer cells by immune means; examples are interferon and monoclonal antibodies.

Informed consent A legal standard (put in writing for all experimental therapies) that states how much a patient must know about the potential risks and benefits of a therapy before being able to knowledgeably participate in a clinical study.

Initiation The first step of carcinogenesis; it takes place at the molecular level.

Interferon Potent natural proteins (alpha, beta, gamma) produced by the lymphocytes of the body as a "front line" defense against viral infections; used as a form of immunotherapy against certain types of cancer and leukemia.

Interleukin-2 A factor that stimulates the growth of specific types of lymphocytes (T).

Intrauterine Within the uterus.

Intravenous   Entering through a vein.

Investigational New Drug (IND)   A drug that has been licensed by the Food and Drug Administration (FDA) for use in clinical trials, but is not yet approved for commercial marketing.

Irradiation   Treatment by radiation.

Kaposi's sarcoma   Cancer of the blood vessel tissues; commonly but not exclusively seen in AIDS patients.

Lesion   A change in the structure of part of an organ or tissue due to any type of disease or injury; a tumor is often referred to as a lesion.

Leukemia   Any of a series of malignant diseases of the blood-forming system. It may be acute or chronic and lymphocytic, myelogenous, monocytic, or erythroid, depending on the cell of orgin.

Leukocyte   White blood cell or corpuscle.

Leukopenia   A decrease in the number of white blood cells.

Local recurrence   A tumor that reappears at the site of the original tumor.

Lumpectomy   Removal of a lump from the breast.

Lymph nodes   Small, bean-shaped structures in the body that act as filters, collecting bacteria and cancer cells that are to be processed by the immune system. When infection or cancer is present, lymph nodes may become enlarged and are commonly called "swollen glands." Nodal involvement in cancer means that cancer cells have spread from the primary tumor site to nearby nodes.

Lymphocytes   White blood cells that are responsible for a variety of immune reactions.

Lymphoma   A tumor originating in lymphatic tissue (neck, groin, armpit); Hodgkin's disease is a particular type of malignant lymphoma. Burkitt's lymphoma is a form of undifferentiated malignant lymphoma usually found in Central Africa, but also seen in other countries, including the United States.

Malignant   "Malignant" usually means cancerous, as opposed to benign.

Mammography Study of the breast by use of soft tissue x-ray techniques.

Mediastinum The area of the chest containing the heart and major blood vessels.

Melanoma A highly malignant form of cancer of the skin; the cells are often pigmented, as derived from a skin mole.

Mesenchyme A diffuse network of cells forming the portion of the embryo that gives rise to connective tissues, blood and blood vessels, the lymphatic systems, et cetera.

Mesothelioma A tumor developed from mesothelial tissue (the layer of flat cells that forms the layer of the epithelium that covers the surface of all true serous membranes). The surfaces of the lung and abdominal organs are among the tissues that can give rise to this tumor.

Metabolite Any substance involved in the chemical process of the body; may be a salt, foodstuff such as a carbohydrate, an organic acid, et cetera.

Metastasis (me-tas'-ta-sis) The migration of cancer cells from the primary tumor site to other parts of the body, thereby producing cancer spread. Metastatic cancer occurs when cancer has spread from its original site to one or more distant sites.

Mitosis The process of cell division by which new cells are formed.

Monoclonal Derived from a single cell or clone (outgrowth) from one cell.

Monocyte One of the white blood cells (leukocytes) involved in host defense mechanisms—against infection, inflammation, cancer.

Multiple myeloma A malignant growth of plasma cells, usually arising in the bone marrow and manifested by bone destruction, pathologic fractures with bone pain, anemia and tendency to infection.

Mutagen Any agent that causes genetic mutations. Many medicines, chemicals and physical agents such as ionizing radiation and ultraviolet light have mutagenic ability.

Mutation In genetics and molecular biology, a sudden change, either in the base sequence of DNA or in the order, number or placement of genes on or across chromosomes, that may result in a change in the structure or function of a protein.

Myelophthisic anemia   A condition in which there is a reduction of the cell-forming functions of the bone marrow because of tumor invasion.

Myelosuppression   A decrease in the ability of bone marrow cells to produce blood cells—including white cells, red cells and platelets.

Necrosis   Death of tissue, usually as individual cells, groups of cells or in small localized areas.

Neoplasm   A new, abnormal growth of cells, also called a tumor, which may be benign or malignant.

Neuroblastoma   Malignant tumor characterized by immature, only slightly differentiated nerve cells of an embryonic type.

Nucleotide   Subunit of DNA or RNA consisting of a sugar molecule, a phosphate molecule and one of four possible base molecules: adenine, thymine, guanine or cytosine (in RNA another base, uracil, is found instead of thymine).

Occult tumor   A concealed or hidden tumor.

Oncogene   Genetic material in viruses that is also found in tumors in various mammalian species.

Oncologist (on-kol'-o-jist)   A physician who specializes in cancer. On-cology is the study of tumors, especially cancerous ones.

Osteosarcoma   A malignant sarcoma of the bone.

Paget's disease of the breast   A cancer of the nipple.

Palliation (pal-ee-ay'-shun)   The act of relieving or soothing a symptom, such as pain, without actually curing the cause.

Pap (cervical) smear   A scraping of cells from the neck of the womb (cervix) for examination under a microscope.

Papillomatosis   The development of multiple benign tumors derived from the epithelium and caused by virus infection.

Pathological   Caused by a diseased condition. A pathological fracture occurs when a bone breaks because it has been weakened by cancer.

Pathologist   A doctor who is specially trained to interpret and diagnose the changes in body tissues caused by disease.

Placebo   An inactive substance or preparation given to satisfy the need for drug therapy, and used in controlled research studies.

Plasma cell   A spherical or ellipsoidal cell that functions in the synthesis of immunoglobulins (proteins that function as specific antibodies). These cells are part of the normal immune system. If plasma cells become malignant, they cause a disease called multiple myeloma.

Platelets   Cells in the blood that help it to clot.

Pleiotropy   The quality of a cell(s) to manifest itself in a multiplicity of ways, i.e., to produce many effects in the phenotype. Pleiotropic drug resistance to one chemotherapeutic drug also causes the cell to be resistant to many other drugs.

Polyp   A benign outgrowth of tissue.

Point mutation   Change in a single nucleotide base, which can alter the message of a codon. This in turn can cause a change in the order of assembled amino acids, resulting in synthesis of an altered or completely different protein.

Premalignancy   An abnormal area in the body that may develop into a cancer but has not as yet done so.

Prognosis   The expected or probable outcome of an illness or disease.

Promoter   In carcinogenesis, a substance that increases the carcinogenic activity of other agents that initiate carcinogenesis.

Prophylaxis   The prevention of disease; preventive treatment.

Protocol   The outline or plan for experimental treatment; also used for standard treatment.

Proto-oncogenes   DNA sequences present in normal cells that are related to oncogenes found in viruses.

Psychotropic drug   Any of a broad category of drugs the primary action of which causes a marked and usually predictable change in mental state; includes tranquilizers, stimulants, antidepressants, barbiturates and hallucinogens.

Radiation therapy   A way of killing or damaging cancer cells by using a beam of radiation.

Radioisotope   An isotope (a chemical element having the same atomic number as another—having the same number of nuclear protons but possessing a different number of nuclear neutrons) with an unstable nucleus, which causes it to give off radioactivity. Radioisotopes are important for diagnostic and therapeutic uses in clinical medicine and research.

Recombinant DNA technology   The methodology and techniques involved in forming hybrid molecules under laboratory conditions by splicing segments of DNA and rejoining them in a novel arrangement.

Recurrence   The return of cancer after its apparently complete disappearance.

Regression   The shrinkage or disappearance of a cancer.

Relapse   The return of a disease after its apparent cessation.

Remission   The decrease or disappearance of all measurable evidence of disease.

Replication   A process that occurs both in self-synthesis of DNA and in synthesis of RNA by DNA. In the latter case, single-strand DNA serves as a template for RNA. DNA reproduces itself by separating into two strands, each of which then synthesizes a complement of itself.

Retrovirus   Any of a class of viruses the genetic material of which is RNA instead of DNA. All viruses must use the genetic machinery of a host cell to reproduce themselves, but retroviruses undergo an extra step in which RNA is converted into DNA.

Reverse transcriptase   An enzyme an RNA virus carries with it that permits viral RNA to be converted into a faithful DNA copy once a cell is infected, providing the infected cells the information to make more RNA for multiplication of additional viruses.

Ricin   A highly toxic protein that can be attached to monoclonal antibodies directed against cancer cells for the purpose of killing them.

Risk factor   An agent or substance that increases an individual's possibility of getting a particular type of cancer.

RNA Ribonucleic acid, which transmits information from DNA to the protein-forming system of the cell.

Roentgen The international unit of x- or gamma-radiation.

Sarcoma A form of cancer arising from cells of nonepithelial tissue, such as connective tissue, lymphoid tissue, cartilage or bone.

Side effect A second, unintentional and usually undesirable effect from a drug or other treatment, in addition to the primary, therapeutic effect. The primary effect of chemotherapy is to control or kill cancer cells; side effects may be hair loss, nausea or suppression of normal bone marrow growth.

Sigmoidoscope A tubular instrument for examination of the sigmoid colon (the lower part of the large bowel).

Single agent chemotherapy Treatment of cancer using one drug rather than a combination of several drugs.

Staging The systematic investigation of the extent of spread of tumor in order to decide what treatment is best. The amount of tumor spread is described as the disease stage.

Steroids A group of synthetic or naturally occurring compounds of a type of chemical structure that may act as hormones.

Supraclavicular Referring to the area above the clavicle (collar bone). Usually used to refer to lymph nodes at this site.

Teratogen A physical or chemical agent that causes a birth defect.

Thrombocytopenia A decrease in the number of platelets in the blood.

Thyrocalcitonin A polypeptide hormone elaborated by the parafollicular cells of the thyroid gland in response to hypercalcemia, which lowers plasma calcium and phosphate levels, inhibits bone resorption and serves as an antagonist to parathyroid hormone.

Titration A method used to determine the smallest amount of a drug or drugs required to bring about a desired effect. In chemotherapy, this adjustment in drug dose is intended to keep the toxicity and side effects to a minimum and the antitumor activity to a maximum.

Toxic Poisonous.

Transcriptase See Reverse transcriptase.

Transcription The first step of protein biosynthesis, in which DNA directs the production of RNA.

Translation The second step of protein biosynthesis, in which RNA directs the assembling of amino acids to form the primary structures of proteins.

Translocation Movement of a gene or genes from one chromosome to another (includes the exchange of genes between chromosomes).

Tumor An abnormal mass of tissue that results from excessive cell division and performs no useful function; a tumor may be benign or malignant.

Tumorigenesis The induction of a benign or malignant growth of abnormal cells.

Tylectomy Partial mastectomy.

Ulcer An erosion in a surface membrane (such as in the stomach) that may be benign or malignant.

Ultrasound test (Ultrasonography) The use of a very high frequency sound (which the ear cannot hear) to look inside the body.

Virus A tiny infectious agent, e.g., EB virus (Epstein-Barr virus), that is associated with probable causation of certain kinds of cancer.

BIBLIOGRAPHY

Works marked with an asterisk (*) were written for health professionals; the other works listed here are intended for a more general audience.

*Abeloff, M. D. (ed.). *Complications of Cancer: Diagnosis and Management.* Baltimore: The Johns Hopkins University Press, 1979. A technical book for health professionals.

American Cancer Society. *Directory of Division Executives.* New York: American Cancer Society, 1984. Describes the objectives and programs of the ACS.

Bruning, N. *Coping with Chemotherapy.* Garden City, NY: The Dial Press, Doubleday & Company, Inc., 1985. Describes the experiences of a patient treated for cancer.

Candlelighters. *Candlelighters.* Washington, D.C.: The Candlelighters Childhood Cancer Foundation, 1986. Describes the program of this group.

*Curran, J. W.; Morgan, W. M.; Hardy, A. M.; et al. "The Epidemiology of AIDS: Current Status and Future Prospects." *Science* 229 (1985): 1352–1357. A technical article for scientists.

*Delong, M. *Practical and Legal Concerns of Cancer Patients and Their Families: A Handbook for Caregivers.* Durham, NC: Duke University Medical Center, 1984. This material was collected to be useful to social workers and other health professionals at the Duke Comprehensive Cancer Center who care for patients with cancer. Its findings are extensively reproduced in Appendix 2, with permission of the authors.

*DeVita, V. T., Jr.; Hellman, S.; and Rosenberg, S. A. (eds.). *Cancer, Principles & Practice of Oncology,* 2nd ed. Philadelphia: J. B. Lippincott Company, 1985. A comprehensive textbook edited by the Director of the National Cancer Institute and two other leading oncologists.

Fiore, N. A. *The Road Back to Health.* New York: Bantam Books, 1984. Written by a psychotherapist to describe his personal battle against cancer; contains many helpful insights for other patients and for health professionals.

*Fischer, D. S.; Knopf, T.; and Welch-McCaffrey, D. *Cancer Chemotherapy: Treatment and Care,* 2nd ed. Chicago: Year Book Medical Publishers, 1984. A well-written text for oncologists.

*Hermann, J. F. "Psychosocial Support: Interventions for the Physician." *Seminars in Oncology* 12 (1985): 466–471. Written for physicians.

Heyden, S., and Pittillo, E. *Sensible Talk about Cancer: A Physician's Program for Prevention.* New York: Delair Publishing, 1980. Dr. Heyden is well known for his work with lay people on the subject of disease prevention. This work is intended for the general public.

Holleb, A. I. (ed.). *The American Cancer Society Cancer Book.* Garden City, NY: Doubleday & Co., Inc., 1986. This is an extensive compendium of information about diagnosis and treatment of specific cancers and steps that can be taken in prevention and cure. Beautifully edited from over forty expert contributors, this book is worth owning for handy reference.

*Howland, W. S., and Carlon, G. C. *Critical Care of the Cancer Patient.* Chicago: Year Book Medical Publishers, 1985. A technical book for physicians and nurses.

Johnson, A. M. *The Ultimate Organizer.* New York: Ballantine Books, 1984. Includes some handy tips pertinent to organizing one's affairs—this woman has thought of everything.

Larschan, E. J., and Larschan, R. J. *The Diagnosis Is Cancer. . . .* Palo Alto, CA: Bull Publishing Co., 1986. A practical psychological and legal resource handbook.

*****Laszlo, J. (ed.).** *Antiemetics and Cancer Chemotherapy.* Baltimore: Williams & Wilkins, 1983. Contains contributions by a number of experts on the subject of vomiting and how it can be controlled.

*****Laszlo, J. (ed.).** *Physician's Guide to Cancer Care Complications.* New York: Marcel Dekker, Inc., 1986. This work on prevention and management of the complications of cancer treatment was written by experts from the Duke Comprehensive Cancer Center and is intended for doctors, nurses, social workers and other health providers. It deals with surgery, chemotherapy, radiation therapy and psychological support.

Leukemia Society of America. "Scope of Assistance" in *Patient-Aid Program.* New York, 1986. Describes the programs of the Leukemia Society.

*****Levy, S. M.** *Behavior and Cancer.* San Francisco: Jossey-Bass Publishers, 1985. A technical and heavily referenced text—the most authoritative book on this difficult subject. A medically sophisticated layperson could follow the discussion.

*****Lynn, J.** "Legal and Ethical Issues in Palliative Health Care." *Seminar in Oncology* 12 (1985): 476–481. Sensible treatment of difficult technical subjects.

Morra, M., and Potts, E. "Choices, Realistic Alternatives." In *Cancer Treatment.* New York: Avon Books, 1980. This is a readable book from experts in cancer education; it provides good supplemental reading for users of this book.

North Carolina Bar Association. *Living Wills: A Declaration of the Desire for a Natural Death.* 1985.

*****Perry, M. C., and Yarbro, J. W. (eds.).** *Toxicity of Chemotherapy.* Orlando, FL: Grune & Stratton, Inc., 1984. Excellent technical book for medical oncologists and nurses who use chemotherapy. Provides detailed information on side effects from all types of cancer drugs.

Quit Smoking Program of the American Cancer Society. *FreshStart: Participant's Guide.* New York: American Cancer Society, 1986. This is a new program to help people who wish to stop smoking. The materials are well prepared for a lay audience.

Rapaport, S. A. *Strike Back at Cancer.* Englewood Cliffs, N.J.: Prentice-Hall Inc., 1978. A nonprofessional has done extensive reading and thinking about the subject of cancer and writes clearly for the public.

Roberts, L. *Cancer Today.* Washington, DC: Institute of Medicine/National Academy Press, 1984.

Rosenbaum, E. H., and Rosenbaum, I. R. *A Comprehensive Guide for Cancer Patients and Their Families.* Palo Alto. CA: Bull Publishing Company, 1980. This book is highly recommended for its extremely practical treatment of hard-to-find information on subjects like how to help patients at home, what to do for feeding, turning in bed, exercise, care of bowel and bladder function, how to be with sick people, and so on. The authors are a very thoughtful and compassionate physician and an excellent nurse.

Shaw, G. B. *The Doctor's Dilemma.* New York: The Trow Press, 1909. This is a sharply critical and witty indictment of doctors and their methods. We might like to think that Shaw's irreverent treatment of doctors is not applicable today, but one occasionally hears similar sentiments even now. If ever I become complacent, I resolve to read this again.

Shimkin, M. B. *Contrary to Nature.* Washington, DC: HEW, 1977. This is a historical review of major developments, scientists and cancer institutions that have been involved in cancer research. It is written for professionals but can be of interest to well-informed lay people also.

Shipley, R. H. *QuitSmart: A Guide to Freedom from Cigarettes.* Durham, NC: J. B. Press, 1985. Dr. Shipley is a psychologist at Duke, and this is a handbook on how to quit smoking—I refer liberally to his work in the chapter on tobacco and cancer.

Siegel, B. S. *Love, Medicine & Miracles.* New York: Harper & Row, 1986. Dr. Siegel is a surgeon who has a nice humanitarian approach to patients with cancer. The book makes for interesting reading—particularly his insights on relationships between patients and their doctors. Not all of his holistic approaches are supportable.

Simonton, O. C.; Matthews-Simonton, S.; and Creighton, J. L. *Getting Well Again.* New York: Bantam Books, 1978. This is the flagship of the self-help or imagery books on what the individual can do to overcome cancer. Some nice ideas on the importance of taking charge are presented, but the book also contains large amounts of pseudo-science.

*Stein, M. "A Reconsideration of Specificity in Psychosomatic Medicine: From Olfaction to the Lymphocyte." *Psychosomatic Medicine* 48 (1986): 3–22. A technical review of psychological influences in determination of disease outcome.

*Twycross, R. G., and Lack, S. A. *Symptom Control in Far Advanced Cancer: Pain Relief.* London: Pitman Publishing Limited, 1983. A good book on pain management, written for professionals.

*Twycross, R. G., and Lack, S. A. *Therapeutics in Terminal Cancer.* London: Pitman Publishing Limited, 1984. Symptom-control, such as pain management, is well described.

U.S. Department of Health and Human Services. *Cancer Prevention.* Washington, DC: Public Health Service, National Institutes of Health, National Cancer Institute, NIH Pub. No. 84-2671, 1984. This free publication deals understandably with a difficult subject—what is known about cancer prevention.

*Wiernik, P. H. (ed.). *Supportive Care of the Cancer Patient.* Mount Kisco, NY: Futura Publishing Company, Inc., 1983. Written for health professionals; includes many practical suggestions about improving the well-being of patients with cancer.

Williams, C. *All about Cancer.* New York: John Wiley & Sons, 1983.

Wilson, J. R. *Non-Chew Cookbook.* Glenwood Springs, CO: Wilson Publishing, Inc., 1985. This privately published book offers excellent eating selections for patients who have sore mouths and/or difficulty in swallowing. A unique type of cookbook for cancer patients. Available from the publisher at P.O. Box 2190, Glenwood Springs, CO 81602.

*Zimmerman, J. M. *Hospice: Complete Care for the Terminally Ill.* Baltimore-Munich: Urban & Schwarzenberg, 1981.

INDEX

acute lymphocytic leukemia, 228, 282
acute myelogenous leukemia, 63
acyclovir, 303
adeno cells, 82
adjuvant chemotherapy, 43, 53, 68
Adriamycin, 222
aflatoxin, 116
Africa, 128–29, 149–51, 201, 278
"Aging, Natural Death, and the
     Compression of Morbidity"
     (Fries), 106
Agriculture Department, U.S., 117, 135
AIDS (acquired immunodeficiency
     syndrome), 2, 86, 123, 128, 279
  causes of, 198–202
  normal state of immunity and,
     204–5
  research on, 205–6, 303–5
  treatment for, 203–4, 227–28

AIDS-related complex (ARC), 201–2
air contamination, 125
alcohol consumption, 113, 134
Alice's Adventures in Wonderland
     (Carroll), 191
alopecia, 68
American Association for Cancer
     Research, 165, 206
American Association of
     Dermatology, 186
American Association of Nutrition
     and Dietary Consultants, 252–53
American Cancer Society (ACS), 71,
     95, 97, 115n, 132–33, 147, 153,
     181, 232, 313–18
  cancer warning signals publicized
     by, 188
  new treatments tracked by, 255
  Public Education Program of, 315

American Cancer Society (ACS) *(cont.)*
    quit-smoking programs of, 156–57,
        162
    recommendations on screening by,
        173–74, 177–78, 183–86
American College of Surgeons, cancer
    programs approved by, 329
American Lung Association, 153
American Heart Association, 153
American Medical Association, 137
Ames test, 164
anatomical gifts, 343–44
angiography, 13
Annals of Internal Medicine, 191
anthracycline drugs, 57
anticipatory nausea and vomiting, 66
antiemetics, 65–67, 191, 196–97
antimetabolites, 52, 56, 242
antioncogenes, 275, 301
anxiety, 7, 13, 70, 270
artificial sweeteners, 116, 136
asbestos, 123–24
asparaginase, 57
Association of Funeral and Memorial
        Societies, 345
attitude:
    imagery and, 77–79, 260
    length of survival and, 258, 260–61,
        269
    likelihood of developing cancer
        and, 258
    mind-body unity issue and, 257–73
    quality of life and, 258–59, 260–61,
        269
    rate of tumor growth related to,
        268
    unconsciously conveyed, by doctors
        to patients, 271
autopsies, 347–48
auto-stimulation, 301
azathioprine, 127
azauracil, 242
azidothymidine (AZT), 203, 206,
    303

Bailar, John, 184
Baltimore, David, 129
bank transactions, 336, 348
Barnum, P. T., 253

basal cell carcinomas, 185–86
Behavior and Cancer (Levy), 268
benign tumors, 83
Benowitz, Neal, 146
benzodiazepines, 270
bills, hospital, 213–16
biofeedback, 259
biopsies, 6, 9–10, 12, 219
Biotherapeutics, 229–30
blacks, cancer death rates in, 96–97
bladder cancer, 127, 248, 306–11
blood banking, 61–62
blood counts, 11–12, 64
blood tests, 11–12
blood transfusions, 25, 61–62
bombesin, 302
Bonadonna, Giovanni, 42
bone cancer, 37, 40, 41, 42, 64, 71, 96,
    119
bone marrow examinations, 11–12
bone marrow transplantation, 48
bowel cancer. *See* colon cancer
brachytherapy, 48
Bradley, Edward, 284
brain tumors, 10, 14, 55
brand-switching programs, 154–56
breast cancer, 10, 11–12, 14, 17–20,
    37, 40, 41, 42, 71, 96, 114, 250,
    269, 279
    amount of surgery for, 43–44
    causes of, 112, 115, 127
    effect of positive attitude on,
        258–59
    in future, 295, 297
    in premenopausal vs.
        postmenopausal women, 42–43
    screening for, 176–81
    statistics on, 102–3
    surgery and chemotherapy for,
        41–42, 67–69
    surgery for, 40–46, 53, 67–68
    tumor metastasis from, 49
breast self-examination (BSE), 176
broiled food, 136
Burchenal, Joseph, 56
Burk, Dean, 204
Burkitt, Denis, 128
Burkitt's lymphoma, 39, 128, 278
Burnett, Sir MacFarlane, 204

Burroughs Wellcome Company, 206, 303, 308

calcium channel blockers, 289
Califano, Joseph, 193
Canadian Cancer Society, 328
cancer:
    definitions and biology of, 81–89
    distinct levels for investigation of, 3–4
    as killer, 89–90
    as personal experience, 306–11
    sources of information on, 313–30
    whom to tell about, 2
cancer cachexia, 92, 302
Cancer Counseling and Research Center, 260
cancer death rates. *See* statistics
Cancer Prevention Study 1 (CPS1), 103
Cancer Research, 170
Candlelighters Childhood Cancer Foundation, 320–21
Cantell, Kari, 71
Capp, Al, 198
carcinogens, 286, 290, 299
carcinomas, 81, 82, 85, 185, 240, 310
Cancer Nursing, 159
Carroll, Lewis, 191
Cassileth, Barrie, 272
catastrophic illness insurance, 235–36
causes, 108–31
    drugs as, 126–28
    environmental factors as, 108–13, 125
    lifestyle as, 113–23
    occupational factors as, 123–26
    role of nutrition in, 113–17, 132–36
    role of viruses in, 128–31
    studies of, 108–13
Centers for Disease Control (CDC), 198
central nervous system (CNS) prophylaxis therapy, 61
cervical cancer, 48, 85, 103–4, 174, 176, 209
    causes of, 122–23, 129
    in future, 298
chemoprevention, 280, 286

chemotherapy, 16, 35, 39, 51–70, 127, 203
    adjuvant, 43, 53, 68
    background of, 51–53, 56–61
    after breast cancer surgery, 67–69
    combination, 59–64, 67
    cost of, 219–20, 221, 226
    counteracting side effects of, 64–67
    experimental, 287–92
    in future, 303–4
    new techniques in blood banking with, 61–62
    practical illustrations of, 67–70
    preoperative, 63
    quantitative research methods for, 57, 59
    radiation therapy with, 48–49
    side effects of, 55–56, 59, 65–66, 67–70, 191–97
    into spinal fluid, 60
    surgery and, 40–43, 67–69
    toxicity and, 67
    as treatment for childhood leukemia, 56–64
    variations in sensitivity to, 55–56
    See also drugs; *specific drugs*
childhood acute leukemia, 53, 56–64, 298
childhood cancer, statistics on, 105–6
"Children of the Zodiac, The" (Kipling), 1
China, People's Republic of, 115, 128–9
cholesterol, 115, 136
choriocarcinoma, 11, 52, 55
chorioembryonic antigen (CEA), 11
chromosomal structures, 84
cigarette smoking. *See* smoking
cisplatin, 222
CMF (cyclophosphamide, methotrexate and fluorouracil) regimen, 68
coffee, 136
Cohen, Stanley, 276
collateral resistance, 287
collateral sensitivity, 287
colon cancer, 11, 43, 55, 114, 186, 278
    in future, 297

colon cancer *(cont.)*
  screening for, 181–85
  statistics on, 104
colonoscopy, 183–84, 186
communication, 22–24
  of bad news, 26–27
  honesty and openness in, 29, 32
  how of, 25
  optimistic, 31
  problems in, 26–34
  restricting information and, 31–34
  setting up goals for, 23–26
  using statistics in, 34
comprehensive cancer centers, 324–26
Comprehensive Smokeless Health
    Education Act (1986), 167
computerized axial tomograph (CT or
    CAT) scans, 12, 219–20
Congress, U.S., 234
constipation, 77
Constitution, U.S., 151
continuous flow centrifugation, 62
Cooper regimen, 42
coping, 269–71
corticosteroids, 127
costs. *See* economic burden
Creagan, Edward, 255
Creighton, J. L., 260
Crick, Francis H. C., 294
cruciferous vegetables, 134
cures, 37–40
  cost of, 228–29
  five-year, 37
Curran, James, 199
cyclophosphamide, 56
cyclosporin A, 127
cystoscope, 307, 311
cytosine arabinoside, 57

Damon Runyon Society, 232
death benefits, 349
debulking, 41, 64
defensive medicine, 225
DeLong, Margaret, 332
depression, 77–78, 258, 268
detection, 3, 186–89
DeVita, Vincent, 63, 319
diagnostic procedures, 9–14
  biopsies as, 6–7, 12

diagnostic procedures *(cont.)*
  blood tests as, 11–12
  cost of, 13, 19, 221
  function served by, 13–14
  monoclonal antibodies in, 280–83
  radiological imaging as, 12–13
diagnostic tests, 4, 6–7
diarrhea, 76–77
diffuse histiocytic lymphoma, 39
dihydrofolate reductase, 288
discrimination, 305
DNA (deoxyribonucleic acid), 82, 84,
    277–78, 294, 301
doctors:
  economic burden of patients and,
    216–23, 226–28, 225–26
  getting information from, 1–2, 4,
    22–34
  mistrust of, 4
  patient communication with, 22–34,
    271
  reasons for going to, 7–9
  second opinions from, 1–2, 3, 14–20
  selection of, 28
drugs, 92
  as causes of cancer, 126–28
  miracle, 251–52
  testing of, on humans, 239–46
  See also chemotherapy; *specific drugs*
Durovic, Marko, 250
Durovic, Steven, 247–49, 250
dysplasia, 85

Early, Joseph, 234
economic burden, 5
  of cancer, 207–38
  of cures, 228–29
  doctors and, 216–23, 225–26, 235
  of experimental therapy, 229–30
  general suggestions for coping with,
    234–38
  hospices and, 223–24, 237
  hospital bills and, 213–16
  lessons learned from, 231–34
  of lung cancer, 168–71, 210–12,
    219–20, 232
  minimization of, 208–12, 216–23
  overview of, 207–8
  society and, 225–28, 236–38

Eddy, David, 183
education, 231–32
Elion, Gertrude, 242
endocrine tumors, 11
endometrial cancer, 103
endoscopes, 9
endotoxin, 302
environmental hazards, 108–13, 125
Environmental Protection Agency,
     126
enzymes, 11, 288, 291
Epidermal Growth Factor (EGF), 276
epithelial cells, 82, 140
Epstein-Barr virus (EBV), 128
Essex, Myron, 279
estates:
   dissent from will and, 351
   legal rights of survivors and,
     350–51
   personal representative for, 350
   probates for, 349–50
   settling of, 349–51
   taxes on, 351
estrogens, 10, 127
ethics, 243, 291
   cost vs., 225–28
European Organization for Research
     on Treatment of Cancer
     (EORTC), 329
exceptional patients, 271
experimental chemotherapy, 287–92
experimental consent forms, 242
experimental therapy:
   paying for, 229–30
   quackery vs., 239–56
   using humans for, 239–46
   See also research

family security, planning for, 342–
     43
Farber, Sidney, 56
fat intake, 114, 115, 117, 133, 298
ferritin, 283
filter cigarettes, 145–47
Fiore, Neil A., 270
Fisher, Bernard, 42, 44–45
five-year cure, 37–38
Folkman, Judah, 87
food additives, 116, 135

Food and Drug Administration
     (FDA), 152, 195–96, 226–28, 230,
     249
formaldehyde contamination, 121
Freeman, Harold, 97
Frei, Emil, III, 63–64, 192
Freireich, Emil, 61, 64
FreshStart program, 156–57
fried food, 136
Fries, James, 106
frustration, 268
funerals, 344–46

Gallo, Robert, 200, 205, 279
gene amplification, 288
generic drugs, 221
Getting Well Again (Simonton,
     Matthews-Simonton and
     Creighton), 260–67
   case reports in, 266–67
   claims made in, 260–61
   critique of, 262–65
   on stress, 267
gifts, 343–44
gliomas, 81
glycoproteins, 289
Gold, Joseph, 93
Goldman, David, 289
Gompertz, Benjamin, 86–87
Gompertz curve, 87
Gompertz equation, 87
Great American Smokeout, 162
Great Britain, 295
growth factors, 275–77
guardianship:
   incompetence and, 337
   of minor children, 339

hairy cell leukemia, 72, 221
Hatch, Orrin, 234
Hawkins, Ralph, 235, 237
head and neck cancer, 18, 48, 63
Health, Education and Welfare
     Department, U.S. (HEW), 193
Health and Human Services
     Department, U.S. (HHS), 299,
     319
health insurance, 224
   for catastrophic illnesses, 235

health insurance *(cont.)*
  economic burden of patients and,
    208–12, 213, 215, 217
Health Insurance Plan of New York,
    180–81
health maintenance organizations
    (HMO's), 236
heart disease, 106, 289
Helsinki Declaration on Human
    Rights, 243
Hemoccult test, 183
hemolytic anemia, 25
Herbert, Victor, 117, 252
Herman, Joan F., 272
Hertz, Roy, 52
high-fiber foods, 115, 117, 133–34, 299
high tech/high touch, 2, 67
Hippocrates, 42, 80
Hippocrates, Oath of, 20, 21
Hodgkin's disease, 36, 39, 40, 63, 228
holistic approaches, 259–60
Holland, James, 247, 272
Holleb, Arthur, 153
homosexuality, 123, 199, 203
hormones, 11, 268
hospices, 223–24, 237
hospitals, economic burden of
    patients and, 213–18, 222, 235
House of Representatives, U.S., Ways
    and Means Committee of, 169
Huang, Andrew T., 63
Hudson, Rock, 227
human chronic gonadotropin (HCG),
    11
human isoantibody, 282
human mortality, law of, 87
human papilloma virus, 129
hybridoma research, 281
hydrazine sulfate, 93
hyperbaric chamber, 87
hyperthermia, 304
hypoxia, 87

imagery, 77–79, 259
immune deficiency conditions, 1–2
immunotherapy, 35, 71–73
  background of, 71–72
  side effects of, 72
  successes of, 72–73

income tax returns, 351
incompetency and guardianship, 337
individual participation associations
    (IPA's), 236
infection, 94
inheritance tax, 351
"Insights on How to Quit Smoking:
    A Survey of Patients with Lung
    Cancer" (Knudsen, et al.), 159
institutional review boards (IRB's), 243
insulin, 11
insurance policies, 208–12, 213, 215,
    217, 224, 235–38, 342–43
interferons, 19–20, 35, 39, 71–73, 203,
    221, 224, 229, 284, 300
interleukins, 35
interleukin-2 (IL-2), 73, 229–30
  research on, 283–85, 303–4
Internal Revenue Service, 351
intraepithelial carcinomas, 310
ionizing radiation, 119–22
Isaacs, Alick, 71
Ivy, Andrew C., 247

Japan, 101, 106, 113, 128–29, 233
Jeune Afrique, 149
Journal of the American Medical Association,
    247
juvenile laryngeal papillomatosis, 71,
    72

Kaposi's sarcoma, 72, 202, 203
kidney cancer, 72, 78
Kipling, Rudyard, 1
Klaidman, Stephen, 151
Knudsen, Nancy, 158
krebiozen, 36, 246–51
Krebiozen Research Foundation,
    248–50

laetrile, 36, 250–51, 252–53
laryngectomies, 47
laser beam therapy, 304–5
Lasker, Mary, 71
Leder, Philip, 279
Legal Aid Offices, 333
legal and practical concerns, 331–51
  anatomical gifts, 343–44
  disposition of body, 347

legal and practical concerns *(cont.)*
  family security, 342–43
  funerals, 344–46
  locating lawyers, 332–33
  managing affairs of another, 335–37
  settling estates, 349–51
  Social Security benefits, 333–35
  whom to notify after death, 346
  wills, 337–42
LeShan, Lawrence, 258
Lesko, Samuel M., 144
leukemias, 12, 14, 18, 25, 37, 38,
    81–82, 84, 208, 217, 224, 279
  causes of, 119–20, 121, 128, 131
  in future, 298
  new drug experiments on, 240, 243,
    255
  statistics on, 105
  See also specific leukemias
Leukemia Society of America, Inc.,
    232, 322–23
Levi-Montalcini, Rita, 276
Levy, Sandra M., 268
Li, M. C., 52
lifestyles:
  hazards of, 113–22
  sexual, 122–23
Lindeman, Jean, 71
Ling, Victor, 289
liver cancer, 11, 82, 128, 130
  research on, 278, 283
Living Wills, 340–42
lorazepam, 66
Love, Medicine & Miracles (Siegel), 271
lumpectomies, 16, 17, 44
lung cancer, 43, 47, 85, 89, 93, 101
  causes of, 115, 124, 137
  economics of, 168–71, 211–12, 219,
    231
  new drug experiments on, 241
  relationship of smoking to, 137–71
  screening for, 181–82
  statistics on, 102, 138–41, 152
lymph glands, 10, 44, 52, 82
lymphocytes, 283–85, 303
lymphokines, 73
lymphomas, 18, 36, 39, 53, 72, 81, 82,
    128, 202, 240
lymphotropic leukemia, 303

McAllaster, Carolyn, 332
McQueen, Steve, 253
Madison, James, 151
magnetic resonance imaging (MRI),
    12
major medical insurance policies, 210
malignant melanomas, 89, 104, 118,
    185, 269
malignant transformations, 84–86
malnutrition, 93, 123
malpractice, 17, 225–26, 235
mammography, 6, 177, 180–81, 187
mastectomies:
  lumpectomies vs., 44
  modified radical, 16, 17, 44, 68
  radical, 44
Matthews-Simonton, S., 260–67, 271
maximum tolerated dose (MTD), 240
Meals on Wheels, 238
Medicaid, 169, 236
Medicare, 170, 210–11, 218, 223, 236
melphalan (Alkeran), 42
megavitamins, 36
mesothelioma, 124
metastases, 41, 49, 83–84, 89, 250, 281
methotrexate, 53, 289
Miami Herald, 252
Mill, John Stuart, 152
mind-body unity, 257–73
  opinions on, 258–60
  programs based on, 260–67
  stress and, 267–70
miracle drugs, 251–52
Moertel, Charles, 183
monoclonal antibodies, 229
  for diagnosis and treatment, 35, 73,
    280–83, 301
Montanier, Luc, 200
multidisciplinary clinics, 221–22
multiple myeloma, 72, 277
mycosis fungoides, 72
myelophthisic anemia, 12
Myers, Charles, 289

Nabilone, 196
Naisbitt, John, 2
Napoleon I, Emperor of France, 192
nasopharyngeal cancer, 128, 278

National Academy of Sciences:
  National Research Council of, 132
  Proceedings of, 255
National Cancer Institute (NCI), 52,
    57, 61–64, 115, 133, 138, 183,
    193–94, 200, 205, 232, 318–20
  Biological Response Modifiers
    Program of, 229
  cancer centers supported by, 326–28
  Cancer Control Branch of, 319
  Cancer Information Services (CIS)
    of, 318–19
  on cancer-related mortality, 294–95
  Clinical Center of, 320
  experimental vs. quack therapies
    and, 245, 248–49, 255–56
  Public Information Office of, 320
  research at, 283, 286, 290
  summary of objectives from, 298–300
national cancer organizations, 313–30
National Hospice Organization, 321
National Institutes of Health (NIH),
    232, 319
National Large Bowel Task Force, 234
National Surgical Adjuvant Breast
    Program (NSABP), 43–44
nausea and vomiting, 64–66, 68, 74,
    75–76
  THC for, 65, 191–97
neoadjuvant chemotherapy, 63
Nerve Growth Factor (NGF), 276
New England Journal of Medicine, 144, 167
New York State Journal of Medicine, 149
New York Times, 151
nicotine, 145
nicotine gum, 154, 155–56
nitrite-cured foods, 135
Nixon, Richard M., 293
NORML (National Organization for
    Reform of Marijuana Laws), 196
nuclear waste exposure, 121
nutritional supplements, 77
nutrition and diet, 2, 73–77, 92–94
  as cause of cancer, 113–17, 132–36
  definition of, 73–74
  preventing cancer with, 113–17,
    132–36, 298–99
  recommendations on, 73–75, 133–35
  topics of general interest in, 135–36

obesity, 113–14, 117, 133, 299
occupational hazards, 123–26, 299
Office of Management and Budget
    (OMB), 234
Office of Technology Assessment
    (OTA), 169
Oldham, Robert K., 229
oncogenes, 277–78
oncologists, 14, 15, 221
"On Liberty" (Mill), 152
oral cancer, 113
  screening for, 185
  statistics on, 105
Order, Stanley, 282
ordinary stresses, 267–68
organ transplantation, 127–28, 204,
    305, 343–44
Orleans, C. S., 162
ovarian cancer, 64

pain, 90–92, 305
palliation, 46, 49
pancreatic cancer, 55
Pap test, 85, 100
  as screening test, 174–76, 187
passive smoking, 164–65
pathological fractures, 49, 277
patients:
  doctor communication with, 22–34
  doctors visited by, 7–9
  economic burden of, 207–38
  exceptional, 271
  as research subjects, 229–31
Paules, Lou, 332
Pauling, Linus, 254
Paulson, David, 307–8, 310
Phase I clinical trials, 241, 243–44
phenacetin, 127
phenothiazines, 65
Philadelphia chromosome, 84
Physician Data Query (PDQ) system,
    319
planning of treatment, 10, 50
plasma cells, 276–77
pleiotropic drug resistance, 84, 289
polypeptides, 302
Pott, Sir Percivall, 112
poverty, 123
power of attorney, 335–36

Practical and Legal Concerns of Cancer Patients and Their Families: A Handbook for Caregivers (DeLong, Paules and McAllaster), 331–32
Prival, Michael J., 132n
probates, 349–50
prostate cancer, 11, 50–51, 102, 297
protein, 75
proto-oncogenes, 130
psychological comfort, 273
psychosocial issues, 5
Public Health Services, 199

quack remedies, 2, 17, 36
  appeal of, 254–55
  definition of, 247
  experimental therapy vs., 239–56
  krebiozen as, 36, 246–51
  laetrile as, 36, 250–51, 252–53
  miracle drugs as, 251–52
  serum therapy as, 36, 252–53
quality of life, 258–59, 260–61, 269
  of successful survivors, 272–73
QuitSmart: A Guide to Freedom from Cigarettes (Shipley), 153–55
quit-smoking programs, 153–64
  of ACS, 156–58, 162
  self-administered, 154–55
  suggestions of lung cancer patients for, 158–59

radiation, as cause of cancer, 117–18
radiation therapy, 10, 35, 46–51, 87
  administration of, 47–48
  as alternative to surgery, 47–48, 49–50
  with chemotherapy, 48
  cost of, 50
  effectiveness of, 51
  for palliation of symptoms, 50
  schedules for, 50
  side effects of, 40, 51
  with surgery, 48
radiological imaging, 12–13
radon gas contamination, 120–21
Ramazzini, Bernardino, 109
randomized controlled studies, 244
Rauscher, Frank, 71
Reach to Recovery, 323–24

Reagan, Nancy, 45, 172, 180
Reagan, Ronald, 104, 172, 183–84, 185, 186, 234
rectal cancer, 64, 104, 297
relapses, 37
research, 5, 274–92
  on cancer cells vs. normal cells, 275–77, 300
  on chemotherapeutic drugs, 287–92
  in future, 293–94, 299–302, 305
  funding for, 233–34
  on lymphocyte stimulation, 283–85, 303–4
  on monoclonal antibodies, 280–83, 301
  new technologies and insights from, 277–80
  patients as subjects for, 229–30
  on turning cancer cells back into normal cells, 285–87, 300
  See also experimental therapy
retinoblastoma, 277
Road Back to Health, The (Fiore), 270
Road to Recovery, 237
Rosen, Richard, 236
Rosenberg, Steven, 283
Roxane Laboratories, 197
Rundles, R. Wayne, 206, 249

safe deposit boxes, 348–49
salt-cured foods, 135
sarcomas, 72, 81, 82, 202, 203
scavenger cells, 302
Schabel, Frank, 59
Schimke, Robert, 288
Science, 117, 199
scientific knowledge, 3
screening, 172–90
  for breast cancer, 176–81
  for colon cancer, 181–85
  detection and, 186–89
  for lung cancer, 181–82
  objectives for, 299–300
  for oral cancer, 185
  Pap tests used in, 174–76, 187
  principles of, 173–74
  for skin cancer, 185–86
  for testicular cancer, 181
scrotum cancer, 112

second opinions, 2, 3, 14–20
  acceptance of, 19–20
  arranging priorities for, 15–16
  consultants for, 17–19
  cost of, 19, 221–22
  differences in, 19
  involving personal doctor in, 18–19
  practical tips on, 15
sedatives, 65
selenium, 136
self-healing techniques, 258–60,
  272–73
serum therapy, 36, 252
sexual lifestyle, 122–23
Shimkin, Michael, 109
Shipley, Robert H., 153–55
short-term stress, 267
Siegel, Bernie S., 271
Silberman, Harold, 228
Simonton, O. C., 260–67, 271
Simonton program, 78
6-mercaptopurine, 56
6-prophylmercaptopurine, 242
skin cancer, 118–19, 209
  screening for, 186
  statistics on, 104
Skipper, Howard, 59, 206
small cell lung cancer (SCLC), 301–
  2
smoked foods, 135
smokeless tobacco, 166–68
smoking, 137–71, 185
  as addiction, 145
  advertising and, 138, 146, 148–53
  beneficial effects of, 144–45
  cancer-causing chemicals and,
    142–44
  cancer mortality rate and, 294–95
  economics of, 168–71
  of filter cigarettes, 145–47
  passive, 164–65
  prevention objectives for, 298
  quit-smoking programs and, 153–64
  recommendations for public policy
    on, 165–66
  relationship of cancer to, 137–71
  warning labels and, 147–48
social and leisure activities, 273
Social Security benefits, 333–35, 349

Social Security checks, representative
  payees for, 336
society, economic burden of patients
  and, 225–28, 235–38
Society for Biological Therapy, 285
Soemmering, Samuel Thomas Von, 112
Sokal, David C., 149–51
Soviet Union, 106
specialists, 14, 221–22
spleen, 25
Sporn, Michael, 301
sputum cytology, 85, 181
squamous cell carcinomas, 82, 185
statistics, 34, 95–107
  on blacks vs. whites, 96–97
  on breast cancer, 102–3
  on childhood cancer, 105–6
  on colon cancer, 104
  as guide, 95–96
  on leukemia, 105
  life expectancy and, 106–7
  on lung cancer, 102, 138–39, 152
  on oral cancer, 105
  on rectal cancer, 104
  on skin cancer, 104
  on uterine cancer, 103–4, 144–45
Stead, Eugene A., Jr., 121
stem cell assay technique, 291
steroids, 11, 25
stomach cancer, 100–101, 116
stool tests, 182–84
Strander, Hans, 71
stress, 267–68
successful survivors, 272–73
sun protection factor (SPF), 118
surgery, 6, 35, 40–46
  for breast cancer, 42–46, 49, 53, 68
  chemotherapy and, 41–43, 67–70
  controversies about, 40–41, 44, 51
  planning strategy for, 40
  radiation therapy as alternative to,
    46–51
  radiation therapy with, 48
Sweden, 106
Szent-Györgyi, Albert, 254

Tamoxifen, 290
technological changes, 2, 277–80
terminal differentiation, 286

terminology, 29
testicular cancer, 39, 55, 228
  in future, 297
  screening for, 181
tetrahydrocannabinol (THC), 65,
    191–97
thorotrast, 121
thyrocalcitonin, 11
thyroid, 10, 11
tobacco. *See* smoking
Todaro, George, 301
treatment:
  for AIDS, 203–4, 227
  attitude and imagery in, 77–79
  for cancer, 1–2, 6, 10, 14, 35–79, 96
  chemotherapy as, 16, 35, 38–39,
    51–70, 127, 191–97, 203, 220,
    222, 226, 287–92, 303–4
  with curative intent, 35–40
  experimental, 37–38
  in future, 295–98, 303–5
  immunotherapy as, 35, 71–73
  monoclonal antibodies for, 35, 73,
    280–83, 301
  nutrition as, 2, 73–77
  planning of, 10, 49
  radiation therapy as, 10, 35, 46, 50, 87
  religious convictions and, 25
  selection of, 35
  successful, 39–40
  surgery as, 6, 35, 40–46, 51, 53,
    67–68
  timeliness of, 35–36, 96
trust funds, 342–43
Tso, C. Y., 265*n*
tumor angiogenesis, 87
tumor necrosis factor (TNF), 73, 285,
    302
tumor promoters, 286
tumors:
  cell growth in, 86–88
  origin of, 87–88
  types of, 81–82
"Type C" person, 269
tyrosine kinase, 276

Unimed, 195, 197
urologic malignancies, 18
uterine cancer, 100, 126
  statistics on, 103–4, 144

venereal warts, 73
veteran's benefits, 236, 336–37, 349
vincristine, 56
vinyl chloride, 123–24
viruses, 128–31, 205
  in animals vs. humans, 279–80
  research on, 279–80, 303
vitamins, 74, 75
  A, 114, 116, 134, 286
  C, 116, 134, 252, 254–55
  E, 116, 136, 286

War Against Cancer, 293
Warner, Kenneth E., 168
Washington Post, 243
water contamination, 125–26
Watson, James D., 294
Wattenberg, Lee W., 132*n*
Waxman, Henry, 234
Weicker, Lowell, 234
Weinberg, Robert, 278
Weinhouse, Sidney, 115*n,* 132*n*
wills, 337–42
  definition of, 337
  dissents from, 351
  guardianship of minor children in,
    339
  kinds of, 338–39
  Living Wills as, 340–42
  making changes in, 339
  safekeeping of, 340
Wise, Noel, 144
women, incidence of lung cancer in,
    138–39
Wyngarden, James, 319

x-rays, 6, 12, 181

Zubrod, C. Gordon, 57

ABOUT THE AUTHOR

Dr. John Laszlo was born in Cologne, Germany, on May 28, 1931. He immigrated to the United States in 1938 and was educated in New York City until graduation from Columbia University in 1952. Thereafter he received his medical degree at Harvard Medical School, interned at the University of Chicago Clinics, spent two and a half years of training and research on cancer and leukemia at the National Cancer Institute in Bethesda, Maryland, completed residency and hematology and oncology training at Duke Medical Center and joined the permanent faculty there in 1960. He became a tenured professor in the Department of Medicine and for five years was Chief of Medicine at the Durham Veterans Administration Hospital. Thereafter, he helped to develop the Duke Comprehensive Cancer Center and served as director of its Clinical Program. He has published over 200 articles on cancer pharmacology and biochemistry, leukemia and blood-related disorders, clinical studies with new drugs, interferon and other research and has pioneered in studies related to comfort of patients who are receiving cancer chemotherapy. He has edited two books about cancer and contributed many chapters to medical textbooks. His most recent textbook for health professionals is entitled *Physicians' Guide to Cancer Care Complications.* In 1986 he left Duke Medical Center to return to New York where he is currently Senior Vice President for Research of the American Cancer Society.

Dr. Laszlo has served on many national committees, on the editorial board of cancer journals, on advisory committees to many of the cancer-related science organizations and is on the Board of Directors of the American Association for Cancer Research, the largest group of cancer researchers in the world. He is interested in teaching, patient care, the use of scarce resources in clinical medicine and research, and in the ethics of animal and human research. He has recently received a national award for volunteer work to the American Cancer Society. An avid tennis player, skier and outdoorsman, he has three children, to whom this book is dedicated.